TREATMENT
EFFICACY
FOR
STUTTERING

A Search for
Empirical Bases

TREATMENT
EFFICACY
FOR
STUTTERING
A Search for Empirical Bases

Edited by
Anne K. Cordes, Ph.D.
Department of Communication Sciences and Disorders
University of Georgia
Athens, Georgia

and

Roger J. Ingham, Ph.D.
Department of Speech and Hearing Sciences
University of California, Santa Barbara

SINGULAR PUBLISHING GROUP, INC.
SAN DIEGO • LONDON

Singular Publishing Group, Inc.
401 West A Street, Suite 325
San Diego, California 92101-7904

Singular Publishing, Ltd.
19 Compton Terrace
London N1 2UN, UK

e-mail: singpub@mail.cerfnet.com
Website: http://www.singpub.com

Typeset in 10/12 Century by Thompson Type
Printed in the United States of America by McNaughton and Gunn

Library of Congress Cataloging-in-Publication Data
Treatment efficacy for stuttering : a search for empirical bases /
    edited by Anne K. Cordes and Roger J. Ingham.
        p.   cm.
    Includes bibliographical references and index.
    ISBN 1-56543-904-X (alk. paper)
    1. Stuttering—Treatment—Congresses.   I. Cordes, Anne K.
II. Ingham, Roger J., 1945–   .
RC424.T698   1998
616.85'5406—dc21   98-5956
                                                        CIP

CONTENTS

Chapter

PREFACE

Is stuttering physical, psychological, both, or neither? Can parents cause it, exacerbate it, cure it, or none of the above? Is it a relatively straightforward speech disorder, or is it an impairment and a disability and a handicap, all of which represent complex interactions of neurological, physiological, anatomical, linguistic, emotional, social, and other characteristics? Can it be treated? Should it be treated? By whom, and when, and how, and why? What treatment results should be expected? What treatment results should be demanded? What constitutes acceptable evidence that a reported result has truly been obtained? What constitutes acceptable evidence that a certain treatment was directly responsible for the obtained results?

Dr. Gerald Siegel, one of the contributors to this volume, expressed some sympathy recently for the alien traveler who, finding herself overwhelmed by such questions, might decide instead to return home to "simpler and more amenable problems, like cold fusion or how to achieve lasting world peace" (Siegel, 1997, p. 439). Siegel also suggested, however, that it is possible to find oneself not overwhelmed, but challenged or even excited by the difficulties that surround our attempts to understand and treat stuttering. The chapters collected here were developed from just such a point of view.

The papers on which these chapters are based were originally presented at a 3-day "State-of-the-Art Conference" held at the University of Georgia in March, 1997. The State-of-the-Art Conferences program, administered by the Vice-President for Academic Affairs of the University of Georgia, allows several faculty members per year to bring up to approximately 15 experts in a well-defined or specialized field to the university for focused discussion. Each participant at a State-of-the-Art Conference presents a relatively long and relatively thorough original work, and each presentation is followed by ample time for the group's thoughtful discussion. In accordance with these guidelines, the authors represented here were originally asked to present or discuss current data or theoretical information about stuttering or its treatment, with the organizing theme of attempting to identify those factors that can be demonstrably related, in a data-based framework, to the effective management of stuttering.

The emphasis on a data-based approach to stuttering and its treatment represented an important theme for the State-of-the-Art Conference on stuttering treatment and, therefore, for this book. This theme was developed from several sources, including two previous small meetings about stuttering research and treatment. The first of these was an informal gathering of approximately 20 people at the University of California, Santa Barbara, in March, 1993. Merrilyn Gow was primarily responsible for that meeting; she and Anne Cordes, both doctoral students at the time, organized it with assistance from their faculty advisors, Roger Ingham and Janis Costello Ingham. The goal of the meeting was to encourage discussion among a group of people with related expertise in the area of stuttering; the journal club or lab meeting format, which functions so well within research groups, was used as a way to allow discussion across research groups. The meeting was successful enough that a second gathering was organized by Dr. Richard Curlee and held at the University of Arizona in March, 1995. These first two meetings were similar to the University of Georgia's State-of-the-Art Conferences, in that they were small gatherings of people with specific interests and expertise, designed to allow the presentation of new data and the open discussion of current issues. Many of the participants at the State-of-the-Art Conference had also attended one or both of the previous meetings, but those meetings were also very different from the State-of-the-Art Conference that led to this book. Most importantly, they remained relatively informal, with presentations that ranged from group problem-solving about proposed research to reports of completed research or literature reviews, and with no organized effort ever made to collect or publish the presentations.

The third meeting, in what has now become a biannual series, was the University of Georgia State-of-the-Art Conference on stuttering treatment. The State-of-the-Art Conference was also motivated by a conference titled "Research and Treatment: Bridging the Gap," which was sponsored by the Special Interest Division for Fluency and Fluency Disorders of the American Speech-Language-Hearing Association and held in May, 1996. During the Bridging the Gap conference, it became relatively clear to a few of us that many of the gaps in our discipline are not between researchers and clinicians at all, but are instead among those who would prefer to approach stuttering from a certain point of view, whether for research or for treatment; thus, we have divisions among those who approach stuttering scientifically, personally, emotionally, socially, behaviorally, cognitively, physiologically, acoustically, or through some combination of these. One of the most disturbing aspects of the Bridging the Gap conference, to those of us who have selected the scientific point of view as one of our perspectives, was that some members of our profession did not seem to consider the scientifically demonstrated effectiveness of a given treatment to be an important element in deciding to recommend or use that treatment. This orientation has actually been increasingly clear at other national and international conferences and in our discipline's publications, and it is, in its own way, extremely compelling: Science obviously has not solved stuttering yet, and people who stutter are real people with real needs that cannot be meaningfully condensed to the production of zero percent syllables stuttered in an experimental setting.

The problem with this point of view, though, is that it is not a complete argument. One possible conclusion to the statement at the end of the previous paragraph would continue ". . . and therefore we should abandon science as a means of developing, testing, or using stuttering treatments." An equally plausible ending, however, reaches the opposite conclusion: ". . . and therefore those who would dare to call themselves stuttering treatment researchers or stuttering clinicians must redouble their efforts to focus all the strongest tools that science has to offer on all the complexities of stuttering and its treatment."

The State-of-the-Art Conference on stuttering, and this, the resulting book, were designed primarily in defense of this second conclusion, as will be clear from the content of the chapters. Of course, the editors can not and do not presume to speak for all who have contributed their work and their energy to these chapters. In fact, as Dr. Siegel's alien might recognize, the strengths and the excitement of this book lie in the continuing conflicts, the unresolved differences, and the many remaining challenges. We do feel safe in speaking for the authors represented here, and for many others, when we say that we are all committed to understanding stuttering and to providing defensible, well-documented, and effective treatments for and with the millions of children and adults who stutter. The pressures imposed on treatment providers in the late 1990s by political, financial, and other forces are numerous, significant, and growing, for stuttering as for most other aspects of health care and education. This book is dedicated to the possibility that appropriate responses to such pressures might be found in that which has been empirically established about the nature and treatment of the condition we are trying to manage.

Anne K. Cordes

REFERENCE

Siegel, G. M. (1997). Afterword. In R. F. Curlee & G. M. Siegel (Eds.), *Nature and treatment of stuttering: New directions* (2nd ed., p. 439). Boston: Allyn & Bacon.

ACKNOWLEDGMENTS

The editors are very pleased to be able to acknowledge the invaluable assistance of many people who contributed directly and indirectly to the State-of-the-Art Conference on stuttering treatment and to this book. Thanks for substantial institutional and financial support to Dr. William Prokasy, Vice-President for Academic Affairs at the University of Georgia; Dr. Russell Yeany, Dean of the College of Education at the University of Georgia; and Dr. George Hynd, Director of the School of Professional Studies in the College of Education. Thanks to Ms. Valerie Franklin and her conference staff at the Georgia Center for Continuing Education at the University of Georgia. Thanks to all the conference participants for scholarly, challenging, and enjoyable presentations and discussions: Edward Conture, Richard Curlee, Susan Felsenfeld, Patrick Finn, James Hillis, Deborah Kully, Mark Onslow, Ann Packman, Bruce Ryan, Gerald Siegel, Scott Yaruss, and Patricia Zebrowski. Thanks to Heather Guger, Bridget Kelly, Steph McGowan, Jenny Nowicki, Kathy O'Keefe, Tracey Samet, Stacy Silverman, Sandy Smith, Jennifer Sullivan, Heather Weintraub, and Paula Woodworth, who were all students in the Department of Communication Sciences and Disorders at the University of Georgia at the time of the conference and who all helped enormously with many details that Anne had foreseen and with many others that they just quietly handled on their own. Thanks to Dr. Shari Campbell, in the Department of Communication Sciences and Disorders at the University of Georgia, for her expert assistance in reviewing manuscripts for this book, and thanks to Ms. Deidra Collier for her dependable help in the final stages of manuscript preparation. Thanks to Dr. Jeffrey Danhauer for connecting this project to Singular Publishing Group, and thanks to everyone at Singular for their thorough and professional guidance and assistance. Anne's personal apologies to Jerry that I missed him in the newsletter, and Anne's personal thanks to the University of Georgia's entire CSD faculty, and especially to Marilyn and Laida, for friendship and support through the conference, this book, and many other past and future projects.

CONTRIBUTORS

Cheryl Andrews, M.A.
Stuttering Unit
Bankstown Health Service
Sydney, NSW, Australia

Edward G. Conture, Ph.D.
Hearing and Speech Sciences
Vanderbilt University
Nashville, Tennesee

Anne K. Cordes, Ph.D.
Department of Communication
    Sciences and Disorders
University of Georgia
Athens, Georgia

Richard F. Curlee, Ph.D.
Department of Speech and
    Hearing Sciences
University of Arizona
Tucson, Arizona

Susan Felsenfeld, Ph.D.
Department of Speech-Language
    Pathology
Duquesne University
Pittsburgh, Pennsylvania

Patrick Finn, Ph.D.
Department of Communicative
    Disorders
University of New Mexico
Albuquerque, New Mexico

Elisabeth Harrison, M.A.
Stuttering Unit
Bankstown Health Service
Sydney, NSW, Australia

James W. Hillis, Ph.D.
Department of Speech and
    Hearing
George Washington University
Washington, DC

Roger J. Ingham, Ph.D.
Department of Speech and
    Hearing Sciences
University of California, Santa
    Barbara
Santa Barbara, California

Jeanne McHugh, M.S.
Department of Speech and
    Hearing
George Washington University
Washington, DC

Mark Onslow, Ph.D.
Australian Stuttering Research
    Centre
University of Sydney
Sydney, NSW, Australia

Ann Packman, Ph.D.
Australian Stuttering Research
    Centre
University of Sydney
Sydney, NSW, Australia

Yingyong Qi, Ph.D.
Department of Speech and
    Hearing Sciences
University of Arizona
Tucson, Arizona

Jill I. Rosenthal, M.S.
Speech-Language Pathology
   Service
National Rehabilitation Hospital
Washington, DC

Bruce P. Ryan, Ph.D.
Department of Communication
   Disorders
California State University, Long
   Beach
Long Beach, California

Gerald M. Siegel, Ph.D.
Professor Emeritus
Department of Communication
   Disorders
University of Minnesota
Minneapolis, Minnesota

Margaret Webber, M.A.
Stuttering Unit
Bankstown Health Service
Sydney, NSW, Australia

J. Scott Yaruss, Ph.D.
Communication Sciences and
   Disorders
University of Pittsburgh
Pittsburgh, Pennsylvania

Patricia M. Zebrowski, Ph.D.
Department of Speech Pathology
   and Audiology
University of Iowa
Iowa City, Iowa

PART I

Current Themes in Research and Theory: Implications for the Treatment of Stuttering

The chapters in this section address some of the important current is-sues in stuttering research: spontaneous recovery; definition and mea-surement; genetics; speech motor control; and the interactive roles of theory, research, and treatment. The authors represented in this section approached their topics in many ways, but always with the implicit or explicit goal of seeking to tie the current knowledge in these areas to the challenges facing stuttering treatment. Patrick Finn explores the spontaneous recovery literature from areas well outside of speech-language pathology, then draws some implications for recovery from stuttering. Ann Packman and Mark Onslow discuss the problems with some current systems for defining or describing stuttered speech, then move beyond current problems to present an alternative and to present data from analyses of that alternative. Susan Felsenfeld adopts some elements from programmed learning texts to engage her readers in a discussion of a timely question for many disorders: What can genetics research teach us about treatment? Roger Ingham attempts to answer a similar question with his review of the speech motor control literature on stuttering: What has this important current perspective taught us about stuttering treatment? Finally, Gerald Siegel turns his well-honed reflective skills on the relationships among theory, research, and treat-ment for stuttering. The chapters in this section do not address stutter-ing treatment directly; instead, they demonstrate that careful analyses of research and theory about the nature of stuttering can form a solid foundation for our efforts to develop effective treatments.

CHAPTER

Recovery Without Treatment: A Review of Conceptual and Methodological Considerations Across Disciplines

PATRICK FINN, Ph.D.

After more than 6 decades of published research on spontaneous recovery from stuttering, much doubt remains about the meaning of these findings. Most of this doubt stems from three issues. First, there is uncertainty about the definition of the term, spontaneous recovery. Second, there are methodological issues concerning the verification of spontaneous recovery. Third, there are opposing models of spontaneous recovery which have resulted in conflicting interpretations of the findings.

These three issues likely account for the diminishing number of studies on spontaneous recovery in the past two decades. In the 20-year period between 1955 and 1975, there were 16 published investigations on the phenomenon. Following this period, several critical reviews (Ingham, 1976, 1983, 1984; Martin & Lindamood, 1986; Wingate, 1976; Young, 1975) raised serious concerns about the validity of these studies' findings. In the following 20-year period, from 1975 to 1995, the number of published studies ($n = 7$) decreased by 56%.

Now there is evidence of renewed scientific interest in spontaneous recovery (see Finn, 1996; Yairi, Ambrose, Paden, & Throneburg, 1996). But before this research advances much further, some direction for resolving these three issues is necessary. One approach that could prove useful is to review the concept of spontaneous recovery across disciplines. It would seem that if spontaneous recovery from stuttering is part of a larger concept that applies to other human problems, then there should be heuristic value in examining what scientists from other clinically related disciplines believe the concept describes, how it should be investigated, and why it should be studied. Therefore, the purpose of this review was to determine if there is sufficient cross-disciplinary consensus concerning the concept of spontaneous recovery to provide a perspective for resolving the issues facing researchers concerned with stuttering.

The remainder of this chapter will be divided into three sections. The first section will briefly expand on the three issues concerning spontaneous recovery from stuttering in order to focus the review on the relevant questions. The second section will outline the scope of the review and then examine the same issues across other clinical disciplines. The final section will summarize the main findings and examine their applicability to stuttering.

SPONTANEOUS RECOVERY FROM STUTTERING

Terminology and Definition

Spontaneous recovery from stuttering is typically defined as the disappearance of the disorder without treatment (Nicolosi, Harryman, & Kresheck, 1996). The terms also connote that the disorder suddenly disappears, without apparent cause, and results in normal fluency (Ingham, 1984). This conventional view, however, is inconsistent with the characteristics of many individuals described as having experienced spontaneous recovery. Some individuals, for example, have described their recovery as very gradual (Wingate, 1976), some have been exposed to past treatment (Sheehan & Martyn, 1966), others describe parent or self-directed behavior changes (Dickson, 1971; Quarrington, 1977), and some still stutter on occasion (Wingate, 1964). Not surprisingly, questions have been raised about whether subjects with these kinds of characteristics should be regarded as valid samples of spontaneous recovery (Ingham, 1984).

Verification of Recovery

The most common designs for studying spontaneous recovery from stuttering are based on retrospective or longitudinal approaches. The retrospective design is often employed because many persons who recover from stuttering without treatment are discovered after their recovery (e.g., Sheehan & Martyn, 1966, 1967). The longitudinal design as used in stuttering is less common because it relies on the chance that a child who stutters will spontaneously recover while, at the same time, the parents will elect not to seek treatment for their child (e.g., Andrews & Harris, 1964). While each design has its strengths and weaknesses, both have been confounded by the same methodological issues. These issues have been based on concerns about the validity of the subject classification as spontaneously recovered (Ingham, 1984; Martin & Lindamood, 1986). In other words, did the subject (a) have a clinically valid stuttering problem (Ingham, 1976; Lankford & Cooper, 1974), (b) recover from stuttering without the benefit of formal treatment (Ingham, 1976; Sheehan & Martyn, 1966), and (c) actually *recover* (e.g., normal fluency) from stuttering (Wingate, 1964)?

Model of Recovery

Two explanatory models have guided and influenced research on spontaneous recovery (Ingham, 1984). The traditional and most influential model views spontaneous recovery as the result of an outgrowing or maturing out of the disorder, especially among children who stutter (Johnson & Associates, 1959). The alternative model views spontaneous recovery as the result of informal corrective factors. These factors are believed to be parent-directed among children who recover and self-directed among adults who recover (Ingham, 1983; Wingate, 1976). These two models have led to diametrically opposed implications for stuttering even when based on the same research findings of spontaneous recovery (Ingham, 1984). The traditional model, for example, has been used to support the recommendation that immediate and direct treatment for children who stutter is not warranted until it is certain that they will *not* outgrow the disorder (Yairi, 1997). In contrast, the alternative model has supported the view that early, direct treatment is essential and delays in intervention are untenable (Onslow, 1992).

A REVIEW OF SPONTANEOUS RECOVERY ACROSS DISCIPLINES

Scope and Focus of This Review

The phenomenon of spontaneous recovery has been described across a surprising variety of clinical areas. In the speech and hearing sciences, recovery without treatment has been documented in aphasia (Davis, 1993), traumatic brain injury (Coelho, DeRuyter, & Stein, 1996), cerebral palsy (Taudorf, Hansen, Melchior, & Pedersen, 1986), otitis media (Ziel-huis, Rach, & Van Den Broek, 1989), expressive language delay (Paul, 1996), articulation problems (Madison, 1982), and voice disorders (Culton, 1986). In other clinically related fields such as psychology, spontaneous recovery has been documented across problems such as alcoholism, cigarette smoking, drug abuse, weight disorders (Mariezcurrena, 1994; Stall & Biernacki, 1986), and depression (Calache & Achamallah, 1991; Pillay & Wassenaar, 1995). The phenomenon occurs frequently enough that it has prompted serious debate about the relative efficacy of many psychologically based treatments (Eysenck, 1952, 1994; Strupp, 1974). In the field of medicine, spontaneous recovery has been recorded across a variety of disorders (O'Regan & Hirshberg, 1993), including infectious diseases (e.g., immunodeficiency virus), circulatory disorders (e.g., hypertension), and respiratory ailments (e.g., asthma). The phenomenon is so well known that medical students were once "congratulated on choosing their profession wisely because a significant proportion of the problems they would be called on to address would take care of themselves" (Institute of Medicine, 1990, p. 152).

Due to the diversity and amount of research on spontaneous recovery, two guidelines were devised to manage the scope of this review. First, the disorders selected were those that could be characterized as chronic, progressive, and difficult to treat. This guideline was used to reasonably insure that the disorder shared some characteristics with stuttering. Second, spontaneous recovery from the disorder needed to have received a sufficient amount of research attention that there was a fair chance that scientists had considered some of the same issues discussed in stuttering. This was determined by obtaining the frequency of published articles on spontaneous recovery for different disorders within a discipline, such as medicine, and examining disorders that received proportionately more publications on the topic.

A subject search of various computer databases (see FirstSearch) yielded two disorders that appeared to meet these guidelines: cancer and alcohol abuse. The following section of this chapter will review the concept of spontaneous recovery across these two disorders. For each disorder, the literature addressing the following issues will be examined and summarized: (1) What is spontaneous recovery? (2) How is spontaneous recovery verified? and (3) What models of spontaneous recovery guide research on the topic?

From this review, it will be concluded that there is a consensus emerging across clinical disciplines concerning the phenomenon of spontaneous recovery. This consensus will provide a perspective for examining current research and providing potential resolutions to the issues identified earlier in studying spontaneous recovery from stuttering.

SPONTANEOUS RECOVERY FROM CANCER

Cancer is a term used to describe various malignant tumors that are characterized by uncontrollable, unstoppable growth of abnormal tissue. While advances in the treatment of some cancers have been made, it is still a widely feared disease that is often resistant to long-term treatment gains (Rosenberg & Barry, 1992). Despite this discouraging picture, numerous cases of spontaneous recovery have been documented over the past 80 years (for an early review see Rohdenburg, 1918). A recent annotated bibliography reported over a thousand cases worldwide (O'Regan & Hirshberg, 1993).

Terminology and Definition

The terms "spontaneous regression" and "spontaneous remission" are the most common descriptors for recovery from cancer without treatment. Though widely used, these terms are often viewed as unsatisfactory because they connote that the cancer will disappear suddenly and without cause (Barasch, 1994; Boyd, 1966; Everson & Cole, 1966; O'Regan & Hirshberg, 1993). Research findings have actually shown that spontaneous recovery gradually occurs and the changes do not necessarily result in complete disappearance of the tumor (O'Regan & Hirshberg, 1993). Furthermore, the evidence suggests that various causal mechanisms may underlie the recovery process, including immunological and psychological factors (Challis & Stam, 1990).

Some of these conditions have been included in the most widely cited definition of the phenomenon. Spontaneous recovery from cancer is defined as:

> the partial or complete disappearance of a malignant tumor in the absence of all treatment or in the presence of therapy which is considered inadequate to exert a significant influence on neoplastic disease. It is not implied that spontaneous regression need progress to complete disappearance . . . nor that spontaneous regression is synonymous with cure. (Everson & Cole, 1966, p. 4)

This definition clearly allows for a wider range of possible cases of spontaneous recovery than might be expected based on conventional wisdom. The drawback is that it may include too many classes of recovery. Therefore, more recent examinations of spontaneous recovery have attempted to subcategorize cases according to factors such as complete or partial remission and the presence or absence of any past treatment (O'Regan & Hirshberg, 1993).

Verification of Recovery

The medical profession has been reluctant to accept that cancer could resolve without treatment (Hirshberg & Barasch, 1995). This reluctance stems from the knowledge that cancer is often difficult to manage. But the main source of doubt can be traced to the frequent criticism that the disorder was not actually cancer in the first place. As a result, scientists have established rigorous standards for supporting their claims that a subject spontaneously recovered from a valid case of cancer (Everson & Cole, 1966).

The most widely accepted evidence that cancer was present is based on a biopsy or histopathological confirmation (see Challis & Stam, 1990; Everson & Cole, 1966; O'Regan & Hirshberg, 1993). This means that a tissue sample removed from the tumor is microscopically examined to confirm that it is comprised of abnormal tissue qualifying as cancer. Technical errors are possible using this procedure, such as obtaining nonrepresentative or insufficient tissue samples, but these errors are more likely to result in false negatives rather than false positives (Molinari, 1988). An advantage of this procedure is that the subject tissue samples can be preserved and stored, thus allowing the diagnosis to be retrospectively confirmed. This allows independent verification of the original diagnosis (Everson & Cole, 1966). In addition to histopathological evidence, researchers have obtained evidence such as subject-reported symptoms and family history of the disease to corroborate the initial diagnosis (Boyd, 1966).

Exposure to treatment has occurred in most cases of spontaneous recovery from cancer (Kent, Coates, Pelletier, & O'Regan, 1989). Usually this has not been a concern because the treatment exposure was considered ineffectual or insufficient to explain the recovery (Boyd, 1966; Everson & Cole, 1966, O'Regan & Hirshberg, 1993). In rare cases where treatment exposure did not occur, it was because the disease had progressed to a stage where it was no longer believed to be amenable to treatment.

Establishing the validity of recovery or remission is usually based on surgical confirmation (Challis & Stam, 1990). This can include visual inspection of the former tumor site, measurement of tumor reduction and, in some cases, histopathological confirmation. Post-recovery interviews with subjects have also been conducted to establish that they are symptom-free and to determine the factors the subjects believed were responsible for their recovery (Hirschberg & Barasch, 1995). Based on these anecdotes, subject determination to beat the cancer has emerged as a common recovery theme (Barasch, 1994; Holzman, 1989).

Model of Recovery

The medical profession has long regarded spontaneous recovery from cancer as implausible largely because it does not conform to the traditional biomedical model of disease (Pincus, 1996). This model posits that the origin and resolution of a disease must be accounted for by an external agent (e.g., bacterial infection and antibiotics). Since spontaneous recovery seemed to occur without an apparent cause, it was believed that the phenomenon was inaccessible to scientific inquiry. In some cases it was somewhat disparagingly described as a "miracle cure" (Barasch, 1994).

Gradually, the medical profession has accepted the possibility of spontaneous recovery from cancer. In the past 30 years, the number of reported cases has doubled (O'Regan & Hirshberg, 1993). This interest has been fueled by findings that suggest spontaneous recovery can be explained by factors that are understandable and possibly replicable. This has led to speculation that knowledge about spontaneous recovery from cancer could lead to the development of alternative treatment approaches (Boyd, 1966; Everson & Cole, 1966; O'Regan & Hirshberg, 1993). This position has appeared more viable in view of new medical research.

Recent advances in molecular oncology (e.g., chemical and genetic bases of cancer) and psychoneuroimmunology (e.g., study of the functional relationship between mind, emotion, and the immune system [see Ader, 1981; Bauer, 1994; Fife, Beasley, & Fertig, 1996]) have provided an empirical foundation for testing mechanisms of recovery (Stoll, 1992). Immunotherapy for cancer has been developed as a result of findings related to spontaneous recovery (Rosenberg & Barry, 1992). Psychoemotional variables have also been of interest because of anecdotal information that a subject's emotional response to the disease may contribute to recovery (Hirshberg & Barasch, 1995; O'Regan & Hirshberg, 1993).

SPONTANEOUS RECOVERY FROM ALCOHOL PROBLEMS

Alcohol abuse is traditionally viewed as a chronic disease characterized by habitual and uncontrolled use of alcohol to a degree that it interferes with physical, personal, and social behavior. While various treatment approaches have been available, two major problems are evident: (1) The most commonly used treatments (Alcoholics Anonymous and drug therapy) have minimal data to support their efficacy or widespread use (Miller & Hester, 1986), and (2) sustainable treatment gains have been unacceptably low and relapse rates have been distressingly high (Annis, 1986; Sobell, Sobell, & Nirenberg, 1988). Despite these problems, there is evidence that a surprising number of problem drinkers recover without the benefit of formal treatment (Smart, 1975, 1976; Tuchfeld, 1981). Recent surveys have reported spontaneous recovery rates as high as 77% (Cunningham, Sobell, Sobell, & Kapur, 1995; Sobell, Cunningham, & Sobell, 1996). This might mean that recovery without treatment is actually more common than recovery with treatment (Tucker & Sobell, 1992).

Terminology and Definition

Various terms, such as "spontaneous remission," "spontaneous recovery," and, more recently, "natural recovery," have been used to describe recovery from alcohol problems without treatment. None of these terms have been considered satisfactory, because they carry the implication that recovery is sudden, unexpected, and occurs for no apparent reason (Institute of Medicine, 1990; Smart, 1975, 1976; Stall & Biernacki, 1986). In contrast, most recognized cases of spontaneous recovery present a range of possibilities that includes persons who still drink moderate amounts of alcohol, might have been exposed to past treatment and, in most cases, attribute their recovery to a conscious decision to change their behavior (Ludwig, 1985; Sobell, Sobell, & Toneatto, 1992; Tuchfeld, 1981). This range has required categorizing recoveries according to factors such as current drinking or nondrinking behavior and exposure or nonexposure to past treatment. The only finding consistent with the conventional view of spontaneous recovery is that almost one-third of the cases judged that their recovery was immediate rather than gradual (Sobell, Sobell, Toneatto, & Leo, 1993).

Verification of Recovery

Knowledge about spontaneous recovery from alcohol problems has been primarily based on retrospective studies and subject self-reports. This has led to doubts about the validity of these findings because they are based on recall of past events (Sobell et al., 1992). The principal issue has involved concerns with the accuracy of subject self-reports (Gladsjo, Tucker, Hawkins, & Vuchinich, 1992). Specific concerns have been raised about the validity of the subjects' former drinking problem, their current nondrinking or drinking behavior, and the factors responsible for their recovery.

To resolve these concerns, researchers have obtained data from multiple sources in order to corroborate the subject's verbal reports. One of the primary sources has been interviews with persons who could confirm that the subject had a drinking problem, had recovered without treatment, and had a stable recovery (Gladsjo et al., 1992; Klingemann, 1991; Sobell et al., 1992; Sobell, Sobell, et al., 1993). Levels of agreement between these collateral reports and subject self-reports have generally been quite acceptable (at least 80%). Additional corroborating evidence has included subject scores on alcoholism screening tests that indicate a past drinking problem, and reports of past behavior (e.g., drunk driving arrests) that are consistent with alcohol dependence (Gladsjo et al., 1992; Sobell et al., 1992).

Exposure to past treatment for alcohol problems has been acceptable as long as there is no reason to believe that the treatment played a role in recovery. Usually this means that the subject regarded the treatment as unrelated to recovery (Gladsjo et al., 1992; Klingemann, 1991; Sobell et al., 1992). In some cases, criteria for the amount and type of treatment exposure have been considered because of evidence that brief interventions can be effective (Heather, 1989; Sobell et al., 1992).

Subject self-diagnosis is the main criterion for determining recovery from alcohol problems. Recovery is based on self-reports of abstinence or levels of nonabstinence that are no longer considered a problem. Nonabstinence is no longer considered a problem when the frequency of reported drinks does not exceed an independent criterion that distinguishes between hazardous and nonhazardous drinking (Sobell et al., 1992). In one study, this level of drinking among nonabstinent subjects who had spontaneously recovered was actually less than levels reported in most controlled drinking treatment studies (Sobell et al., 1992). The subject's level of recovery, abstinent or nonabstinent, must be confirmed by a person who knows the subject in everyday life (Sobell et al., 1992). Finally, subjects must also demonstrate a zero blood alcohol level, at least at the time of the study.

Model of Recovery

The traditional definition of alcoholism as a chronic, progressive, and incorrigible disease (Jellinek, 1960) has been a longstanding and highly influential view of the disorder (Morse & Flavin, 1992). This view has had an especially negative effect on the credibility of spontaneous recovery.

Based on the disease model, treatment (e.g., Alcoholics Anonymous, drug therapy) is viewed as the only viable pathway to recovery (Prugh, 1986; Roizen, Cahalan, & Shanks, 1978), a belief that is also widely accepted among the general public (Cunningham, Sobell, & Sobell, 1996; Fingarette, 1988). Furthermore, it has led to the belief that abstinence from alcohol is the only treatment outcome that could qualify as recovery (see for review: Marlatt, 1983; Marlatt, Larimer, Baer, & Quigley, 1993). From this view, the idea that recovery could occur without treatment was considered highly improbable and, as a result, the phenomenon was largely ignored (Cooke, 1980; Prugh, 1986; Sobell et al., 1992).

There are some cases where spontaneous recovery has been accepted as a valid phenomenon. In these cases, the recovery has usually been explained as the result of subjects growing out of their drinking problem (Klingemann, 1991; Smart, 1975, 1976). The supporting evidence for this view is the decrease in the frequency of alcohol problems that has been found across progressively older population samples (Institute of Medicine, 1992). In other words, it appeared that as problem drinkers grew older, they would either die from the negative health consequences of drinking or they would simply lose their desire to compulsively drink.

In recent years, another perspective of spontaneous recovery has emerged. This alternative perspective views spontaneous recovery as a phenomenon that can be explained by understandable factors that might also inform formal treatment (Institute of Medicine, 1990; Prugh, 1986). A considerable number of studies now suggest that spontaneous recovery may be associated with several significant variables such as (a) negative life events (e.g., heightened health concerns), (b) conscious evaluation of drinking (e.g., pros and cons of continued drinking), (c) support from significant others, and (d) self-monitoring of drinking behavior (Cunningham, Sobell, Sobell, & Kapur, 1995; Humphreys, Moos, & Finney, 1995; Ludwig, 1985; Sobell, Cunningham, Sobell, Toneatto, 1993; Sobell, Sobell, et al., 1993; Tucker, Vuchinich, & Gladsjo, 1994). These research findings have led to the development of a treatment approach (Sobell & Sobell, 1993) designed to foster self-change among problem drinkers by getting them to view their drinking problem from a different perspective (e.g., health risks associated with drinking). Recent studies have described the preliminary stages of a control group treatment study to evaluate its effectiveness (Sobell, Cunningham, Sobell, Agrawal, et al., 1996).

APPLICATIONS TO STUTTERING

The purpose of this chapter was to determine if there was a cross-disciplinary consensus on conceptual and methodological issues concerning spontaneous recovery that could provide a perspective for examining the same issues in stuttering. From this review, it is apparent that scientists studying spontaneous recovery from other human disorders have struggled with several issues similar to those that have interfered with an understanding of spontaneous recovery from stuttering. It is also fairly obvious that scientists have attempted to resolve these issues using broadly similar approaches. This consensus should be instructive for developing solutions to the same issues in the area of stuttering as explained in the remainder of this chapter.

Terminology and Definition[1]

It is clear from this review that the conventional view of spontaneous recovery has been abandoned across disciplines because the connotation of a sudden and unexplained return to normal contradicts the empirical evidence about this phenomenon. Instead, the alternative view sees recovery as an oftentimes gradual process with knowable factors underlying the process. This alternative view is still based on the notion that recovery occurs without treatment, but there is a wide range of possibilities that are acceptable within that framework. First, the fact that recovery has occurred without treatment does not exclude any past exposure to treatment, as long as there is no reason to believe that treatment was responsible for improvement. Second, recovery does not mean that signs of the disorder are absent nor that the resulting condition is

---

[1] During the research for this review, it was found that various terms have been used across disciplines to label the phenomenon of recovery without treatment. It appeared that the most common included combinations of the words "spontaneous," "natural," "recovery," "remission," and "regression." It is possible that these words have been used in the literature in ways that depart from their originally intended meaning. In order to explore this possibility the definitions of these terms were separately examined.

Looking through the *Oxford English Dictionary* (Simpson & Weiner, 1989), it was found that the term spontaneous refers to a natural process, occurring without apparent external cause, or having a self-contained cause or origin. Natural is defined as being in accordance with nature or with minimal medical or technological intervention. Remission is described as a diminution of force or effect. Recovery is viewed as the restoration or bringing back of a person to a healthy or normal condition and, finally, regression is defined as returning to a particular condition or state.

The original meanings of these words appear to be generally consistent with a conventional understanding of recovery without treatment. However, as this review revealed, there has been immense dissatisfaction with these terms because they have implied meanings (e.g., sudden or rapid change) that have led to confusion and misunderstanding about the phenomenon. Or they imply a condition (e.g., return to a normal state) that is inconsistent with the empirical findings. Despite this dissatisfaction, no one has yet offered an alternative set of descriptors that have gained any less notoriety or greater acceptance. As a result, some researchers (Everson & Cole, 1966; Stall & Biernacki, 1986) have suggested that the term spontaneous recovery, or its variants, be retained simply because they are the most widely used and best known. For this reason, and also to maintain some consistency in terminology throughout the chapter, this author decided to also use the term spontaneous recovery. In other writings, this author has preferred the term unassisted recovery (see Finn, 1996) to describe recovery without treatment. But since this term appeared very rarely across the literature reviewed for this chapter, it was decided not to introduce yet another set of descriptors.

completely normal. It does mean, however, that improvement has occurred to a degree that the disorder is no longer considered to be a problem or a handicap by the recovered individual. Third, and perhaps most
important, while recovery may have occurred without treatment, it nonetheless occurred for a reason, a reason that is understandable and possibly replicable. These three characteristics could be readily incorporated
into an alternative view of spontaneous recovery from stuttering.

As described at the beginning of this chapter, there has been uncertainty about the conventional definition of spontaneous recovery from
stuttering because it has been contradicted by empirical observations.
With the added support of this cross-disciplinary consensus, it is obvious
that this conventional view is no longer viable and should be replaced by
the alternative view outlined above. As a result, there is a need for reev-
aluating previous concerns about cases of spontaneous recovery where
past treatment exposure or an occasional tendency to stutter was evident.
This reevaluation, however, should be conducted with some caution.

From the alternative view, subjects who have had stuttering treatment in the past are acceptable cases of spontaneous recovery if the
recovery was reasonably independent of treatment. Based on current
research, there is no evidence that past treatment that was subject-
judged as ineffective would have delayed ameliorative effects or could
confound a classification of spontaneous recovery. It also seems reasonable to consider that subjects who report an occasional tendency to
stutter may still be viewed as recovered from their problem, at least to
some degree, especially since the speech parameters that might define
recovery from a chronic disorder have never been fully established
(Finn, 1996). Besides, if subjects—or parents in the case of children—
are not concerned about speech fluency at this level, then self-judged
acceptability of fluency might serve as an acceptable operational definition of a significant level of recovery, treated or untreated (Baer, 1988;
Ingham & Cordes, 1997).

This cross-disciplinary review also revealed that accepting a wider
range of cases will likely result in a more heterogeneous sample of spontaneous recovery. In order to manage this heterogeneity, scientists from
other disciplines have usually subgrouped their subjects according to
relevant distinguishing factors. In stuttering, this means that subjects
who have experienced spontaneous recovery could be subgrouped according to factors such as whether or not they report a tendency to still
stutter (Finn, 1997) or have been exposed to any treatment in the past.

In the final analysis, this alternative definition of spontaneous recovery is appropriate because it is consistent with empirical observations of the phenomenon. But this does not mean that any subject who
appears to satisfy these characteristics of spontaneous recovery is necessarily a valid sample of spontaneous recovery. In order to establish

the validity of the sample, an appropriate verification methodology is needed.

Verification of Recovery

As seen across disciplines, a frequent criticism of research on spontaneous recovery is that the findings are based on persons who did not have the actual disorder. This is oftentimes bolstered by the belief that the disorder can only improve with formal treatment. As a result, the most challenging methodological issue across disciplines has been establishing that subjects are valid samples of spontaneous recovery. This means verifying that they actually had the disorder, recovered without the benefit of treatment, and reasonably satisfy a set of criteria for recovery. To resolve this issue, a verification methodology has emerged that requires obtaining data from an essential source (e.g., tissue biopsy, subject self-report) and then cross-validating that source so that a conclusion can be founded on a convergence of mutually corroborative data.

In stuttering, there have also been doubts about the authenticity of some cases of spontaneous recovery. These doubts have an empirical basis because research has shown that some subjects who claimed to have spontaneously recovered probably never had a valid stuttering problem (Lankford & Cooper, 1974).

An early method for verifying that subjects used to stutter was conducted by examining the consistency between subject reports and generally accepted characteristics of stuttering (Sheehan & Martyn, 1966; Wingate, 1964). This method was problematic because the reports were not cross-validated by an independent source or supported by relevant speech samples.

More recent studies of spontaneous recovery from stuttering have described a verification methodology that is comparable to the methodology evident across other disciplines in this review. This more sophisticated methodology has included corroborating data from multiple sources. The two methods that have been used in stuttering, however, have varied depending on the age range of the subjects and whether the research design was longitudinal or retrospective. Both methods have strengths and weaknesses that deserve some comment.

In longitudinal studies investigating children who recovered from stuttering, Yairi and colleagues (Yairi, Ambrose, Paden, & Throneburg, 1996) have usually reported that they verified their subjects had spontaneously recovered based on three sets of criteria. First, the diagnosis of the child's initial stuttering problem was based on the judgments of the parents and two speech-language pathologists and a set of criterion speech behavior measures obtained from videotaped speech samples recorded in a "treatment room" prior to recovery. Second, based on the parents' report, the child did not receive any formal treatment for stuttering. However, the parents did receive general information about the nature of stuttering, the probability of spontaneous recovery ("65–75%" see Yairi, Ambrose, & Niermann, 1993), and were advised to reduce their speaking rate with the child. Third, the child's recovery from stuttering was based on the judgments of the parents and two speech-language pathologists and a set of criterion speech behavior measures obtained from videotaped speech samples obtained in the "treatment room" after recovery.

This verification method has several strengths. First, it is based on speech samples obtained before and after recovery. Second, there is agreement between parents and professionals about the child's speech status. Third, the child's recovery cannot be attributed to treatment since the parents chose not to seek treatment for their child. There are several problems, however, that warrant mention. First, the parents were exposed to an information session about stuttering. Although there is no evidence that this would have a direct ameliorative effect on the child's stuttering, it is unclear what effect this information might have on the parents' behavior or, more importantly, their decision not to seek treatment in the first place. Second, the absence of recorded speech samples from the child's home setting is a serious concern because there was no independent confirmation that the child was no longer having speech difficulty in everyday speaking situations. Although the parents' reports are important, there is evidence that parents' judgments of improvements in their child's stuttering are sometimes contradicted by objective speech samples recorded in the home (Ingham, 1997).

In retrospective research investigating adults who recovered from stuttering, Finn (1996) verified that subjects had spontaneously recovered based on data obtained from two sources. First, interview data were obtained from subjects describing their past stuttering, exposure to past treatment, and factors they believed contributed to their recovery. These interviews were analyzed by independent judges for their consistency with characteristics of stuttering, the degree of benefit (if any) received from past treatment, and the potential role of factors contributing to recovery. The duration between the last treatment exposure and the estimated spontaneous recovery was also estimated (average = 9 years). Second, each subject named a corroborator who was familiar with their past stuttering problem. The corroborators were contacted and asked to verify the subject's past stuttering problem and identify the types of speech behaviors that were evident. Finally, recorded speech samples were obtained so that the subjects' recovered speech behavior could be examined (Finn, 1997).

Since a subject's past speech problem cannot be directly verified, the main strength of this method is the concurrence of information from two sources, the subject self-report and corroborator judgment. This provides a basis for inferring that the subject once had a valid stuttering problem. For several reasons, this method also provides a basis for inferring that the subject's recovery was independent of any past treatment. First, based on the subjects' self-report, independent judges determine if there were any benefits received from the past treatment. Second, these judges also determine if subjects attribute their recovery to factors other than any past treatment. This is informative because numerous studies have suggested that many subjects, or parents in the case of children who stutter, credit their recovery to informally, self-managed or parent-managed activities (Finn, 1996; Johnson, 1950; Quarrington, 1977; Sheehan & Martyn, 1966; Wingate, 1964). Third, the estimated time between the age when treatment was received and the age of reported recovery was used to determine if it was sufficiently long enough that the probability of a treatment effect was unlikely. Finally, recorded speech samples obtained after recovery provide a basis for objectively evaluating the subject's recovery.

One of the drawbacks of this retrospective method is the absence of a criterion for deciding how much elapsed time is sufficient to insure that any treatment that might have been received was not the responsible change agent. In other words, how long after treatment has ended is it likely that treatment benefits might dissipate and significant levels of stuttering would have returned so that the spontaneous recovery occurred relative to a relapsed stuttering problem?

A possible answer could be developed from examining treatment studies that report follow-up data on the time elapsed before subjects clearly showed signs of relapse. Boberg and Kully (1994), for example, reported in a 2-year follow-up study that the amount of time the majority of their treated adult subjects ($n = 7$) demonstrated at least 50% relapse in their frequency of stuttering occurred within 4 to 12 months posttreatment. Therefore, at least 1 year between the age when treatment was last received and the age of reported spontaneous recovery might be a credible guideline. This should at least insure that spontaneous recovery was from a clinically meaningful level of stuttering, even though this stuttering was the result of a relapse from treatment.

Another drawback of this method is that the subject's recovery has been objectively evaluated only from recorded speech samples obtained in a laboratory setting (Finn, 1997). Since many subjects report that they still have a tendency to stutter (Finn, 1997; Wingate, 1976), it would be useful to also obtain speech samples from the subjects' everyday settings since it is unclear to what extent the speech behavior in the laboratory is typical of speech in other settings. It would also be informative to follow subjects across time in order to objectively evaluate the longevity of their recovery.

In summary, these two methods from longitudinal and retrospective studies for verifying spontaneous recovery from stuttering appear to be sufficient for reasonably establishing the validity of these kinds of cases. But, at the same time, it is also clear that both will require additional refinements in order to further strengthen them.

Model of Recovery

It is evident from this review that spontaneous recovery has been traditionally viewed across disciplines either as an improbable occurrence, because it does not conform to a conventional view of the disorder, or as the result of the person maturing out of the problem. However, it appears that neither explanation is currently regarded as having much credibility. Instead, an alternative model has emerged across disciplines that explains spontaneous recovery as the result of naturally occurring remedial factors. The credibility of this model has been strengthened by the development of treatment hypotheses based on findings from this model.

A similar contrast is apparent between traditional and alternative views of spontaneous recovery from stuttering. The traditional model, as mentioned earlier, describes spontaneous recovery as the result of a maturation process, especially among young children who stutter. The high rate of recovery among preschool and early school-age children (Andrews et al., 1983) is usually cited as supporting evidence. But the mechanism of recovery that might underlie the maturation process has never been clear. One possibility is that the child's stuttering is the reflection of an immature speech and language system that with time sufficiently matures to overcome the disability (Perkins, 1992). Recent evidence suggests that this is unlikely because children who spontaneously recover had normal language skills prior to their recovery (Watkins & Yairi, 1997).

Another suggested mechanism that might account for children outgrowing stuttering is a genetic-based factor (Yairi, Ambrose, & Cox, 1996). The most convincing evidence so far is that children who spontaneously recover are more likely to have a family history of recovery than children who continue to stutter (Yairi, Ambrose, Paden, & Throneburg, 1996). Much of this evidence has emerged from longitudinal research on children who stutter conducted by Yairi and his colleagues. Caution is needed in interpreting this evidence, however, because there may be a self-selection bias influencing the formation of subject groups (Felsenfeld, see Chapter 3). In this research, as described earlier, children who spontaneously recovered did not receive help because their parents chose not to seek treatment. When parents first entered the study they were told by the researchers that as many as 65–75% of children may recover without treatment. The parents, who were surely aware of their family history of recovery, were probably influenced by this information about recovery rates in their decision to withhold treatment for their child. Whereas, parents who were not aware of any family history of recovery would probably be less influenced by this information. Thus, the difference in distribution of family history may be an artifact that ironically resulted from the parents learning more about spontaneous recovery.

Another potential drawback of the genetic explanation is that it does not readily account for recovery in adolescence and adulthood. As many as 50% of adults who used to stutter report that they spontaneously recovered during adolescence or adulthood (Johnson, 1950; Sheehan & Martyn, 1966; Wingate, 1964). It is not clear how a genetic factor that accounts for recovery in preschool children is also a mechanism for recovery in later years.

In contrast to the traditional model, the alternative model explains spontaneous recovery from stuttering as the result of informal corrective factors that were either parent-directed among children or self-directed among adults. This view clearly resembles the alternative model discussed in this cross-disciplinary review. The most convincing evidence supporting this model is the finding that parents of children who spontaneously recover sometimes corrected their child's stuttering with suggestions to slow down or stop and start over (see Ingham, 1983). Similarly, adults who spontaneously recover have reported self-modifying their speech behavior by slowing down their speech rate or by stopping and thinking before speaking (Finn, 1996; Wingate, 1964). The significance of these reports is that they describe factors that resemble documented fluency-inducing techniques (Ingham, 1984). Therefore, this model provides a reasonable account of recovery across the life span. But, at the same time, it does not adequately explain why some children and adults who have been exposed to similar conditions do not spontaneously recover.

The credibility of this model has been further strengthened by the formal treatment hypotheses that have been developed from these findings. Onslow and colleagues' clinician-guided, parent-directed program for young children who stutter, for example, was developed from spontaneous recovery findings based on this model (see Onslow, Costa, & Rue, 1990). Several studies have since demonstrated the efficacy of this approach (Lincoln & Onslow, 1997; Onslow, Andrews, & Lincoln, 1994). Wingate (1976) has also suggested potential treatment applications of spontaneous recovery findings to adult populations, but these suggestions have not yet been formally tested.

In summary, from the perspective of this cross-disciplinary review, the alternative model of spontaneous recovery from stuttering is more consistent with current conceptualizations of the phenomenon. Moreover, this model has been indirectly supported by the positive outcomes from treatment studies that were based on factors described in the spontaneous recovery literature. This strongly suggests that serious attention to the alternative model is warranted in future discussions of this phenomenon.

CLOSING REMARKS

This chapter provided a cross-disciplinary view of spontaneous recovery in order to apply an alternative perspective to three issues that have confounded our understanding of this phenomenon in the area of stuttering. This perspective was useful for suggesting possible directions for resolving some of these problems. But the point should be made that even though spontaneous recovery from stuttering is part of a larger phenomenon, in the final analysis, it behooves researchers and practitioners within our own discipline to determine how this phenomenon will contribute to our understanding of the nature and treatment of stuttering.

ACKNOWLEDGMENT: This chapter was based on a paper read at the Athens State-of-the-Art Conference on Stuttering in Athens, Georgia, March 1997.

REFERENCES

Ader, R. (1981). *Psychoneuroimmunology*. New York: Academic Press.

Andrews, G., Craig, A., Feyer, A. M., Hoddinott, S., Howie, P., & Neilson, M. (1983). Stuttering: A review of research findings and theories circa 1982. *Journal of Speech and Hearing Disorders, 48*, 226–246.

Andrews, G., & Harris, M. (1964). *The syndrome of stuttering*. London: Heinemann.

Annis, H. M. (1986). A relapse prevention model for the treatment of alcoholics. In W. R. Miller & N. Heather (Eds.), *Treating addictive behaviors: Processes of change* (pp. 407–434). New York: Plenum Press.

Baer, D. M. (1988). If you know why you're changing a behavior, you'll know when you've changed it enough. *Behavioral Assessment, 10*, 219–223.

Barasch, M. (1994). A psychology of the miraculous. *Psychology Today, 27*, 54–63.

Bauer, S. M. (1994). Psychoneuroimmunology and cancer: An integrated review. *Journal of Advanced Nursing, 19*, 1114–1120.

Boberg, E., & Kully, D. (1994). Long-term results of an intensive treatment program for adults and adolescents who stutter. *Journal of Speech and Hearing Research, 37*, 1050–1059.

Boyd, W. (1966). *The spontaneous regression of cancer.* Springfield, IL: Charles C. Thomas.

Calache, M. J., & Achamallah, N. S. (1991). Spontaneous remission of depression after attempted suicide by hanging: A case report and literature review. *International Journal of Psychosomatics, 38*, 89–91.

Challis, G. B., & Stam, H. J. (1990). The spontaneous regression of cancer: A review of cases from 1900 to 1987. *Acta Oncologica, 29*, 545–550.

Coelho, C. A., DeRuyter, F., & Stein, M. (1996). Treatment efficacy: Cognitive-communicative disorders resulting from traumatic brain injury. *Journal of Speech and Hearing Research, 39*, S5–S17.

Cooke, D. J. (1980). Spontaneous recovery or statistical artifact? *British Journal of Addiction, 75*, 323–324.

Culton, G. L. (1986). Speech disorders among college freshmen: A 13-year survey. *Journal of Speech and Hearing Disorders, 51*, 3–7.

Cunningham, J. A., Sobell, L. C., & Sobell, M. B. (1996). Are disease and other conceptions of alcohol abuse related to beliefs about outcome and recovery? *Journal of Applied Social Psychology, 26*, 773–780.

Cunningham, J. A., Sobell, L. C., Sobell, M. B., & Kapur, G. (1995). Resolution from alcohol problems with and without treatment: Reasons for change. *Journal of Substance Abuse, 7*, 365–372.

Davis, G. A. (1993). *A survey of adult aphasia and related language disorders* (2nd ed.). Englewood Cliffs, NJ: Prentice Hall.

Dickson, S. (1971). Incipient stuttering and spontaneous remission of stuttered speech. *Journal of Communication Disorders, 4*, 99–110.

Everson, T. C., & Cole, W. H. (1966). *Spontaneous regression of cancer.* Philadelphia, PA: W. B. Saunders Company.

Eysenck, H. J. (1952). The effects of psychotherapy: An evaluation. *Journal of Consulting Psychology, 16*, 319–324.

Eysenck, H. J. (1994). The outcome problem in psychotherapy: What have we learned? *Behaviour Research and Therapy, 32*, 477–495.

Fife, A., Beasley, P. J., & Fertig, D. B. (1996). Psychoneuroimmunology and cancer: Historical perspectives and current research. *Advances in Neuroimmunology, 6*, 179–190.

Fingarette, H. (1988). *Heavy drinking: The myth of alcoholism as a disease.* Berkeley, CA: University of California Press.

Finn, P. (1996). Establishing the validity of recovery from stuttering without formal treatment. *Journal of Speech and Hearing Research, 39*, 1171–1181.

Finn, P. (1997). Adults recovered from stuttering without formal treatment: Perceptual assessment of speech normalcy. *Journal of Speech, Language, and Hearing Research, 40*, 821–831.

Gladsjo, J. A., Tucker, J. A., Hawkins, J. L., & Vuchinich, R. E. (1992). Adequacy of recall of drinking patterns and event occurrences associated with natural recovery from alcohol problems. *Addictive Behaviors, 17*, 347–358.

Heather, N. (1989). Psychology and brief interventions. *British Journal of Addiction, 84*, 357–370.

Hirshberg, C., & Barasch, M. I. (1995). *Remarkable recovery: What extraordinary healings tell us about getting well and staying well.* New York: Riverhead Books.

Holzman, D. (1989). Chasing answers to miracle cures. *Insight on the News, 5,* 52–53.

Humphreys, K., Moos, R. H., & Finney, J. W. (1995). Two pathways out of drinking problems without professional treatment. *Addictive Behaviors, 20,* 427–441.

Ingham, R. J. (1976). "Onset, prevalence, and recovery from stuttering": A reassessment of findings from the Andrews and Harris study. *Journal of Speech and Hearing Disorders, 41,* 280–281.

Ingham, R. J. (1983). Spontaneous remission of stuttering: When will the emperor realize he has no clothes on? In D. Prins & R. J. Ingham (Eds.), *Treatment of stuttering in early childhood* (pp. 113–140). San Diego: College-Hill Press.

Ingham, R. J. (1984). *Stuttering and behavior therapy: Current status and experimental foundations.* San Diego: College-Hill Press.

Ingham, R. J. (1997, March). *Stuttering treatment efficacy: Why haven't we solved this one yet?* Paper presented at the University of Georgia State-of-the-Art Conference, Athens, GA.

Ingham, R. J., & Cordes, A. K. (1997). Self-measurement and evaluating stuttering treatment efficacy. In R. F. Curlee & G. M. Siegel (Eds.), *Nature and treatment of stuttering: New directions* (2nd ed., pp. 413–437). San Diego, CA: Singular Publishing Group.

Institute of Medicine. (1990). Is treatment necessary? *Broadening the base of treatment for alcohol problems* (pp. 152–162). Washington, DC: National Academy Press.

Jellinek, E. M. (1960). *The disease concept of alcoholism.* New Haven, CT: Hillhouse Press.

Johnson, P. A. (1950). *An exploratory study of certain aspects of the speech histories of twenty-three former-stutterers.* Unpublished master's thesis. University of Pittsburgh, Pittsburgh, PA.

Johnson, W., & Associates (1959). *The onset of stuttering.* Minneapolis, MN: University of Minnesota.

Kent, J., Coates, T. J., Pelletier, K. R., & O'Regan, B. (1989). Unexpected recoveries: Spontaneous remission and immune functioning. *Advances, 6,* 66–73.

Klingemann, H. K. H. (1991). The motivation for change from problem alcohol and heroin use. *British Journal of Addiction, 86,* 727–744.

Lankford, S. D., & Cooper, E. B. (1974). Recovery from stuttering as viewed by parents of self-diagnosed recovered stutterers. *Journal of Communication Disorders, 7,* 171–180.

Lincoln, M. A., & Onslow, M. (1997). Long-term outcome of early intervention for stuttering. *American Journal of Speech-Language Pathology, 6,* 51–58.

Ludwig, A. M. (1985). Cognitive processes associated with "spontaneous" recovery from alcoholism. *Journal of Studies on Alcohol, 46,* 53–58.

Madison, C. (1982). Spontaneous remission of misarticulations. *Perceptual and Motor Skills, 54,* 135–142.

Mariezcurrena, R. (1994). Recovery from addictions without treatment: Literature review. *Scandinavian Journal of Behaviour Therapy, 23*, 131–154.

Marlatt, G. A. (1983). The controlled-drinking controversy. *American Psychologist, 38*, 1097–1110.

Marlatt, G. A., Larimer, M. E., Baer, J. S., & Quigley, L. A. (1993). Harm reduction for alcohol problems: Moving beyond the controlled drinking controversy. *Behavior Therapy, 24*, 461–504.

Martin, R. R., & Lindamood, L. P. (1986). Stuttering and spontaneous recovery: Implications for the speech-language pathologist. *Language, Speech, and Hearing Services in Schools, 17*, 207–218.

Miller, W. R., & Hester, R. K. (1986). The effectiveness of alcoholism treatment: What research reveals. In W. R. Miller & N. Heather (Eds.), *Treating addictive behaviors: Processes of change* (pp. 121–174). New York: Plenum Press.

Molinari, R. (1988). The biopsy. In G. Bonadonna & G. Robustelli della Cuna (Eds.), *Handbook of medical oncology* (3rd ed., pp. 55–62). Chicago, IL: Year Book Medical Publishers, Inc.

Morse, R. M., & Flavin, D. K. (1992). The definition of alcoholism. *Journal of the American Medical Association, 268*, 1012–1014.

Nicolosi, L., Harryman, E., & Kresheck, J. (1996). *Terminology of communication disorders* (4th ed.). Baltimore, MD: Williams & Wilkins.

Onslow, M. (1992). Choosing a treatment procedure for early stuttering: Issues and future directions. *Journal of Speech and Hearing Research, 35*, 983–993.

Onslow, M., Andrews, C., & Lincoln, M. (1994). A control/experimental trial of an operant treatment for early stuttering. *Journal of Speech and Hearing Research, 37*, 1244–1259.

Onslow, M., Costa, L., & Rue, S. (1990). Direct early intervention with stuttering: Some preliminary data. *Journal of Speech and Hearing Disorders, 55*, 405–416.

O'Regan, B., & Hirshberg, C. (1993). *Spontaneous remission: An annotated bibliography.* Sausalito, CA: Institute of Noetic Sciences.

Paul, R. (1996). Clinical implications of the natural history of slow expressive language development. *American Journal of Speech-Language Pathology, 5*, 5–21.

Perkins, W. H. (1992). *Stuttering prevented.* San Diego, CA: Singular Publishing Group.

Pillay, A. L., & Wassenaar, D. R. (1995). Psychosocial intervention, spontaneous remission, hopelessness, and psychiatric disturbance in adolescent parasuicides. *Suicide & Life-Threatening Behavior, 25*, 386.

Pincus, T. (1996). A rationale for studies of spontaneous remission. *Advances: The Journal of Mind-Body-Health, 12*, 64–69.

Prugh, T. (1986). Recovery without treatment. *Alcohol Health and Research World, 11*, 24, 71–72.

Quarrington, B. (1977). How do the various theories of stuttering facilitate our therapeutic approach? *Journal of Communication Disorders, 10*, 77–83.

Rohdenburg, G. L. (1918). Fluctuations in the growth energy of malignant tumors in man, with especial reference to spontaneous recession. *Journal of Cancer Research, 3*, 193–225.

Roizen, R., Cahalan, D., & Shanks, P. (1978). "Spontaneous remission" among untreated problem drinkers. In D. B. Kandel (Ed.), *Longitudinal research on drug use: Empirical findings and methodological issues* (pp. 197–221). New York: John Wiley & Sons.

Rosenberg, S. A., & Barry, J. M. (1992). *The transformed cell: Unlocking the mysteries of cancer.* New York: G. P. Putnam's Sons.

Sheehan, J. G., & Martyn, M. M. (1966). Spontaneous recovery from stuttering. *Journal of Speech and Hearing Research, 9,* 121–135.

Sheehan, J. G., & Martyn, M. M. (1967). Methodology in studies of recovery from stuttering. *Journal of Speech and Hearing Research, 10,* 396–400.

Simpson, J. A., & Weiner, E. S. C. (1989). *Oxford English Dictionary* (2nd ed.). Oxford: Clarendon Press.

Smart, R. G. (1975/1976). Spontaneous recovery in alcoholics: A review and analysis of the available research. *Drug and Alcohol Dependence, 1,* 277–285.

Sobell, L. C., Cunningham, J. A., & Sobell, M. B. (1996). Recovery from alcohol problems with and without treatment: Prevalence in two population surveys. *American Journal of Public Health, 86,* 966–972.

Sobell, L. C., Cunningham, J. A., Sobell, M. B., Agrawal, S., Gavin, D. R., Leo, G. I., & Singh, K. N. (1996). Fostering self-change among problem drinkers: A proactive community intervention. *Addictive Behaviors, 21,* 817–833.

Sobell, L. C., Cunningham, J. A., Sobell, M. B., & Toneatto, T. (1993). A life-span perspective on natural recovery (self-change) from alcohol problems. In J. S. Baer, G. A. Marlatt, & R. J. McMahon (Eds.), *Addictive behaviors across the life span: Prevention, treatment, and policy issues* (pp. 34–66). Newbury Park, CA: Sage Publications.

Sobell, L. C., Sobell, M. B., & Nirenberg, T. D. (1988). Behavioral assessment and treatment planning with alcohol and drug abusers: A review with an emphasis on clinical application. *Clinical Psychology Review, 8,* 19–54.

Sobell, L. C., Sobell, M. B., & Toneatto, T. (1992). Recovery from alcohol problems without treatment. In N. Heather, W. R. Miller, & J. Greeley (Eds.), *Self control and the addictive behaviours* (pp. 198–242). New York: Maxwell Macmillan.

Sobell, L. C., Sobell, M. B., Toneatto, T., & Leo, G. I. (1993). What triggers the resolution of alcohol problems without treatment? *Alcoholism: Clinical and Experimental Research, 17,* 217–224.

Sobell, M. B., & Sobell, L. C. (1993). *Problem drinkers: Guided self-change treatment.* New York: Guilford Press.

Stall, R., & Biernacki, P. (1986). Spontaneous remission from the problematic use of substances: An inductive model derived from comparative analysis of the alcohol, opiate, tobacco, and food/obesity literatures. *International Journal of the Addictions, 21,* 1–23.

Stoll, B. A. (1992). Spontaneous regression of cancer: New insights. *Biotherapy, 4,* 23–30.

Strupp, H. H. (1974). "Spontaneous remission" and the nature of therapeutic influence. *Psychotherapy and Psychosomatics, 24,* 389–393.

Taudorf, K., Hansen, F. J., Melchior, J. C., & Pedersen, H. (1986). Spontaneous remission of cerebral palsy. *Neuropediatrics, 17,* 19–22.

Tuchfeld, B. S. (1981). Spontaneous remission in alcoholics: Empirical observations and theoretical implications. *Journal of Studies in Alcohol, 42,*
626–641.

Tucker, J. A., & Sobell, L. C. (1992). Influences on help-seeking for drinking
problems and on natural recovery without treatment. *Behavior Therapist,*
15, 12–14.

Tucker, J. A., Vuchinich, R. E., & Gladsjo, J. A. (1994). Environmental events
surrounding natural recovery from alcohol-related problems. *Journal of*
Studies on Alcohol, 55, 401–411.

Watkins, R. V., & Yairi, E. (1997). Language production abilities of children
whose stuttering persisted or recovered. *Journal of Speech, Language, and*
Hearing Research, 40, 385–399.

Wingate, M. E. (1964). Recovery from stuttering. *Journal of Speech and Hearing*
Disorders, 29, 312–321.

Wingate, M. E. (1976). *Stuttering: Theory and treatment.* New York: Irvington.

Yairi, E. (1997). Disfluency characteristics of childhood stuttering. In R. F. Curlee
& G. M. Siegel (Eds.), *Nature and treatment of stuttering* (2nd ed., pp. 49–78).
Boston, MA: Allyn & Bacon.

Yairi, E., & Ambrose, N. (1992). A longitudinal study of stuttering in children:
A preliminary report. *Journal of Speech and Hearing Research, 35,*
755–760.

Yairi, E., Ambrose, N., & Cox, N. (1996). Genetics of stuttering: A critical review.
Journal of Speech and Hearing Research, 39, 771–784.

Yairi, E., Ambrose, N., & Niermann, R. (1993). The early months of stuttering: A
developmental study. *Journal of Speech and Hearing Research, 36,* 521–528.

Yairi, E., Ambrose, N., Paden, E. P., & Throneburg, R. N. (1996). Predictive factors of persistence and recovery: Pathways of childhood stuttering. *Journal*
of Communication Disorders, 29, 51–77.

Young, M. A. (1975). Onset, prevalence, and recovery from stuttering. *Journal of*
Speech and Hearing Disorders, 40, 49–58.

Zielhuis, G. A., Rach, G. H., Van Den Broek, P. (1989). Screening for otitis media
with effusion in preschool children. *Lancet, 333,* 311–314.

CHAPTER

The Behavioral Data Language of Stuttering

ANN PACKMAN, Ph.D.,
and
MARK ONSLOW, Ph.D.

A behavioral data language underpins a behavioral science. It enables scientists to report their observations and to communicate with each other about the behavior or condition being studied (Zuriff, 1985). Objectivity and "empiricalness" (Zuriff, 1985, p. 48) are necessary conditions for inclusion in a data language, although interjudge agreement is also an important criterion. This chapter will examine the current data language in stuttering and draw attention to its shortcomings. We suggest that descriptors of stuttering in our current literature are illogical and imprecise and do not, in the main, operationalize the behaviors that characterize the disorder. We suggest that this situation is not conducive to effective communication about stuttering. We present a new behavioral data language of stuttering that incorporates many of the features of current and historical descriptive systems and which, we argue, is more logical, valid and reliable. The benefits for our scientific community of developing a valid and reliable behavioral data language for stuttering are discussed.

DEVELOPMENT OF THE BEHAVIORAL DATA LANGUAGE OF STUTTERING

The current stuttering literature contains numerous descriptors of stuttering, the origins of which are diverse. Many writers have contributed to this terminology over many years and these contributions typically reflect their particular bias or theoretical position. Thus, while some descriptors are behavioral, others incorporate underlying assumptions about the nature of stuttering. There is little doubt that the most influential and lasting contribution to the data language of stuttering was made over 40 years ago by Johnson, who proposed eight disfluency categories (see Johnson & Associates, 1959): *word repetition, sound/syllable repetition, phrase repetition, interjection, revision, incomplete phrase, broken word,* and *prolongation.* Johnson used these categories to describe the disfluencies of normally fluent children as well as the disfluencies of children thought to be stuttering, because he believed that stuttering arises when so-called normal disfluencies are judged to be aberrant. The descriptors formed the data base of a set of landmark studies into the disfluencies of stuttering and nonstuttering children and indeed, subsequent research has confirmed that Johnson's categories can be applied to the speech of both groups of children (for a review see Onslow, 1992).

Johnson's disfluency types marked a departure from previous attempts to describe stuttering, such as *clonic and tonic* (see Van Riper, 1982; Wingate, 1976) and *primary and secondary* (Bluemel, 1932). These descriptors were simplistic in that they divided stuttering events into two categories only. For example, clonic stuttering refers to repetitive movements while in tonic stuttering the speech organs are static. This taxonomy reflects medical terminology for certain types of muscle activity and is not used today; however, the terms clearly describe the kinematic status of the speech mechanism in the two types of stuttering. Bluemel (1932) suggested that sound and syllable repetitions comprise the simple speech disturbance of *primary* stuttering and that *secondary* stuttering occurs when the child becomes aware of this primary disturbance and attempts to force the words out. Both taxonomies include assumptions about the underlying nature of the disorder.

Many writers have revised and added to Johnson's categories, and Table 2–1 shows the contribution of some prominent scholars. These contributions come from both empirical studies and general discussions of stuttering. *Interjection, incomplete phrase,* and *revision* are included because they were part of Johnson's data language, even though they do not typically distinguish between stutterers[1] and normally fluent speakers and hence are typically thought of as normal disfluencies (see Bloodstein, 1995).

---

[1] For stylistic reasons we use the term "stutterer" in this chapter in preference to "person who stutters" (for a discussion of this issue see Manning, 1996, p. xviii). We only use the term "stutterer" in scientific discourse and we do not identify individuals, in any other context, by the way they speak.

Table 2–1. Descriptions of Stuttering Contributed by Prominent Scholars. These Descriptions Come from Both Empirical Studies and General Discussions About Stuttering.

	Johnson & Associates (1959)	Bloodstein (1960); Bloodstein & Grossman (1981)	Williams, Silverman, & Kools (1968)	Wingate (1976)	Van Riper (1982)	Yairi & Lewis (1984)	Conture (1990a)	Lewis (1991)	Zebrowski (1991)
Syllable repetition		X			X			X	
Part-word repetition			X			X			
Word repetition	X	X	X		X	X	X	X	X
Single-syllable/ Monosyllabic word repetition							X		X
Multisyllabic/Polysyllabic word repetition						X			
Sound/Syll repetition	X						X		X
Sound repetition		X						X	
Audible elemental repetition				X					
Silent elemental repetition				X					
Phrase repetition	X	X	X			X		X	
Sound prolongation	X	X					X	X	X
Inaudible/silent prolongation				X	X		X		
Audible prolongation				X	X		X		X
Broken word	X						X	X	
Disrhythmic phonation			X			X			
Hard contact		X							
Hard attack		X							
Block(age)		X			X			X	
Tense pause			X			X		X	
Inappropriate pause		X							
Silent fixation					X				
Fixed (articulatory) posture							X		
Interjection	X		X			X			
Incomplete word/phrase	X		X					X	
Revision	X		X			X		X	

It is well known that stuttered speech disfluencies are frequently accompanied by nonverbal behaviors such as facial, head, and torso movements (for a review see Zebrowski, 1995). These behaviors are typically thought of as associated rather than essential features of the disorder (see Bloodstein, 1995; Van Riper, 1982).

PROBLEMS WITH THE CURRENT DATA LANGUAGE OF STUTTERING

The differences among experts in describing stuttering (see Table 2–1) convey an impression of disarray, suggesting that scientists within the field may not be communicating with each other as effectively as they might. It also suggests that the wider readership of the stuttering literature may be confused about interpreting reports and how best to describe stuttering. We submit that the source of this current disarray is in the nature of the data language, which is inconsistent, illogical, and imprecise and frequently does not portray the behavioral characteristics of the disorder. Below we present some support for this submission.

The shortcomings of Johnson's data language were highlighted in a recent study (Onslow, Bryant, Stuckings, Gardner, & Knight, 1992) in which listeners were instructed to assign the disfluencies of preschool-age children to Johnson's disfluency types (as modified by Williams, Silverman, & Kools, 1968). Five experienced speech-language pathologists listened to an audiotape that contained 200 examples of disfluencies. These were selected from the speech of children judged to be normally fluent and children judged to be stuttering. The disfluency types were *part-word repetition, whole-word repetition, phrase repetition, dysrhythmic phonation,*[2] *tense pause, revision, interjection,* and *incomplete phrase.* The judges were also instructed to judge whether each disfluency was stuttered or not stuttered. Onslow et al. found a low level of agreement among the judges in assigning the eight categories. The findings also supported previous findings (Boehmler, 1958) that one disfluency may be assigned to more than one category; the judges did so for the majority of disfluencies. Onslow (1995) underscored this phenomenon with spectrographic evidence of a repetition and a sound prolongation during the same instance of stuttering. Onslow et al. (1992) also reported that all disfluency types were used to describe disfluencies judged to be stuttered and disfluencies judged not to be stuttered. In other words, the data language appeared to have doubtful capacity to

---

[2] Defined by the investigators as *prolongation.*

provide useful descriptions of normal and stuttered speech. Indeed, Onslow et al. concluded that Johnson's categories do not have sufficient descriptive power and that the validity of the data language must be seriously questioned.

Another problem with our current data language is that it appears inconsistent, the terminology being derived from various sources. Both the word and the syllable are used as the frame of reference. Some writers use *whole-word repetition* and *part-word repetition*, while others use *syllable repetition* and *sound repetition*. Because a word is a unit of meaning, using the word as the frame of reference for stuttering invokes the idea that semantics is implicated in the disorder. On the other hand, the syllable is not a semantic unit but rather is regarded as a unit of speech production. Syllables are the basis of speech timing and of prosodic and phonological organization (Bernhardt & Stoel-Gammon, 1994); thus, using the syllable as the frame of reference invokes the idea that stuttering is a speech disorder. Still other descriptors have their origins in other disciplines or fields of study. For example, *sound repetition* and *sound prolongation* are derived from phonetics, and the word "phonation" in *disrhythmic phonation* describes a physiological phenomenon involving vibration of the vocal folds.

The stuttering descriptors in our current data language are also imprecise. Although *syllable repetition* is commonly used, it is not always the case that syllables are repeated in their entirety during stuttering, the vowel in repeated syllables frequently being perceived as a schwa (see Van Riper, 1982). This perception is apparently due to the failure of the vowel to reach its target duration (Howell, Williams, & Vause, 1987; Howell, Williams, & Young, 1991). Thus, because the target vowels in these repeated syllables are truncated, it is more accurate to describe the disfluencies as the repetition of an incomplete syllable. This is an important distinction because it has been suggested that "part-sound part-syllable repetitions" (Stromsta, 1987, p. 268) distinguish preschool-age children who develop chronic stuttering from their normally fluent peers (see also Stromsta, 1986).

Sound repetition also fails to reflect the true state of affairs in most instances. While the repetition of a speech sound on its own may occur in some contexts (see Viswanath & Neel, 1995), the repeated element is more likely to consist of a consonant and a short portion of the following vowel. To illustrate this, it would be more usual to hear "su-su-su-simply great!" than "s-s-s-simply great!." Thus, it could be argued that in such cases the target syllable has also been truncated, but to a greater extent than in the example in the previous paragraph. Thus we also regard the repeated elements currently classified as *sound repetition* as the repetition of an incomplete syllable, unless, of course, that element constitutes a syllable and is repeated in its entirety, such as in "a-a-a-bout."

The meaning of *disrhythmic phonation* is also not immediately clear, probably because phonation is always disrhythmic, at least in normal conversational or monologue speech. *Audible prolongation* and *silent prolongation* are also not self-explanatory, leaving the reader to assume the referent. It is also not clear if *audible prolongation* is synonymous with *sound prolongation*, whether *silent prolongation* is synonymous with *fixed articulatory posture*, and whether *block*, *tense pause*, and *broken word* all refer to the same phenomenon, although they all apparently refer to cessation of speech of some sort. The term *broken word* is particularly problematic, because of the absence of criteria that an observer would use to judge that a spoken word is "broken."

In short, our current data language fails to facilitate effective communication about the disorder. The following examples of usage, by prominent scholars, of *disrhythmic phonation, prolongation*, and *block* illustrate this.

Disrhythmic phonation has been defined as *sound prolongation* and *block* (see Yairi & Ambrose, 1992).[3] However, *prolongation* has been defined as audible or silent fixation (Van Riper, 1982). This contradicts Yairi and Ambrose since phonation cannot be silent. *Prolongation* has also been described as "sound or airflow continues but movement of one or more articulators is stopped" (Peters & Guitar, 1991). This is incompatible with Van Riper because in Peters and Guitar's definition sound or airflow continues, so the stoppage or fixation cannot be silent (as suggested by Van Riper). Peters and Guitar defined *block* as an inappropriate stoppage of the flow of air or voice and sometimes the articulators. This use of *block* cannot be reconciled with Yairi and Ambrose's term *disrhythmic phonation*, because phonation always involves airflow. In contrast to Peters and Guitar (1991), Conture (1990b) indicated that *block* need not incorporate a stoppage in airflow or voice, because it may involve an audible sound prolongation. And this is consistent with suggestions by Wingate (1976) and Van Riper (1982) that *block* should actually be subsumed by *prolongation*!

Language is a socially constructed device that reflects perceptions of reality. One example is the way we describe the repetitions of early stuttering, in that confusion in the use of descriptors reflects confusion in our understanding of the role of repetitions at the onset of stuttering. Not only are *word repetition* and *part-word repetition* imprecise, but they are interchangeably used with *syllable repetition* (see Wingate, 1976). Clearly, a word may consist of one or more syllables. Thus, in the case of a single-syllable word, *word repetition* and *syllable repetition*

---

[3] *Dysrhythmic phonation* was previously defined by Yairi and Lewis (1984) as "sound prolongations within words, unusual stress or broken words" (p. 156).

are interchangeable. Similarly, *part-word repetition, syllable repetition,* and even *sound repetition* are interchangeably used to refer to the repetition of part of a multisyllabic word. The failure of these components of our data language to reflect the behavioral characteristics of stuttering at its most critical stage—its onset—is illustrated in the following examples.

Bluemel (1932) characterized the onset of stuttering as the repetition of the first word of a sentence and Froeschels (1964) stated that the repetition of syllables and words are the first signs of stuttering. Johnson's categories, which were intended to describe both normal disfluencies and early stuttering, distinguished between *syllable and sound repetition,* and *word repetition.* Van Riper (1982) suggested that in most cases (Track 1 stutterers) *multiple syllable repetition* characterizes the onset of stuttering. Van Riper stated that these repetitions are either of single syllable words or of one syllable of a multisyllabic word. In reviewing the findings of studies that have investigated the speech characteristics of early stuttering, Bloodstein (1995) used *word repetition* and *part-word repetition.* Conture (1990b) distinguished between *single-syllable word repetition* and *sound/syllable repetition,* suggesting that the former may reflect "pure expressive language delays" (p. 60) rather than stuttering. Yairi considered the repetitions of single-syllable words to be elemental in the development of stuttering and included *monosyllabic word repetition* in his *stuttering-like disfluency* category (see Yairi, 1997).

Two statements by Starkweather exemplify this equivocation about the role of repetitions in the onset of stuttering. Starkweather stated that "the stutterer typically begins repeating whole words and then goes on to repeat parts of words" (Starkweather, 1987, p. 120). But later, when discussing "whole-word and whole-syllable repetitions" he stated:

> I don't consider these early behaviors to be stuttering, at least not in the sense that they are a disorder and a problem. I see the problem of stuttering as the extraneous effort, the reactions, and the struggles that can develop in response to those disfluencies. On the other hand, I don't believe that those early, easy repetitions are normal either. (Starkweather, 1997, p. 79)

It seems that further empirical research is needed before we understand what type of repetitions have a role in the onset of stuttering and what that role might be. However, we submit that a prerequisite to further understanding is a consistent data language. The word and the syllable are frequently ambiguously used, even though this issue has been addressed by Wingate (1976) and Van Riper (1982). And, as Yairi (1997) pointed out, at around the age of the onset of stuttering, about 80% of children's words consist of a single syllable anyway. Therefore, it would seem that, in this context, distinguishing between the repetition of a single-syllable word and the repetition of a single syllable in a multisyllabic word is unnecessary. We agree with Van Riper that when a syllable is repeated, regardless of whether it constitutes a whole word or part of a multisyllabic word, it should be regarded simply as the repetition of a syllable, until there is evidence to suggest that there is some benefit in doing otherwise.

Not only does a data language reflect perceptions of reality but it may also influence how we conceptualize the phenomena it describes. We suggest that this is the case with the widely used *block*, to the extent that the term reflects the long-held idea that anatomical structures block the flow of air during stuttering. This perception of a "blockage" appears to be related to the fact that during stuttering the speech mechanism is frequently static and that these "fixations" are typically accompanied by signs of effort. For example:

> It is immediately apparent that the stutterer has closed off his airway. The closure may be produced by pressing the lips together, or by the tongue being pressed firmly against the teeth or roof of the mouth, or by closing the true or false vocal folds. (Van Riper, 1982, p. 121)

And:

> The stutterer blocks off the airway at the glottis or in the mouth, tries to force through this blockage by pushing from the abdomen, but simultaneously increases the pressure at the blockage. (Starkweather, 1987, p. 124)

However, the idea that the stutterer is trying to force the speech airflow past a blockage is not supported by recent research. Zocchi et al. (1990) found that, in adults, subglottic pressure excessively fluctuated during stuttered speech and was frequently below atmospheric pressure. Negative subglottic pressure is incompatible with speech production and is certainly inconsistent with the idea that stutterers are trying to force the speech airflow past an obstruction; if that were the case, subglottic pressure would be consistently above atmospheric pressure. An alternative explanation for the processes underlying speech events described as a "block" is that speech is not progressing because there is insufficient subglottic pressure to produce the airflow that is necessary for that progression.

We have argued that *block* has perpetuated a possibly erroneous perception of the nature of stuttering, because *block* is not a behavioral descriptor but rather invokes an image of the physiological processes thought to underlie the cessation of speech during instances of stuttering that are so labeled. We submit that *fixed posture*, which is a description of the speech mechanism during this type of stuttering, is more accurate because it describes observable behavior, independent of assumptions about the intention or nature of that behavior.

It is logical to assume that the data language of stuttering has been constructed to describe the behavioral features of the disorder. However, an investigation of the origins of the data language suggests this is not always the case. As noted earlier, Johnson intended that his categories describe all disfluencies, not only those of children judged to be stutterers. This is also the case in the so-called "new wave" (Zebrowski, 1995, p. 77) studies of early stuttering. For example, in a landmark study of the disfluencies that typify the speech of young children who do and do not stutter, Yairi and Lewis (1984) assigned all disfluencies from both groups to categories similar to those of Johnson. Naturally, the stuttering group was found to have more disfluencies, the most common of which were *part-word repetition, dysrhythmic phonation,* and *single-syllable word repetition*. Although these disfluency types occurred much more frequently in the stuttering group than in the control group, there was overlap between the groups.

Considering this overlap and the fact that none of the disfluencies were independently identified as stuttered or not stuttered, these disfluencies do not define stuttering or identify individuals as stutterers. Yet these categories are now used for that purpose, particularly with children. For example, Yairi's *stuttering-like disfluencies* (SLDs) incorporate *part-word* and *monosyllabic word repetitions, disrhythmic phonation,* and *tense pause* (see Yairi, 1997), and Yairi and colleagues use three or more SLDs per 100 syllables as a criterion for identifying an individual as a stutterer. This is despite the fact that three or more SLDs per 100 words accounted for only 80% of the children that were judged to be stutterers in Johnson's study (see Yairi, 1997). *Within-word disfluency* and *between-word disfluency* are also used to distinguish between stuttering and normal disfluencies (for a discussion of this issue see Cordes & Ingham, 1995b). Based on Johnson's descriptors, Conture (1990b) has defined *within-word disfluencies* (WWDs) as *sound/syllable repetitions, broken words,* and *sound prolongations* (and possibly monosyllabic whole-word repetitions). Conture (1990b; 1997) suggested that three or more WWDs per 100 words be used as a criterion for identifying an individual as a stutterer, despite the fact that this criterion accounted for only about 60% of the children that were judged to be stutterers in Johnson's study (see Conture, 1990b).

The fact that SLD and WWD do not categorically distinguish stutterers from nonstutterers is acknowledged by their protagonists (see Conture, 1990a, 1990b; Yairi, 1997). Thus, when these categories are used in empirical studies, they typically comprise one of two or more criteria for identifying subjects as stutterers. Zebrowski (1991) allocated children to the stuttering group on the basis of (1) "quantitative criteria" (p. 484) which were three or more WWDs per 100 words, and (2) parental concern about the child's fluency or the "belief that the child was stuttering or a stutterer" (p. 484). Similarly, Yairi, Ambrose, Paden, and Throneburg (1996) allotted children to the stuttering group if they (1) had three or more SLDs per 100 syllables, (2) had stuttering severity ratings of at least 2, and (3) were judged by parents and two investigators as having a "stuttering problem" (p. 53). In short, criterion frequencies of SLD and WWD are considered necessary but not sufficient in identifying a person as a stutterer.

However, it can be argued that criterion frequencies of certain types of verbal disfluencies are not necessary for such identification. The logic underlying them is circular because, in both the Johnson and the Yairi and Lewis studies, children were allocated in the first instance to either a stuttering group or a nonstuttering group on the basis of a perceptual judgment. That is, in those studies, the groups whose membership SLD and WWD are designed to predict were determined on the basis of parental judgment. And because WWD and SLD do not predict membership of those groups with a high degree of accuracy, it can be argued that consensus diagnosis[4] is sufficient to identify an individual as a stutterer. We do not mean to imply that it is not important to explore the distribution and types of disfluency that are found in the speech of young children, or to investigate why observers judge some individuals to be stutterers and others not; we simply argue that the role of a behavioral data language is to describe stuttering rather than to define it.

As noted earlier, aberrant nonverbal behaviors are frequently observed during stuttering. For this reason, descriptions of verbal disfluencies alone are insufficient to describe the range of behaviors that typify the disorder. The complexity of stuttering is reflected in some stuttering protocols (for a review see Gordon & Luper, 1992). For example, Curlee (1980) takes facial and body movements into account along with type, frequency, and duration of verbal disfluencies in a protocol designed to identify the incipient stutterer. These nonverbal behaviors may be critical in making a perceptual judgment that a person is a stutterer. For example, brief pauses that infrequently occur during speech but are accompanied by signs of effort might prompt such a judgment. We suggest that, if the role of a behavioral data language is to describe

---

[4]A consensus diagnosis of stuttering rests on agreement that the child is a stutterer by two or more of the following: parents, investigators, clinicians, and other people in the child's environment (see Ingham, 1993; Onslow, 1992).

stuttering, then that language should include descriptors of nonverbal behaviors that are part of the disorder.

THE DATA LANGUAGE OF STUTTERING AND TREATMENT RESEARCH

Although disfluency descriptors have been used in discussions about the nature of stuttering and to investigate differences between stutterers and normally fluent speakers, they are rarely used in treatment research. This is probably because such research typically relies on perceptual judgments of stuttering and because the goal of behavioral treatments is typically the elimination of stuttering.

To date, efficacy research in stuttering has been predominantly behavioral, and severity measures based on stutter counts are usually the main dependent variable. These measures rely on perceptual judgment rather than on a standard behavioral definition of stuttering (see Martin & Haroldson, 1981). In other words, they rely on a categorical judgment that stuttering is, or is not, present. For example, on-line measures of percent syllables stuttered (%SS) depend on a listener judging each syllable spoken to be either stuttered or not stuttered. Interval-based measures of stuttering (see Cordes & Ingham, 1995a) also rely on categorical judgments, in that intervals of speech rather than syllables or words are judged to be either stuttered or not stuttered. Another commonly used severity measure, the Stuttering Severity Instrument (SSI; Riley, 1972), reflects the frequency and duration of instances of stuttering and the severity of associated nonverbal behaviors. In all these behavioral measures, the observer is not required to describe or classify the stuttering behaviors.

The primary goal of behavioral programs is typically zero, or near zero, levels of stuttering, and in such cases passage through the program is contingent on attaining that criterion level. Thus, there is an implication that type of stuttering is irrelevant in assessing treatment outcome. However, there are grounds for arguing that such an assumption is unfounded. Although eliminating stuttering is a worthy goal of treatment, that goal is rarely achieved by clients, particularly adults. For example, in treatments based on novel speech patterns such a goal would be achieved by only a small proportion of clients and even they may relapse to some extent after treatment (Martin, 1981). For example, 0%SS was an infrequent finding in a recent outcome study (Boberg & Kully, 1994) of treatment based on prolonged speech. In that study, 17 adult clients were assessed at regular intervals after their clinic-based treatment. Although low levels of posttreatment stuttering were reported for the group, particularly immediately after treatment, of 58 data points ranging from immediately posttreatment to 12 months posttreatment, 50 indicated residual stuttering. In the Lidcombe Program (Lincoln, Onslow, & Reed, 1977; Lincoln, Onslow, Wilson, & Lewis, 1996; Onslow, Andrews, & Lincoln, 1994; Onslow, Costa, & Rue, 1990), which is a treatment for early stuttering, very low levels of stuttering frequency have been detected some years after the cessation of treatment, more so in school-age than in preschool-age children (Lincoln & Onslow, 1997). Indeed, the criterion for progression to the maintenance phase of this program is typically set at below 1%SS, rather than at 0%SS. This criterion means that a very low level of mild, probably normal, disfluency in a child's speech is an expedient goal of treatment.

If it is the case that residual stuttering is commonplace after behavioral treatments, albeit at low levels, it can be argued that severity measures alone are insufficient grounds for assessing outcome (see Ingham & Andrews, 1971). Take the example of an adult whose stuttering frequency reduces by, say, 75% as a result of treatment. In terms of existing outcome data this would be regarded as a poor outcome. However, that outcome might be evaluated differently if before treatment the client's stuttering consisted of long speech stoppages accompanied by signs of effort, and after treatment it consisted of syllable repetitions with no signs of effort. Similarly, outcomes of the Lidcombe Program can only be evaluated comprehensively if we can accurately describe the nature of the remaining disfluencies. Reports of the Lidcombe Program have not addressed this issue to date because Onslow et al. (1992) concluded that the existing data language was not sufficiently valid or reliable.

This issue of the importance of the nature of residual stuttering was addressed in a study (Ingham & Andrews, 1971) of outcomes of two behavioral treatments for adults based on novel speech patterns, one based on rhythmic speech and one based on prolonged speech. Although %SS was the main dependent variable, the nature of residual disfluencies was also investigated. The residual stuttering of subjects who received the prolonged-speech treatment consisted of simple repetitions while that of the rhythmic speech group still contained blocks and prolongations. This finding apparently contributed to the decision of the authors to replace rhythmic speech with prolonged speech in that treatment program. According to Andrews and Ingham (1972) "assessment of outcome can be approached with increased sophistication if the quality of resulting fluency and the nature of any residual stuttering are considered" (p. 299). Certainly, descriptions of residual stuttering would enable a more sophisticated assessment of outcome in the Lidcombe Program. For instance, it may be the case that the typology of residual stuttering in that program differs as a function of age.

A valid and reliable data language also has implications for outcome research into treatments other than those based on behavioral principles. A recent study of the effects of drugs on stuttering (Stager, Ludlow, Gordon, Cotelingham, & Rapoport, 1995) used length of disfluency as the dependent variable. Only one of the drugs was reported to have an effect on this variable. However, it is possible that changes in the topography of subjects' stuttering might have been detected if stuttering types had been included as a dependent variable, as reported by Prins, Mandelkorn, and Cerf (1980). Identifying changes in stuttering topography may lead to interesting insights into the effects of drugs on the neurophysiology of speech. Indeed, a valid and reliable data language may have implications for wider physiological experimental research, although perhaps only when experimental conditions do not completely eliminate stuttering.

There are other areas of treatment research that could benefit from a valid and reliable data language. For example, it is possible that topography of stuttering predicts response to treatment. In other words, certain types of stuttering may be more amenable to certain treatments and/or may be associated with more durable treatment effects. This idea was integral to Brutten and Shoemaker's (1967) Two-Factor Theory of stuttering. According to that theory, the repetitions and prolongations of stuttering, which are classically conditioned, should be treated with reciprocal inhibition while other behaviors, which are instrumentally conditioned (and not considered to be stuttering), should be treated with massed practice. However, the efficacy of this treatment approach was never satisfactorily established (see Ingham, 1984). Given the pervasive and serious nature of relapse after behavioral treatments based on novel speech patterns, the possibility of a relationship between type of stuttering and treatment outcome seems worth investigating.

The idea that stuttering type may predict responsiveness to treatment has implications for matching subjects in controlled treatment trials, particularly where a treatment is compared with other treatments and/or with a control group. If there is such a relationship, then stuttering severity alone is insufficient grounds for matching subjects and stuttering type may be an important variable in studies where treatments are replicated across clinical sites. For example, it may be inappropriate to attempt to replicate findings of successful outcome in the Lidcombe Program with children whose stuttering differs in topography from those in the original studies.

THE LIDCOMBE DATA LANGUAGE

We have outlined the importance of a behavioral data language for theoretical and empirical investigations into stuttering, including treatment research, and we have briefly explored the validity and reliability problems with our existing data language. Accordingly, we suggest that it is

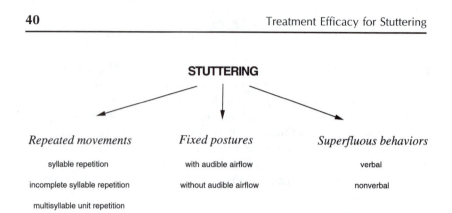

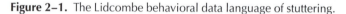

Figure 2–1. The Lidcombe behavioral data language of stuttering.

timely to develop a more accurate, logical, and reliable way of describing the behavioral features of stuttering. In this section we describe a data language that we believe incorporates those criteria but, at the same time, does not introduce any new concepts about stuttering. All the stuttering descriptors in the proposed data language have been previously used in the literature; we have simply extracted those that are consistent with the above criteria and organized them into a logical and parsimonious taxonomy. The stuttering descriptors reflect audible and visible behaviors and are consistent with the idea that stuttering presents as a speech disorder. The proposed data language, which is known as the Lidcombe data language, is presented in Figure 2–1.

The stuttering descriptors fall into three classes: *repeated movements, fixed postures*, and *superfluous behaviors*. The first two classes reflect the kinematic status of the speech mechanism. In the first, the speech mechanism is moving, albeit in a repetitive fashion. In the second, the speech mechanism is primarily fixed and any movements that occur are not functional for speech production. The behaviors of *repeated movements* and *fixed postures* occur during the production of the target utterance, while those of the third class, *superfluous behaviors*, are related, but not integral, to the perceived target utterance.

Repeated Movements

The syllable is the frame of reference for these repetitive speech movements. *Syllable repetition* refers to the repetition of a syllable in its entirety. The repetitions in "on-on-on a chair" and in "un-un-under a chair" would both be included in *syllable repetition*, despite the fact that the former is the repetition of a single-syllable word and the latter is the repetition of a syllable that is part of a multisyllabic word. We argue that in both examples the speaker is repeating a unit of speech production, namely the syllable.

Incomplete syllable repetition refers to the repetition of a syllable that has not reached its potential. This includes instances where (1) the vowel of the syllable is not fully realized, regardless of whether this is because it does not reach the target duration or because it does not reach the target formant structure, and (2) a consonant or consonant cluster without the vowel is repeated. This means that the extent to which a syllable is incomplete is a perceptual continuum.

Distinguishing between *syllable repetition* and *incomplete syllable repetition* may be problematic on some occasions because of the nature of syllabification. In spoken English there is a preference for syllables to be produced in CV form (see Tuller & Kelso, 1991); thus the syllables in the word "passing" are "pa" and "ssing," despite the fact that the morphological structure of the word is "pass" and "ing." Thus, "pa-pa-pa-passing" contains a single-syllable repetition, not a part-syllable repetition, as might appear to be the case.

Multisyllable-unit repetition refers to instances where more than one syllable is repeated as a unit. This includes multisyllabic words such as "over-over-over the top . . . ," a cluster of words such as "in the-in the-in the end . . . ," or syllables that form part of a word such as ". . . photo-photo-photographic"

Fixed Postures

The defining feature of this class of stuttering behaviors is that the structures of the vocal tract are stationary during attempts to speak. The structures assume a posture (that is, they are not at rest) but then movement is arrested. These fixed postures may or may not be accompanied by airflow and that judgment is perceptually made . That is, the listener either hears or does not hear airflow. Airflow may be voiced, for example in "aaaaaaaaaaafter lunch . . ." or it may be unvoiced, for example "hhhhhhhhhhhhe's over here." These stuttering behaviors would have been previously described as *sound prolongation* or *audible prolongation*. Of course, when no airflow is perceived, there will be no noise accompanying the fixed posture. This type of stuttering would previously probably have been described as *silent prolongation, block, tense pause*, and so on. Some or all of the stuttering behaviors included in *fixed postures* may have been previously categorized as *disrhythmic phonation*. In summary, *fixed postures* captures the feature that underpins a number of previous descriptors, namely that the articulators are not moving in a way that is essential for speech to proceed. *Fixed postures* is used rather than *fixed articulatory postures* in order to specify that the immobility is related to the production of all speech sounds, not only consonants.

Although by definition *repeated movements* and *fixed postures* are mutually exclusive, behaviors belonging to both classes may sequentially occur within an instance of stuttering (see Onslow, 1995).

Superfluous Behaviors

The salient feature of the stuttering behaviors in this descriptor class is that, unlike those in the two previous ones, they are superfluous to the final utterance (as it would normally be spoken). The characterization of these stuttering behaviors as superfluous was prompted by the definition by Johnson and Associates (1959) of interjection as "extraneous syllables, sounds, words or phrases that were distinct from sounds and words associated with the fluent or meaningful text" (p. 202). Superfluous behaviors consist of (1) verbal behaviors currently classified as *interjection, incomplete phrase*, and *revision*, and which are usually considered to be normal disfluencies but which have been incorporated into the stuttering, such as "I went-oh well-oh well-um, I-well . . ."; and (2) visible or audible nonverbal behaviors such as facial, head, and torso movements, speaking on inspiratory air, grunts, and other inappropriate noises and aberrant fluctuations in pitch and loudness. All of these behaviors are typically highly idiosyncratic (Van Riper, 1982; Wingate, 1976) and may be described in detail for individual speakers.

A PRELIMINARY STUDY

We believe that the Lidcombe data language has considerable face validity because it is consistent with many existing observations and descriptions of stuttering behaviors. However, we wanted to know whether these descriptors could actually be applied to the speech of stutterers and how well judges would agree when they did so. We conducted a small study to collect some preliminary data on the usefulness of the proposed data language.

Method

A videotape was constructed with 47 short speech samples, each of which contained an instance of stuttering. An independent clinician selected the samples and the first investigator agreed that the disfluencies contained in the samples were stutterings. The samples were selected from videorecordings of 16 speakers who had been previously identified as stutterers. The speakers ranged from preschool-age to adult and were as stutterers. The speakers ranged from preschool-age to adult and were judged to display a range of type and severity of stuttering. Two to three samples were selected from each speaker. The samples were dubbed in random order onto the master tape and separated by a 10-second silence. Each sample was preceded by the sample number.

Five speech-language pathologists who were experienced in treatment and research in stuttering served as judges. All had worked together and routinely used variations of Johnson's data language to describe stuttering. Judges viewed the videotape alone. They were given one page of information about the Lidcombe data language, including a description and an example of each stuttering descriptor. They were also given a response form, which listed the sample numbers down the left hand side and the seven descriptors across the top. Judges were instructed to watch the videotape and to assign each sample to one or more of the descriptors by ticking one or more of the seven cells next to the sample number. They were instructed to replay samples as often as they wished before assigning them. There was an eighth column on the response sheet labeled Other/Comments and judges were instructed to note in this column any stuttering behavior that they could not assign to any of the seven descriptors and to write any comments they might have about any of the descriptors. They were instructed to write down, upon completing the task, any comments they had about the task in general. The first investigator interviewed each judge after he or she completed the task.

Results

There were 329 opportunities to agree that a behavior was, or was not, present (47 samples times 7 descriptors). Of these, 198 (60%) attracted unanimous agreement. Four out of five judges agreed on 69 (21%) of these occasions and there was no agreement (that is, the judges were split 2–3) on 62 (19%) of these occasions. Interestingly, of the occasions where there was no agreement, over half involved *syllable repetition* and *incomplete syllable repetition*. In other words, over 50% of the error was accounted for by two descriptors.

All the samples were assigned to one or more descriptors and all descriptors were used with about the same frequency. Descriptors were used about as often as they were not used. There were no other behaviors noted in the eighth column.

At the exit interview, all judges reported that they found the task difficult. They said they felt they needed more information about the data language and that they would have liked to view examples of the descriptors and discuss them before attempting the task. However, all judges reported that they felt the data language made sense.

Interestingly, judges reported that doing the task was like learning a new language. For example, they reported thinking "This is a block, what is it called in the new data language?" However, they reported that as the task progressed they started to directly process auditory and visual information without needing to "translate" from the old data language to the new one.

DISCUSSION

We have presented an alternative data language for stuttering that we believe is potentially useful for describing the behavioral features of the disorder. Although all observations are theory-laden (Zuriff, 1985), the Lidcombe data language is not derived from a theoretical position about the nature of stuttering, other than that we view stuttering as a speech disorder. We have argued elsewhere (see Packman, Onslow, Richard, & van Doorn, 1996) that, regardless of the underlying deficit in stuttering, that deficit is mediated through speech. In other words, regardless of whether the aberrant process underlying stuttering is in the area of phonological encoding, lexical retrieval, anticipatory struggle, or at some level of speech motor control, that deficit manifests itself through speech. The syllable is the frame of reference for stuttering in the Lidcombe data language because the syllable, rather than the word, is the unit of speech production.

The Lidcombe data language has considerable face validity. The results of the preliminary study suggest that the data language is comprehensive and that none of the descriptors is redundant. It does not introduce any new concepts about stuttering but simply takes existing descriptions of, and ideas about, stuttering and reorganizes them into a more logical, consistent, and parsimonious descriptive system. The three descriptor classes in the Lidcombe data language resemble, to some degree, the classificatory system proposed by Wingate (1976), who categorized stuttering into *repetitions*, *prolongations*, and *associated features*, although Wingate regarded only the first two categories as "core" behaviors in stuttering. In our view, all the observable behaviors of stuttering *are* stuttering. Thus, a stuttering behavioral data language should reflect all of the aberrant audible and visible behaviors, both verbal and nonverbal, that comprise the disorder.

To some extent the Lidcombe data language also reflects the early stuttering classification systems of *primary and secondary* and *tonic and clonic*, in that the Lidcombe data language's *repetitive movement* obviously distinguishes between repetitions and other stuttering behaviors. Conture (1990b) also distinguished between repetitive or *beta* behaviors and fixed or *gamma* behaviors, the latter being described as a response to *beta* behaviors. However, the Lidcombe data language does not ascribe any intention to the three descriptor classes. That is, it does not *a priori* suggest that the behaviors of *fixed posture* and *superfluous movement* are a progression from, or a reaction to, repetititive movements. However, a valid and reliable behavioral data language would lay the foundation for investigating empirically the long-held view that chronic stuttering develops along such a course.

Although there are grounds to believe that the Lidcombe data language has the potential to be a valid and reliable system for describing stuttering, further research is required to establish just how useful the language will be. One aspect of the data language that needs further investigation is the independence of the descriptors. That is, it will be necessary to demonstrate that two or more descriptors are not always used together. There was no evidence of this in the preliminary study, but this will need to be established in further research. Another aspect that needs to be investigated is the construct validity of the data language. It is essential that the descriptors typify the speech of persons identified as stutterers but not the speech of individuals who are judged to be normally fluent.

We have argued that the Lidcombe data language has considerable validity as a system for describing the behavioral features of stuttering in both children and adults. However, that will count for little without acceptable reliability. The present findings suggest that listeners can achieve reasonable agreement when using the data language; however, comparative research is needed to investigate whether it is more reliable than existing classification systems.

The results of the preliminary study suggest a number of ways that the reliability of the Lidcombe data language may be increased. The first is to simplify the task. The judges reported that it took up to an hour to complete the task, which suggests that there were too many speech samples. The fact that the judges were unfamiliar with the data language would have added to task demands. Thus, it is likely that reducing the number of judgments made simultaneously would simplify the task. This could involve fewer speech samples per task or applying fewer descriptors. In the latter case, instructing judges to apply, say, *repetitive movements* first, then replay the video and apply *fixed postures*, and then replay the video and apply *superfluous behaviors*, may increase interjudge agreement.

Applying the Lidcombe data language is a novel task that requires a considerable reconceptualization of what one is observing when a person stutters, and all judges suggested that more information about the descriptors and experience in assigning disfluencies to them may have improved their performance. Thus, a second way of attempting to improve interjudge agreement would be training judges. The finding that *syllable repetition* and *incomplete syllable repetition* accounted for more than half the disagreement suggests that distinguishing between these descriptive categories would be one target of that training. It is also likely that practice in using the new data language would increase interjudge agreement.

It should be noted that there are two levels at which agreement may be reached. Thus, if it is not possible to obtain acceptable agreement for a particular individual on the seven descriptors, it might be possible to obtain acceptable agreement on the three descriptor classes.

It needs to be emphasized that the Lidcombe data language is simply a way of talking about stuttering. It provides a logical and consistent way of describing the behaviors that typify stuttering but does not predict stuttering or identify individuals as stutterers. The authors favor a perceptual definition of stuttering rather than a behavioral one. That is, we accept that stuttering is present if two or more experienced judges agree that it is present. The Lidcombe data language is a way of describing disfluencies that have already been judged to be stuttering.

Further, the Lidcombe data language is not a stuttering severity instrument. It does not suggest that one descriptor or descriptor class represents a more severe form of stuttering than another. Rather, the Lidcombe data language would be used in conjunction with a measure of severity such as frequency counts, interval judgments, duration of stutterings, or the SSI. Again, the Lidcombe data language is simply a way of describing the features of stuttering.

So why is it important to have a valid and reliable behavioral data language for stuttering? We have argued that our data language underlies much of how we understand stuttering; we use it to describe features of the disorder and as a data base for empirical investigations into the nature of the disorder. Clearly, a valid and reliable data language would contribute to research into the nature of stuttering by providing a more accurate and precise tool for describing the observable features of the disorder. For the same reasons, a valid and reliable data language is likely to enhance treatment research. The observable features of stuttering may predict responsiveness to treatment and maintenance of treatment effects, and accurate and reliable descriptions of posttreatment residual stuttering could provide an added perspective on treatment outcome.

Language is never static; it changes over time as perceptions of reality change. The data language of stuttering is no exception; it has been altered and added to over the years as empirical and theoretical developments contributed to our understanding of the disorder. We submit that it is timely to reconsider the data language we currently use and to modify it to ensure that it validly reflects the behaviors of stuttering. A valid and reliable behavioral data language may lead to new insights into stuttering by enabling accurate reporting of behavior and behavior change. We have presented a new data language that describes stuttering in behavioral terms and which we believe is consistent, logical, and valid. Further research is needed to investigate the usefulness of the Lidcombe data language and to establish whether it facilitates more effective communication about stuttering.

REFERENCES

Andrews, G., & Ingham, R. (1972). An approach to the evaluation of stuttering therapy. *Journal of Speech and Hearing Research, 15*, 296–302.

Bernhardt, B., & Stoel-Gammon, C. (1994). Nonlinear phonology: Introduction and clinical applications. *Journal of Speech and Hearing Research, 37*, 123–143.

Bloodstein, O. (1960). The development of stuttering. I: Changes in nine basic features. *Journal of Speech and Hearing Disorders, 25*, 219–237.

Bloodstein, O. (1995). *A handbook on stuttering* (5th ed.). San Diego, CA: Singular Publishing Group.

Bloodstein, O., & Grossman, M. (1981). Early stuttering: Some aspects of their form and distribution. *Journal of Speech and Hearing Research, 24*, 298–302.

Bluemel, C. S. (1932). Primary and secondary stammering. *The Quarterly Journal of Speech, 18*, 187–200.

Boberg, E., & Kully, D. (1994). Long-term results of an intensive treatment program for adults and adolescents who stutter. *Journal of Speech and Hearing Research, 37*, 1050–1059.

Boehmler, R. M. (1958). Listener responses to nonfluencies. *Journal of Speech and Hearing Research, 1*, 132–141.

Brutten, G. J., & Shoemaker, D. J. (1967). *The modification of stuttering.* Englewood Cliffs, NJ: Prentice Hall.

Conture, E. (1990a). Childhood stuttering: What is it and who does it? In J. A. Cooper (Ed.), *Research needs in stuttering: Roadblocks and future directions. ASHA Reports, 18*, 2–14.

Conture, E. (1990b). *Stuttering* (2nd ed.). Englewood Cliffs, NJ: Prentice Hall.

Conture, E. (1997). Evaluating childhood stuttering. In R. F. Curlee & G. M. Siegel (Eds.), *Nature and treatment of stuttering: New directions* (2nd ed., pp. 239–256). Needham Heights, MA: Allyn & Bacon.

Cordes, A., & Ingham, R. J. (1995a). Judgments of stuttered and nonstuttered intervals by recognized authorities in stuttering research. *Journal of Speech and Hearing Research, 38*, 33–41.

Cordes, A., & Ingham, R. J. (1995b). Stuttering includes both within-word and between-word disfluencies. *Journal of Speech and Hearing Research, 38*, 382–386.

Curlee, R. F. (1980). A case selection strategy for young disfluent children. *Seminars in Speech, Language, and Hearing, 1*, 277–287.

Froeschels, E. (1964). *Selected papers of Emil Froeschels.* Amsterdam, Holland: North-Holland Publishing Co.

Gordon, P. A., & Luper, H. L. (1992). The early identification of beginning stutter-
    ing. I: Protocols. *American Journal of Speech-Language Pathology, May,*
    43–53.
Howell, P., Williams, M., & Vause, L. (1987). Acoustic analysis of repetitions in
    stutterers' speech. In H. F. M. Peters & W. Hulstijn (Eds.), *Speech motor dy-
    namics in stuttering* (pp. 372–380). New York: Springer–Verlag.
Howell, P., Williams, M., & Young, K. (1991). Production of vowels by stuttering
    children and teenagers. In H. F. M. Peters, W. Hulstijn, & C. W. Starkweather
    (Eds.), *Speech motor control and stuttering* (pp. 409–414). Amsterdam, Hol-
    land: Excerpta Medica.
Ingham, J. C. (1993). Behavioral treatment of stuttering children. In R. F. Curlee
    (Ed.), *Stuttering and related disorders of fluency* (pp. 68–100). New York:
    Thieme.
Ingham, R. J. (1984). *Stuttering and behavior therapy: Current status and ex-
    perimental foundations.* San Diego, CA: College-Hill Press.
Ingham, R. J., & Andrews, G. (1971). Stuttering: The quality of fluency after
    treatment. *Journal of Communication Disorders, 4,* 289–301.
Johnson, W., & Associates (1959). *The onset of stuttering.* Minneapolis, MN:
    University of Minnesota Press.
Lewis, K. E. (1991). The structure of disfluency behaviors in the speech of adult
    stutterers. *Journal of Speech and Hearing Research, 34,* 492–500.
Lincoln, M., & Onslow, M. (1997). Long-term outcome of an early interven-
    tion for stuttering. *American Journal of Speech-Language Pathology, 6,*
    51–58.
Lincoln, M., Onslow, M., & Reed, V. (1997). Social validity of an early interven-
    tion for stuttering: The Lidcombe Program. *American Journal of Speech-
    Language Pathology, 6,* 77–84.
Lincoln, M., Onslow, M., Wilson, L., & Lewis, C. (1996). A clinical trial of an
    operant treatment for school-age stuttering children. *American Journal of
    Speech-Language Pathology, 5,* 73–85.
Manning, W. H. (1996). *Clinical decision making in the diagnosis and treat-
    ment of fluency disorders.* Albany, NY: Delmar.
Martin, R. (1981). Introduction and perspective: A review of published research.
    In E. Boberg (Ed.), *Maintenance of fluency.* New York: Elsevier.
Martin, R. R., & Haroldson, S. K. (1981). Stuttering identification: Standard
    definition and moment of stuttering. *Journal of Speech and Hearing Re-
    search, 46,* 59–63.
Onslow, M. (1992). Identification of early stuttering: Issues and suggested strat-
    egies. *American Journal of Speech-Language Pathology, September,* 21–27.
Onslow, M. (1995). A picture is worth more than any words. *Journal of Speech
    and Hearing Research, 38,* 586–588.
Onslow, M., Andrews, C., & Lincoln, M. (1994). A control/experimental trial of
    an operant treatment for early stuttering. *Journal of Speech and Hearing
    Research, 37,* 1244–1259.
Onslow, M., Bryant, K. M., Stuckings, C. L., Gardner, K., & Knight, T. (1992).
    Stuttered and normal speech events in early childhood: The validity of a
    behavioral data language. *Journal of Speech and Hearing Research, 35,*
    79–87.

Onslow, M., Costa, L., & Rue, S. (1990). Direct early intervention with stuttering: Some preliminary data. *Journal of Speech and Hearing Disorders, 55,* 405–416.

Packman, A., Onslow, M., Richard, F., & van Doorn, J. (1996). Syllabic stress and variability: A model of stuttering. *Clinical Linguistics and Phonetics, 10,* 235–263.

Peters, T., & Guitar, B. (1991). *Stuttering: An integrative approach to its nature and treatment.* Baltimore, MD: Williams & Williams.

Prins, D., Mandelkorn, T., & Cerf, F. A. (1980). Principle and differential effects of haloperidol and placebo treatments upon speech disfluencies in stutterers. *Journal of Speech and Hearing Research, 23,* 614–629.

Riley, G. (1972). A stuttering severity instrument for children and adults. *Journal of Speech and Hearing Research, 37,* 314–322.

Stager, S. V., Ludlow, C. L., Gordon, C. T., Cotelingham, M., & Rapoport, J. L. (1995). Fluency changes in persons who stutter following a double blind trial of clomiprimine and desiprimine. *Journal of Speech and Hearing Research, 38,* 516–525.

Starkweather, C. W. (1987). *Fluency and stuttering.* Englewood Cliffs, NJ: Prentice Hall.

Starkweather, C. W. (1997). Therapy for younger children. In R. F. Curlee & G. M. Siegel (Eds.), *Nature and treatment of stuttering: New directions* (2nd ed., pp. 257–279). Needham Heights, MA: Allyn & Bacon.

Stromsta, C. (1986). *Elements of stuttering.* Oshtemo, MI: Atsmorts Publishing.

Stromsta, C. (1987). Acoustic and electrophysiologic correlates of stuttering and early developmental reactions. In H. F. M. Peters & W. Hulstijn (Eds.), *Speech motor dynamics in stuttering* (pp. 268–277). New York: Springer–Verlag.

Tuller, B., & Kelso, J. A. S. (1991). The production and perception of syllable structure. *Journal of Speech and Hearing Research, 34,* 501–508.

Van Riper, C. (1982). *The nature of stuttering* (2nd ed.). Englewood Cliffs, NJ: Prentice Hall.

Viswanath, N. S., & Neel, A. T. (1995). Part-word repetitions by persons who stutter: Fragment type and their articulatory processes. *Journal of Speech and Hearing Research, 38,* 740–750.

Williams, D. E., Silverman, F. H., & Kools, J. A. (1968). Disfluency behavior of elementary-school stutterers and nonstutterers: The adaptation effect. *Journal of Speech and Hearing Research, 11,* 622–630.

Wingate, M. E. (1976). *Stuttering: Theory and treatment.* New York: Irvington Publishers, Inc.

Yairi, E. (1997). Disfluency characteristics of childhood stuttering. In R. F. Curlee & G. M. Siegel (Eds.), *Nature and treatment of stuttering: New directions* (2nd ed., pp. 49–78). Needham Heights, MA: Allyn & Bacon.

Yairi, E., & Ambrose, N. (1992). Onset of stuttering in preschool children: Selected factors. *Journal of Speech and Hearing Research, 35,* 782–788.

Yairi, E., Ambrose, N. G., Paden, E. P., & Throneburg, R. N. (1996). Predictive factors of persistence and recovery: Pathways of childhood stuttering. *Journal of Communication Disorders, 29,* 51–77.

Yairi, E., & Lewis, B. (1984). Disfluencies at the onset of stuttering. *Journal of Speech and Hearing Research, 27,* 145–154.

Zebrowski, P. M. (1991). Duration of the speech disfluencies of beginning stutterers. *Journal of Speech and Hearing Research, 34*, 483–491.

Zebrowski, P. M. (1995). The topography of beginning stuttering. *Journal of Fluency Disorders, 28*, 75–91.

Zocchi, L., Estenne, M., Johnston, S., del Ferro, L., Ward, M. E., & Macklem, P. T. (1990). Respiratory muscle incoordination in stuttering speech. *American Review of Respiratory Diseases, 141*, 1510–1515.

Zuriff, G. E. (1985). *Behaviorism: A conceptual reconstruction.* New York: Columbia University Press.

CHAPTER

What Can Genetics Research Tell Us About Stuttering Treatment Issues?

SUSAN FELSENFELD, Ph.D.

A book about treatment and treatment efficacy for stuttering might seem an unlikely place to find a chapter on genetics. Although it is widely understood that genetics research can answer important questions about the etiology of a condition, it is less obvious how the results of these studies contribute to the day-to-day clinical management process. In reality, good behavioral genetics research enhances our understanding of disorders at many levels, most of which have no direct connection with gene-finding or genetic modeling activities. Thus, although behavioral genetics work usually does not directly focus on clinical process or outcome variables, many of the issues that must be resolved for genetics work to proceed (e.g., issues of case selection and phenotypic definition) turn out to have direct and important clinical implications.

Probably the most obvious interface between these two research domains is the shared notion that family history status (i.e., the presence or absence of a positive family history for disorder) is a relevant variable to examine. On the surface, this variable is straightforward to conceptualize and measure. You ask a person who stutters, or his or her parents in the case of a child, whether anyone else in their immediate or extended family ever stuttered. If the answer is yes, that person has a positive family history (i.e., they are an [FHP] or familial case). If the answer is no, the person is considered a family history negative (FHN) or sporadic case. Implicit in this classification is the idea that these two groups are fundamentally different; they stutter for different reasons and might therefore be genetically "programmed" to *behave* differently in a number of clinically relevant ways, including responsiveness to therapeutic management, probability of spontaneous recovery, and long-term outcome. These are profoundly important hypotheses that, if true, will likely change the way we assess and treat our stuttering clients. Can genetic studies, particularly those examining family history status, fulfill this promise? Can they help to resolve some of the most fundamental puzzles surrounding stuttering etiology, pathogenesis, and treatment? Has behavioral genetics research already made significant advances in these areas? These are the questions that will be addressed, in a preliminary manner, by the present chapter. It is worth noting that this chapter is not a comprehensive review of previous behavioral genetic (i.e., twin and family) studies of stuttering. For these, the reader is directed to Felsenfeld (1997) and Yairi, Ambrose, and Cox (1996). Instead, the chapter will focus on a critical examination of the family history design in general and as applied to stuttering, and will end with some personal reflections about the responsible use of current family-genetic data in the management of stuttering clients.

WHAT CLINICIANS WANT TO KNOW ABOUT FAMILY HISTORY AND STUTTERING

Many professionals who treat and/or study persons who stutter have an intuition that family history status is a significant case history constituent. When clinicians are asked to identify ways in which the results of genetic studies have been helpful in their management of clients, family history is often mentioned as the one variable whose contribution is clear and understandable; a positive family history is "known" to be prognostically unfavorable, particularly for children. The family history variable has received recent attention in the research literature as well. Zebrowski (1997), for example, has suggested that the presence of other persistent stutterers in a child's family may be "the first potentially clear indicator of stuttering risk" (p. 20), and Curlee and Yairi (1997) indicate that recent empirical findings provide "strong support for using genetic information in predicting the remission or persistence of stuttering" (p. 12). This optimism about the family history variable may well spark a flurry of clinical studies designed to answer important clinical questions such as the following:

- Are children who are FHP less likely to spontaneously improve than children with no known family history?

- Is a disfluent child more likely to persist in stuttering if he or she has relatives who are persistent stutterers?
- Do stutterers who are FHP show more benefit from a certain type of treatment (e.g., fluency shaping approaches) than stutterers who are family history negative?
- Are clients who are FHP more likely to require a longer interval of direct intervention to reach a fluency criterion than clients who are FHN?
- Are clients who fail to maintain treatment gains at follow-up more often those with a positive family history of stuttering?
- Do FHP clients require more structured or lengthier maintenance programs than clients who are FHN?
- Do FHP stutterers experience more severe or prolonged intervals of relapse following successful treatment than persons who are FHN?
- Is the long-term treatment outcome for FHP stutterers less favorable than for stutterers with a negative family history?

Keep these questions in mind as you proceed through the remainder of this chapter; they will be referred to later as the "fundamental clinical questions." As an exercise, create one or two additional questions of particular interest to you that use family history as a main effect variable for grouping subjects.

IT'S ALL IN THE FAMILY: USING FAMILY HISTORY STATUS AS A GROUPING VARIABLE

As it turns out, the practice of dividing affected cases into those with a positive versus a negative family history is far from new. More than a century ago, scholars wrote about the unfavorable consequences associated with a positive family background for various disorders. In 1860, Morel (cited in Bleuler, 1978) summed up the sentiment of the time quite succinctly when he wrote that "a familial hereditary taint (for psychosis) is cause for an unfavorable prognosis." To these early writers, familial meant inherited, and inherited meant immutable to change. Rosenthal (1963) was one of the first of several contemporary psychologists to challenge this rigid precept about family history. In so doing, he developed a simple model which has been credited with providing one of the theoretical cornerstones for current multifactorial models of disorder etiology (Monroe & Simons, 1991). Specifically, in his "diathesis-stress model," Rosenthal argued that genetic predisposition and environmental stress interact to "activate" disorders, with varying levels of stressors needed depending on the extent of the (genetic) diathesis. In its elegant simplicity, this small paper challenged two of the most widely accepted doctrines of the day: (1) that a high genetic diathesis was both necessary and sufficient to precipitate the expression of a disorder, and (2) that a strong (genetic) diathesis invariably presaged a poor prognosis.

More recently, Eaves, Kendler, and Schulz (1986) made more explicit the relationship between Rosenthal's (1963) etiologic continuum and the family history status variable. They noted that, in its strongest form, this model creates two etiologically distinct subgroups that are distinguished by family history. Eaves et al. wrote that

> On one end of the continuum are patients in whom genetic factors appear overwhelmingly important, and in whom little evidence can be found for any substantial environmental stress [familial cases]. On the other end of this continuum are patients for whom environmental factors appear to play a major etiologic role in their disorders, and in whom there is no apparent evidence for the operation of genetic factors [sporadic cases]. (p. 115)

It should be noted that, in this model, *some* intrinsic diathetic loading is presumed to be necessary for a disorder to develop, although the loading may be minimal. If the diathesis is completely absent, the disorder is (theoretically) not possible, irrespective of the level of stress. (In other words, one could not produce a stutterer solely by introducing the relevant stress variables unless some intrinsic predisposition to stutter existed.) When the diathesis is present, the probability that the disorder will be expressed is a function of the interaction between the degree of stress (low to high) and the corresponding diathesis loading (Monroe & Simons, 1991). Relatively more stress is presumed to be needed to activate a disorder when the diathesis (predisposition) is low. In contrast, for individuals with a high diathesis, less stress may be necessary for activation to occur. This model is only relevant for disorders such as stuttering whose transmission appears to be a function of both genetic and nongenetic factors. (Thus, both a multifactorial-polygenic transmission model and a single major locus model with incomplete penetrance are theoretically compatible with a diathesis-stress orientation.) Figure 3–1 is a simplified schematic of the diathesis-stress model as it might be applied to the development of stuttering.

Some support for this conceptual view of stuttering etiology was reported by Poulos and Webster (1991). In this investigation, 169 adult and adolescent stutterers were retrospectively divided into cases reporting a positive family history of stuttering and cases with no known fam-

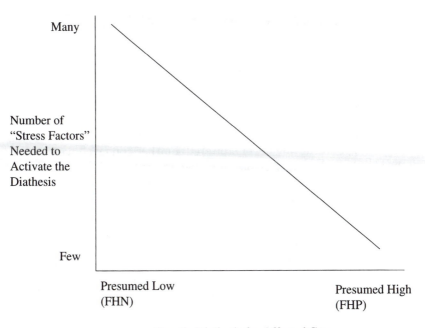

Figure 3–1. Simplified schematic of the diathesis-stress model.

ily history. Although both groups were similar in terms of reported age of stuttering onset, dysfluency characteristics, and emotional concomitants, group differences were found for the number of nongenetic (stress) factors that "were thought to be associated with stuttering onset or that potentially might have precipitated stuttering" (p. 5). Consistent with the predictions of the diathesis-stress model, stutterers who were classified as sporadic (nonfamilial) reported a significantly greater number of physically traumatic events at birth or in early childhood than did the familial cases (37% vs. 2% respectively). On the basis of these findings, the authors concluded that there might be two etiologically distinct groups of adult stutterers: one group consisting of "individuals with a genetically inherited predisposition for stuttering, and the second of individuals without such a predisposition but who may have sustained some form of early brain damage" (p. 5). Notably, 21% of the stuttering subjects in this investigation were "unclassifiable," in that they had neither a positive family history (high genetic diathesis) nor evidence of early neurological trauma (high nongenetic stress). The authors themselves point out that this investigation had methodological weaknesses common to many retrospective self-report studies. Nevertheless, the

Poulos and Webster study is of considerable interest because it is one of the only theoretically motivated studies of the family history variable in the stuttering literature.

A recent study by Ambrose, Cox, and Yairi (1997) used an interesting variant of the traditional family history status design to test the hypothesis that *recovery* from stuttering is genetically mediated. In this investigation, the extended family members of 66 stuttering children were coded as having persistent stuttering, as having recovered from stuttering, or as having never stuttered. Further coding conventions for the affected relatives were not provided. For example, it is not known if recovered cases were only those who had recovered without formal treatment (spontaneous recovery), or whether treatment successes (even into adulthood) were coded as "recovered" if so labeled by the informant. The coded pedigrees from the 22 children in the sample who were reported to have persisted in stuttering for 36 months or more postonset, and the 44 children who had recovered from stuttering at some point within this time period, were then compared. As they had predicted, Ambrose and colleagues found that the children who persisted in stuttering had significantly more affected relatives in their immediate and extended families who were reported to be persistent as opposed to recovered stutterers (about 5% vs. 2%), while, in contrast, the recovered children had a significantly higher proportion of recovered than persistent relatives in their pedigrees (about 4% vs. 1%, respectively). Based on these proportional differences, these investigators concluded that recovered stuttering tends to run in families and persistent stuttering tends to run in families. In conceptualizing how the "recovery diathesis" might be transmitted, Ambrose and colleagues offer the hypothesis that "a unitary liability to stuttering is transmitted (genetically), but some individuals also inherit an additional factor that prompts persistence" (p. 577). In other words, they suggest that in addition to inheriting a genetic vulnerability to express the disorder in the first place (the etiological diathesis), individuals inherit a predisposition toward either recovery or persistence (with persistence requiring additional deleterious genetic material). Implicit in their theory is the hypothesis that individuals with a high recovery diathesis should require less aggressive treatment efforts than those with a low recovery (i.e., a persistence) diathesis, since the former are believed to be "preprogrammed" to recover, and therefore less dependent upon external (nongenetic) interventions to effect a positive change.

Two related assumptions about the construct of recovery are important to note when interpreting the results of this interesting study. The first assumption is that recovery status is unambiguous and is easily documented. Considerable experience, however, tells us that people differ in their internal definitions of recovery: for some, it is the absolute freedom from all stuttering moments and all affective concerns about stuttering in all situations. For others, recovery would be endorsed if there was a significant improvement in speech fluency. The question of who should determine recovery, the person being interviewed or a professional judge examining multiple indicators, is quite important. To concretely highlight this point, here are examples of responses from four (hypothetical) relatives of a stuttering child. You decide whether you would code each as "unaffected," "recovered," or "persistent." For fun, compare your decisions with those made independently by a colleague.

- Grandma Sophie indicates that she stuttered when she was a little girl, and still stutters mildly when she is fatigued or under stress. She does not report any fluency-related speaking anxieties.
- Uncle Arnold indicates that he was told by his parents that he stuttered when he was a child, but has no personal recollection of having ever stuttered.
- Brother Jed recalls receiving some form of therapy that may have been for stuttering when he was 4 or 5. He denies having any problems with stuttering now.
- Cousin Stanley produces several "stutter-like" (less typical) dysfluencies during your interview with him, but claims that he is and has always been a normally fluent speaker.

A second and related assumption about recovery is that it is stable over time within individuals. However, as the above examples illustrate, responses may be time-dependent and may therefore have poor retest stability. For example, a mother may be interviewed about her affected child at Time 1, when the child is 9, and report that he is "completely recovered." At some subsequent point in time, perhaps when that child reaches adolescence, some relapse may occur. If interviewed then, the same mother may report that her son still "occasionally stutters" (i.e., is persistent). By early adulthood, it is anybody's guess how that young man will report on his own recovery status. He may consider himself "recovered" if he has again attained reasonable fluency, or he may reflect on his ups and downs and report that he "still stutters now and again." At present, we do not have the longitudinal retest data on a group of subjects that would enable us to establish the seriousness of this classification problem. However, given the notoriously cyclical nature of stuttering, it is possible that intraindividual shifts in recovery status may be a rather common occurrence over the course of the lifespan.

FAMILY HISTORY STATUS: MEANINGFUL GROUPING VARIABLE OR METHODOLOGICAL MORASS?

One of the first indicators that family history status might be problematic for studying client outcomes is the virtual absence of these studies in other clinical domains. Given the inherent attractiveness of family history status as a predictor variable, one would expect to find multiple examples of family history × treatment interaction studies in, for example, the psychiatric treatment literature. Certainly, one would assume that fundamental clinical questions such as those posed earlier for fluency have occurred to others dealing with complex human problems such as depression or alcoholism. Although there are examples of studies (primarily from the 1980s) that have examined various *etiological* markers in FHP and FHN cases (e.g., neurochemical or electrophysiological differences between groups), there has been very limited study of epidemiological or treatment variables using this design.[1]

One exception to this generalization is schizophrenia. For this disorder, several studies in the 1970s and 1980s analyzed patient outcome as a function of family history status. Table 3–1 presents a summary of several of these investigations. Although these studies differed from one another in methodological particulars, all employed multiple outcome measures, both subjective and standardized, to establish performance in daily living domains after dismissal from treatment for schizophrenia.

Contrary to what had been hypothesized, statistically significant outcome differences between adults with a positive versus a negative family history were found in only one of the studies reviewed here. These essentially negative but contradictory results are in accord with the literature in general in this area, which has been unevenly divided between a small number of prognostic studies that show some effect as a function of family history status and a larger group of studies in which family history status was found to be of no prognostic import (Kendler & Hays, 1982). Perhaps because of these disappointing early results, studies that employ the family history design as a predictor of outcome for schizophrenia and related psychiatric disorders have been diminishing in the psychiatric treatment literature.

In addition to such "concerns by omission," there have been recent "direct attacks" on the validity of the family history status design. Although a number of conceptual and methodological concerns have been

---

[1] Another possible exception is Tourette syndrome where there has been some interesting work examining the role of family history in the onset and expression of this condition (see Shapiro, Shapiro, Young, & Feinberg, 1988, for a review).

Table 3–1. Summary of Schizophrenia Studies Assessing Outcomes for Family History Positive [FHP] and Family History Negative [FHN] Probands.

Study	Subjects	Outcome Differences as a Function of FH Status
Bleuler, 1978	208 hospital patients	NS* outcome differences
Ciompi, 1980	284 hospital patients	NS outcome differences
Huber, Gross, Schuttler, & Linz, 1980	502 hospital patients	NS outcome differences
Kendler & Hays, 1982	113 DSM-III schizophrenics	NS outcome differences, although there was a trend for increased relapse for FHP probands
McGlashan, 1986	163 DSM-III schizophrenics	Probands who were FHP had "significantly poorer work records and global outcomes" than probands who were FHN

*NS = nonsignificant

cited, three will be the focus of discussion here: (1) family history status is complex to establish, (2) family history classification is imprecise for genetic reasons, and (3) the family history design lacks statistical power.

Family History Status Is Complex to Establish

Somewhat surprisingly, there are no established rules for determining what constitutes a positive versus a negative family history for disorder. A conservative convention, advocated by Eaves and colleagues (1986), is to define a familial case as "one in which a first-degree relative (or co-twin) is affected with the same disorder suffered by the patient," and a sporadic case as "one in which no first-degree relative (or co-twin) is [similarly] affected" (p. 116). Although assessing extended family members (e.g., second- and third-degree relatives) has some benefit for increasing statistical power, this practice can introduce some uncertainties. For example, if a proband from a large extended family has a cousin, a niece, or a great-uncle who stuttered at some point in time, is he a "familial" or a "sporadic" stutterer? Should he be considered as "strongly familial" as a proband with an affected first-degree relative? Does this ambiguous case actually lie in the middle of a diathesis continuum, being neither clearly familial nor clearly nonfamilial? Or, conversely, should *any* positive case in the family tree, irrespective of family size and genetic remoteness, be sufficient for classification as FHP? This practical dilemma underscores one of the conceptual problems with the family history design. Because few measurement alternatives have presented themselves, researchers and clinicians have continued to treat genetic diathesis as a dichotomous variable, despite the fact that this diathesis is far more likely to be "quasi-continuous" for complex disorders (Monroe & Simons, 1991).

In addition to problems of definition and conceptualization, the family history design is known to be particularly sensitive to methodological biases, particularly those involving sample size (Eaves et al., 1986; Kendler & Hays, 1982). The simple fact is that the more relatives that are assessed, the more likely it is that a family will be classified as FHP. A mathematical simulation by Eaves and colleagues (1986) nicely makes this point. For this exercise, assume that you assess *one* relative for each of several stuttering probands, and code a certain percentage of families as FHP on this basis. If you subsequently increase the number of relatives you assess to *two* per family, a shift from sporadic to familial will occur for approximately 7% of these cases. In fact, as Eaves and his colleagues (1986) note:

> For all but the most extremely heritable case, the number of familial probands is approximately a multiple of the number of relatives studied. For example, the examination of three first-degree relatives will generate nearly three times the proportion of familial probands as the examination of one first-degree relative. (p. 125)

Although pedigree-based studies set out to obtain uniform family history data from all participants (by administering a standard interview protocol), in reality it is difficult to recruit equal numbers of familial and sporadic (or recovered and persistent) probands and to match these families for family size, socioeconomic status, or any other potentially relevant variable (Eaves et al., 1986). By way of example, assume you assess two proband (stuttering) adults, Proband A and Proband B, to determine if there is a positive family history for the presence of stuttering (or recovery from it). Proband A has one sibling, no children, and no living parents or grandparents for whom valid information about stuttering can be obtained. Proband B, on the other hand, has four siblings, two school-aged children, both parents, and three of four grandparents available for assessment. If no stuttering relatives were found in either family, we would code both probands as FHN, despite the considerable difference in the informativeness of the two pedigrees. If samples are very large, it is less likely that there will be systematic group differences in family size. However, for the modest sample sizes like those typically seen in the family-genetic literature for speech disorders (fewer than 50 families per group), the potential for bias due to imbalanced family sampling is a reasonable concern.

Family History Classification Is Imprecise for Genetic Reasons

The family history design is built upon the premise that family history status and genotypic status are meaningfully related, with the former serving as a convenient proxy for the latter. That is, if no overtly affected relatives are found in the family of an affected individual, a *prima facie* case is made for "low genetic diathesis" for that individual. Although this is tidy, it is inaccurate. In fact, geneticists have long understood that a positive genetic diathesis may be present in an individual with no overtly affected relatives. In fact, both of the two most current genetic models of stuttering, the single major locus model with incomplete penetrance, and the polygenic model, would predict that individuals who have a high genetic diathesis for stuttering could easily be found in a family with no overtly stuttering relatives other than the proband (Eaves et al., 1986; Kendler & Hays, 1982). Similarly, it is possible that, in some families, multiple family members might stutter for entirely nongenetic reasons, even for disorders that are known to be heritable in the population (Eaves et al., 1986; Kendler & Hays, 1982). Although the practice of identifying families as high versus low in genetic diathesis on the basis of pedigree information alone *may* be reasonable, there is no direct empirical evidence from the field of genetics to support the validity of this practice.

The Family History Design Lacks Statistical Power

One final and very important methodological limitation of the family history design concerns its lack of statistical power. Inadequate power is a problem that plagues many researchers who study disorders such as stuttering that are of relatively low frequency in the population. The temptation is to publish preliminary work with inadequate sample sizes (particularly if the findings are positive), in the hopes that these findings will gain in strength through replication. However, as consumers of such research, it is important to recognize that the family history design and its variants rely on mathematical assumptions that are easily violated in small samples.

The question of "how large a sample is large enough" was addressed in a seminal paper by Eaves et al. (1986). In this paper, a series of mathematical simulations were presented to demonstrate the importance of performing power calculations when using the familial versus sporadic classification design. To illustrate the power problem, Eaves and his colleagues created hypothetical cases in which relevant assumptions (e.g., heritability, family size, etc.) were varied. In one such simulation, a case was created in which the disorder liability was assumed to be .75 (a heritability value that has been reported in the literature for stuttering), with the remaining 25% of the variation in liability attributed to a risk factor that was entirely environmental. The results of this simulation, presented here as an example, revealed that

> Under these circumstances, we would still need 430 probands, each with three relatives on whom valid psychiatric assessments can be made, in order to have an 80% chance of detecting heterogeneity . . . using the familial vs. sporadic classification [method] (p. 126).

In summarizing their conclusions about the power of the familial versus sporadic design for psychiatric research, Eaves and his colleagues concluded that

> If the [simulation] model employed in this report is a reasonable first approximation of reality, the findings suggest that, as routinely used, the familial vs. sporadic design is not very powerful. Little justification can be offered for its use with first-degree relatives in small sample sizes where negative results are nearly meaningless. Only with large sample sizes of nuclear families or with monozygotic twins does this method provide a reasonable chance of detecting etiologic heterogeneity. These results show that, although somewhat difficult to determine, power calculations can be as important in designing "genetic" as biological studies in psychiatry. (p. 129)

FINAL THOUGHTS AND FUTURE DIRECTIONS: CAN BEHAVIORAL GENETICS RESEARCH CONTRIBUTE TO THE MANAGEMENT OF STUTTERING?

The present discussion of the family history design has been cautionary, to say the least. However, despite its shortcomings, there are ways to improve on and to supplement the traditional family history design so that answers to the "fundamental clinical questions" can be pursued. I believe that behavioral genetics research has much to offer the clinical management of stuttering, although, ironically, some of these initial contributions may have more to do with mapping the complexities of the stuttering phenotype than mapping the genotype in the search for stuttering genes.

As a first step in this process, researchers should develop better methods for measuring stuttering diatheses using family history information. It is quite possible that the dichotomous groups we favor (e.g., FHP vs. FHN, recovered vs. persistent, etc.) are fundamentally inaccurate, and will need to be replaced by other (perhaps polychotomous) classifications. In addition, in order to obtain the requisite sample sizes, researchers who are interested in these issues should consider establishing collaborative longitudinal projects to pool family and treatment data. Ideally, these studies should be designed to collect multiple measures on subjects and their immediate family members over time, including measurements of fluency status and outcome variables. Although expensive and logistically difficult, the potential payoffs in information from such a project might outweigh the practical disadvantages. Finally, and perhaps most importantly, it should be emphasized that questions about the importance of heritability (genetic factors) in the pathogenesis of stuttering can be more directly answered using an alternative behavioral genetic design (the twin design). Specifically, for addressing questions such as, "How heritable is recovery? How heritable is relapse? How heritable are high levels of affective involvement?" and so forth, the twin design is the superior choice. Although it may not be feasible to initiate a prospective twin study of stuttering, again for reasons of sample size, it may be possible for researchers in stuttering to collaborate with one of the international research teams who have large longitudinal twin studies in progress.

For clinicians who work with stuttering clients every day, reading this chapter has, I imagine, been a rather discouraging experience. I have not, after all, provided specific advice about how to use family history information to make diagnostic decisions or how to counsel families with a positive history of stuttering. First, let me point out that there is presently no consensus about these matters, and there is likely to be a good deal of healthy debate among professionals about the significance of family history information in the coming months and years. However, for what it is worth, I will offer my personal thoughts about the role of family history status in the management of stuttering given our present state of knowledge.

First, I believe that the results of the current family history and familial aggregation studies must be very cautiously applied to individuals. Although it is true that stuttering is familial in the population, and it may be true that there is a familial tendency for recovery, we still do not have sufficient empirical justification to use a family history profile to predict outcome for any given client. Precise risk estimates can be made only for those disorders that are inherited as single-gene dominant, recessive, or sex-linked (Mendelian) conditions. For more complex transmissions such as those proposed for stuttering (polygenic, mixed major locus, etc.), we have no way to make mathematical predictions for *individuals*. Thus, even though we know that, on average, 15% of the first-degree relatives of stuttering clients will have stuttered at some point in their lifetime (Felsenfeld, 1997), it does not follow that each child born into an FHP family has a "15% chance" of becoming a stutterer. The fact is, we don't know what the risk of stuttering is for a particular FHP child, other than it is probably greater than the risk for a child selected at random from the population, and may (or may not) be somewhat greater than the risk for a child who is (outwardly at least) family history negative.

Although we tend to focus on the predictive importance of the *presence* of affected relatives when diagnosing stuttering cases, it is worth recalling that there are a sizeable number of clients who have no family history and yet still stutter. Poulos and Webster (1991), for example, reported that over one-third (37%) of the 169 persistent adolescent and adult stutterers who came to their clinic for treatment (and participated in their pedigree study) had no history of stuttering in their immediate or extended families. Clearly, for this large subset of cases, being FHN did not assure a more favorable outcome. Predicting the likelihood of recovery from stuttering from family history data may also be difficult for many of the clients we see. In their recent study of the familiality of recovery, for example, Ambrose et al. (1997) found that 24% of the children in their sample (16/66) came from families containing a mix of recovered and persistent stutterers. Since both recovery and persistence diatheses are presumably represented in these families, the recovery outcome in these cases would be impossible to predict.

These two examples are provided to emphasize a point I hope I have made clearly throughout this chapter: Family history (and recovery) status are complex, noncategorical phenomena. Consequently, it must be understood that our attempts to establish "family history" in the clinic through a very cursory interview are of questionable sensitivity and are almost certainly inaccurate. Although I am not suggesting that clinicians should stop collecting family history data during assessments, I am arguing that clinical decisions that are based in large part on these constituents should be avoided until we have stronger empirical evidence to support their predictive value. We know precious little about the genetic diathesis, and even less about the "stressors" that we know must be relevant for this diathesis to be activated. The following quotation by Monroe and Simons (1991) is a succinct expression of our state of affairs in this area, and serves as an excellent closing statement. These authors wrote, and I agree, that

> In our present world of incomplete concepts and imperfect measures, it would seem that the intensive focus on concepts, measures, and interactions most closely exemplifies the spirit—and may help to realize the promise—of diathesis-stress concepts in . . . research. (p. 422)

ACKNOWLEDGMENT: This chapter is based on a presentation delivered at the University of Georgia's "State-of-the-Art" Conference, March 1997.

REFERENCES

Ambrose, N. G., Cox, N., & Yairi, E. (1997). The genetic basis of persistence and recovery in stuttering. *Journal of Speech, Language, and Hearing Research, 40*, 567–580.

Bleuler, M. (1978). *The schizophrenic disorders: Long-term patient and family studies.* New Haven: Yale University Press.

Ciompi, L. (1980). Catamnestic long-term study on the course of life and aging in schizophrenics. *Schizophrenia Bulletin, 6*, 606–618.

Curlee, R., & Yairi, E. (1997). Early intervention with early childhood stuttering: A critical examination of the data. *American Journal of Speech-Language Pathology, 6*, 8–18.

Eaves, L., Kendler, K., & Schulz, C. (1986). The familial vs. sporadic classification: Its power for the resolution of genetic and environmental etiologic factors. *Journal of Psychiatric Research, 20*, 115–130.

Felsenfeld, S. (1997). Epidemiology and genetics of stuttering. In R. F. Curlee & G. M. Siegel (Eds.), *Nature and treatment of stuttering: New directions* (2nd ed., pp. 3–23). Boston: Allyn and Bacon.

Huber, G., Gross, G., Schuttler, R., & Linz, M. (1980). Longitudinal studies of schizophrenic patients. *Schizophrenia Bulletin, 6*, 592–605.

Kendler, K., & Hays, P. (1982). Familial and sporadic schizophrenia: A symptomatic, prognostic, and EEG comparison. *American Journal of Psychiatry, 139*, 1557–1562.

McGlashen, T. (1986). The prediction of outcome in chronic schizophrenia: The Chestnut Lodge follow-up study. *Archives of General Psychiatry, 43*, 167–176.

Monroe, S., & Simons, A. (1991). Diathesis-stress theories on the context of life stress research: Implications for the depressive disorders. *Psychological Bulletin, 110*, 406–425.

Poulos, M., & Webster, W. (1991). Family history as a basis for subgrouping people who stutter. *Journal of Speech and Hearing Research, 34*, 5–10.

Rosenthal, D. (1963). *The Genain quadruplets: A case study and theoretical analysis of heredity and environment in schizophrenia* (pp. 505–511). New York: Basic Books.

Shapiro, A., Shapiro, E., Young, J., & Feinberg, T. (1988). *Gilles de la Tourette syndrome* (2nd ed., pp. 289–312). New York: Raven Press.

Yairi, E., Ambrose, N., & Cox, N. (1996). Genetics of stuttering: A critical review. *Journal of Speech and Hearing Research, 39*, 771–784.

Zebrowski, P. (1997). Assisting young children who stutter and their families: Defining the role of the speech-language pathologist. *American Journal of Speech-Language Pathology, 6*, 19–28.

CHAPTER

On Learning From Speech-Motor Control Research on Stuttering

ROGER J. INGHAM, Ph.D.

For almost two decades a Speech Motor Control (SMC) perspective on stuttering has held tremendous sway over stuttering research. It has been largely responsible for promoting the view that stuttering is best understood as a neurophysiological disorder that directly affects the speech motor system. It has also generated a massive amount of research, most of which has been directed at the level of control that stutterers exert over motor behaviors in their speech, rather than toward any "underpinning" neurological variables (see Bloodstein, 1995; Peters & Hulstijn, 1987; Peters, Hulstijn, & Starkweather, 1991). Of course, SMC has also been intimately associated with the promotion of the "demands and capacities" concept of stuttering (Adams, 1990; Andrews et al., 1983; Starkweather, 1987).

Given SMC's sustained dominance, it is fair to ask whether it has actually led to any major advance in either knowledge about stuttering or, more importantly, its treatment. In the Introduction to their 1991 text, Hulstijn, Starkweather, and Peters also expressed some concern with this question when they made the following observation: "If a speech motor control approach to stuttering really goes to the heart of the disorder, then it ought to foster the development of new and useful methods of diagnosis and treatment" (1991, p. xxi). Yet none appeared then, nor, it seems, since then (see, for example, Curlee & Siegel, 1997). Indeed, it is very difficult to identify any product of SMC research that has altered the way stutterers are diagnosed or treated.[1] Why should that be?

The SMC perspective certainly seemed to be well conceived when it appeared. In the late 1970s reports of stutterers' timing and coordination problems were almost cluttering the *Journal of Speech and Hearing Research's* pages, and emerging evidence of unusual hemispheric processing of speech by stutterers (e.g., Moore & Haynes, 1980) certainly added credibility to SMC's neurophysiological connections. So, what went wrong? One possibility is that SMC's lack of influence on diagnosis and treatment may have been due to a mode of research that almost disavowed procedures that might identify the most *powerful and functional* "speech motor" variables that serve to control stuttering—and then directly manipulate those variables. In fact, it is hard to find any serious attempt to relate the variables investigated under the SMC rubric to treatment. Another possibility is that SMC's research agenda was largely focused at the peripheral level of what many were beginning to accept was a more central neural processing problem. Both of these possibilities are at least worth some consideration, especially now that potentially powerful methods for investigating stuttering at that more central level are beginning to be used by stuttering researchers. Indeed, the recent history of SMC research may offer an emerging neuroscience perspective on stuttering a useful lesson on how to avoid falling into a clinical wasteland.

---

[1] At a conference in Banff in 1989, Dick Curlee and this author attempted to float this issue with respect to stuttering assessment (Curlee, 1993) and treatment (Ingham, 1993). It is probably fair to say that it did not receive a warm reception. A well-crafted critique, embodying this same issue, was offered by Martin Young (1994) who noted that a vast amount of speech motor research is essentially designed to determine the level of correlation between target variables and stuttering, thereby excluding any endeavor to identify causal variables. Perkins (1997) has made a similar argument, albeit from his particular theoretic perspective.

Some of the pitfalls of the descriptive research methods that have so characterized SMC studies are also central to Armson and Kalinowski's (1994) critique of studies comparing the fluent speech of stutterers and nonstutterers. However, they argued that any differences emerging from these studies are likely to be confounded by the effects of stuttering "spreading" to the surrounding "fluent" intervals, and that these intervals might also be confounded by "subperceptual stuttering." Interestingly, they do not then propose that the isolated variables might have been directly manipulated in order to determine if they do indeed directly control stuttering.

THE ARTICULATORY DYNAMICS MODEL: INFLUENCE ON SMC

The origins of the SMC perspective are debatable. They could reside in Lee Travis's (1934) early EMG facial muscle experiments that were designed to test the Orton-Travis theory. They might also be traced to Wingate's seminal (1969, 1970) papers that spawned the Modified Vocalization Hypothesis which, in turn, prompted a rash of studies that sought to relate laryngeal activity to stuttering. Those studies clearly revived interest in a much more physiological view of the disorder. However, history may ultimately show that the SMC perspective most obviously emerged from three papers that Jerry Zimmermann published in 1980 (Zimmermann, 1980a, 1980b, 1980c). If citations mean anything then Zimmermann's (1980c) Articulatory Dynamics (AD) model quickly became *the* driving force within the SMC approach.

One strength of Zimmermann's (1980c) AD model was its appearance. It displayed a relatively clear set of seemingly well-founded postulates that lent themselves to experimental investigation. The model's main premise was that excessively variable articulatory kinematics and timing caused alterations to the excitability level of the motoneuron pools in the various brain stem nuclei via peripheral afferent pathways. This altered excitability level was then supposed to make it difficult to modulate reflexive interactions properly within the cranial system, which, in turn, would cause the oscillatory and tonic movement patterns associated with stuttering. It followed, then, that stutterers *should* display asynchronous articulatory movements and unusual timing patterns during speech, plus evidence of orofacial muscle oscillations in conjunction with stuttering. It is not clear how or why this *should* be the case, but it was hypothesized that unusual timing patterns and oscillations would definitely characterize the speech of stutterers. The model also predicted that reduced variability among timing patterns and an absence of tremorlike oscillations would enhance fluency.

Zimmermann's model actually emerged from the arena of muscle stimulation research and two of his own empirical investigations. The first investigation (Zimmermann, 1980b), and possibly the most influential, compared seven adult normal speakers, four males and three females aged 22 to 31 years, and six adult male stutterers, whose ages ranged from 22 to 61 years. They produced fluent tokens while measures were made of lower lip and jaw movement duration, displacement, and velocity. The result: The stutterers displayed *longer* durations than the nonstutterers, but the stutterers also displayed *smaller* lower lip and jaw displacements and *lower* velocities within these articulators than the normals. There was also evidence of asynchrony in lip and jaw onset. In short, even during fluent productions, the stutterers' articulatory dynamics were considered nonnormal. The second study (Zimmermann, 1980a), compared the articulatory movements of four adult male stutterers and one female nonstutterer and confirmed the finding of asynchronous articulatory patterns during fluent productions by the stutterers, and that they did not resemble the movement patterns of the sole normal speaker. Thus emerged three cornerstones of the AD model:

1. Stutterers display asynchronous articulatory movements during their stutter-free speech.
2. Stutterers display unusual timing and variability in their stutter-free speech.
3. Stutterers display tremorlike muscle oscillations in conjunction with stuttering.

Any overview of stuttering research since the 1980s will show that it has been the search for these features, especially the second, that has driven a huge amount of SMC research (see Starkweather, 1987; Peters et al., 1991).

Viewed from the present it is surprising, even instructive, that Zimmermann's initial papers should have been greeted so enthusiastically (they even received the 1980 *JSHR* Editor's award). In fact, Howard Goldsmith, one of Mike McClean's students, may have been a solitary skeptic at the time. In 1983 he published a prophetic and much overlooked critique of Zimmermann's (1980b) initial study. He simply pointed out the obvious: Why should so much importance be given to differences emerging from a comparison between two groups of speakers who were, quite literally, matched on no obvious factor other than that they were adults? For instance, as he observed, the lowest velocities and displacement values were from two stutterers aged 51 and 61, raising the possibility that the lower displacement values in the stutterers could have been due to their age (about twice the age of the oldest control) rather than their disorder. Also, because orofacial structure size (usually larger in males than females) may influence articulatory displacement and velocity, the sex differences between the groups may have easily accounted for the relatively longer duration scores among the stutterers.[2] Hindsight is 20/20, but if Goldsmith's critique had been

---

[2]Indeed, data from Bennett (1981), for instance, suggest that males may use smaller jaw openings and/or more lip rounding during speech, thereby accounting for the smaller lip and jaw displacements among the predominantly male stutterers. It is also known that males and females use different articulatory strategies in producing low vowels (Fant, 1966).

Zimmermann (1983) partially acknowledged the issues raised by Goldsmith, but basically responded by suggesting that it should be the responsibility of other researchers to endeavor to replicate the findings reported in his study.

taken more seriously then perhaps some of the pitfalls of descriptive research, seemingly the preferred methodology of SMC researchers, might have been avoided.[3]

In the early 1980s Zimmermann's propositions were so influential that, arguably, they literally absorbed a then burgeoning interest in the role of phonation in stuttering and its treatment.[4] For instance, Adams and Hayden's (1976) report that stutterers were on average slower than normally fluent speakers in voice initiation, and termination time became synonymous with the timing problems associated with the speech of stutterers. A frenzy of studies (see Bloodstein, 1995) then clearly demonstrated that this average reaction time (RT) effect was replicable, but did it have any clinical value? Subsequently the effect was teased apart to the point where it is generally accepted that production planning time and laryngeal adjustment variables differentially contribute to the slightly slower RT effects among adult stutterers (Peters, Hulstijn, & Starkweather, 1989; Watson & Alfonso, 1983, 1987). Bakker and Brutten (1990) did try to argue that the RT effect (actually, the laryngeal adjustment time) might be a diagnostic indicator of stuttering, though they readily conceded that it might simply be part of the compensatory adjustments made by a handicapped individual. Of course, that suggestion was aided by the less consistent evidence of an RT effect among young stutterers (e.g., Cullinan & Springer, 1980; also see Adams, 1987). Like the adaptation effect, however, nothing whatsoever emerged from this research that has aided or improved treatment in any way. At best, the history of this research emerges as an interesting testimonial to SMC's preoccupation with theoretically seductive but clinically impotent variables.

There were many other studies in the acoustic domain that also appeared to enhance the validity of a SMC perspective. There were reports that adult stutterers exhibit increased pause time (Love & Jeffress, 1971), longer voice onset time (e.g., Agnello, 1975; Healey & Gutkin, 1984; Hillman & Gilbert, 1977), longer segment durations (Colcord & Adams, 1979; Di Simoni, 1974; Starkweather & Myers, 1979), and decreased articulatory rate (Borden, 1983; Ramig, Krieger, & Adams, 1982).

---

[3] Actually, in the same year Zimmermann and Hanley (1983) reported findings from a study that contradicted the AD model. They reported that during an adaptation task stutterers' and normals' articulators showed an *increased* velocity. This might seem to be supportive of the model, but Zimmermann and Hanley concluded that according to Zimmermann's (1980c) prediction, articulatory movement velocities should decrease during fluency inducing conditions.

[4] In fact, Zimmermann, Smith, and Hanley (1981) made this quite explicit when they advanced their "unifying conceptual framework" for stuttering in 1981 based on motor control processes.

All of these differences related to speech production, but the reported differences were never shown to be reflective of an unstable system. In fact, as Ingham and Cordes (1997) have noted, none of those differences has ever been demonstrated to be a feature that is experientially or empirically antagonistic to normal speech. Furthermore, with the possible exception of articulatory rate (see Prosek & Runyan, 1982, 1983), none has ever been experimentally manipulated in order to determine if it exerted any functional control over stuttering.[5]

WHITHER THE AD MODEL?

So, what is now known about the three cornerstones of the AD Model?

Whatever Happened to "Asynchrony"?

Some really serious concerns about the strength of these cornerstones began to emerge among studies that sought to test whether stutterers' articulatory movements are characterized by asynchrony. The SMC position was clearly bolstered by Caruso, Abbs, and Gracco's (1988) finding that six adult stutterers displayed inconsistent upper lip, lower lip, and chin peak velocity sequencing when they repeatedly uttered "sapapple." By contrast the movement sequences of their six normally fluent controls seemed stable. However, much less significance has been accorded evidence this effect was unreplicable. Studies by McClean, Kroll, and Loftus (1990), Alfonso (1991) and, ultimately, by Jäncke, Kaiser, Bauer, and Kalveram (1995) essentially failed to replicate the Caruso, Abbs, and Gracco (1988) finding.

The McClean et al. (1990) study is particularly significant because it really dealt a powerful blow to one of the most important cornerstones of the original AD model. In this reasonably well-controlled descriptive study, McClean et al. could also find *no* differences between measures of movement duration, amplitude, and velocity of the articulatory movements of untreated stutterers and nonstutterers. Moreover, this finding

---

[5]Incidentally, no claim is being made that the experimental manipulation of variables that control the presence and absence of stuttering will necessarily isolate causal variables. The fact that stuttering can be reduced by rhythmic stimulation or loud noise does not mean that stuttering is caused by the absence of rhythmic stimulation or the absence of loud noise. However, this methodology does at least offer a way to identify those sources of variance that might be functionally controlling behavior.

actually replicated a similar and generally ignored result within the Caruso et al. (1988) study.

It is rather curious that so little attention seems to have been given to the implications of the lack of support for this cornerstone of the AD model.[6] For instance, no SMC researcher or theorist appears to have speculated that perhaps stutterers' kinematic systems are reasonably stable after all!

What About "Variability"?

Another AD model cornerstone and an enduring SMC proposition is that fluency hinges on a speech motor system that displays limited variability. However, some recent findings may have turned this assumption on its head. Research conducted by Wieneke and Janssen in the late 1980s (Janssen & Wieneke, 1987; Wieneke & Janssen, 1987; Wieneke & Janssen, 1991) set the stage. They based their research on the orthodox SMC claim that "reduced temporal variability reflects a more stable motor system and therefore is related to enhanced fluency" (1991, p. 330). Of course, the corollary is that greater variability reflects an unstable and dysfunctional neuromotor system that will be associated with stuttering.

Initially, Janssen and Wieneke (1987) tested whether adult stutterers showed greater temporal variability of voiced and voiceless segments (using electroglottography [EGG]) than matched nonstutterers during fluent productions. They then tested if that difference disappeared during certain fluency-inducing conditions. In fact, their stutterers did display higher segment variability during perceptually fluent productions, but the fluency-inducing (FI) conditions produced both increased *and* decreased within-subject segment variability; a similar pattern appeared among the nonstutterers' data. Wieneke and Janssen (1991) then conducted a systematic replication and this time the FI conditions actually failed to reduce segment variability. In short, their studies may have shown that stutterers display greater speech segment variability, but they also showed that *reduced variability was not* a prerequisite for their stutter-free speech, let alone for normally fluent speech.

Mark Onslow, Ann Packman, and colleagues also studied this issue, but in a therapy context. In a study testing the results of an operant-based treatment of children who stutter, they (Onslow, van Doorn, & Newman, 1992) reported that vowel durations and articulatory rate

---

[6]McClean et al.'s study is unmentioned in recent chapters by Denny and Smith (1997) and Smith and Kelly (1997). Even McClean et al. (1990) failed to observe that their findings almost fatally damage the AD model.

showed reduced variability following treatment. Subsequently another group (Packman, Onslow, & van Doorn, 1994) reported almost similar effects as a result of a prolonged speech treatment program with four adult stutterers. Reduced variability did occur in the data from three subjects, but a reverse trend actually occurred in the other subject's data. More recently, Onslow, Packman, Stocker, van Doorn, and Siegel (1997) reported that one of two children (10 and 11 years old) showed reduced vowel duration variability when stuttering was reduced during time-out conditions. The overall data trends in these studies certainly fit the orthodox position, but they also included some incompatible findings. It is also possible that the reported effects reflect treatment-induced adjustments rather than demonstrating a necessary condition for fluency.[7]

A dramatically different perspective regarding variability emerged from a study by McClean, Levandowski, and Cord (1994) in which they measured the duration and variability of intersyllabic articulatory events, using kinematic measures of the lips, among treated and un-treated stutterers ($n = 31$). They found that the untreated stutterers who displayed most stuttering (on a conversational task) actually displayed *least* variability in timing durations during fluent productions. They then deduced that perhaps reduced variability might *not* be com-patible with normally fluent speech production. They argued that, at a wider physiological level, reduced variability is now considered to be a possible sign of pathology (Goldberger, Rigney, Mietus, Antman, & Greenwald, 1988). Conceivably, Wieneke and Janssen's studies could have included similar findings; unfortunately that cannot be deduced from their reports.

In short, the concept of variability has become an almost crumbling cornerstone within the original AD model.[8] Segment and kinematic var-iability are yet to be shown as functionally related to stuttering. Further-more, there is now some suggestion that reduced rather than increased variability characterizes a dysfunctional speech motor system.

---

[7] Ultimately, Packman, Onslow, Richards, and van Doorn (1996) may have moved away from an SMC-based argument by proposing a model in which the variability with which stutterers produce syllabic stress is conceptualized as a source of vulnerability to speech disruption. Reductions in syllabic stress vari-ability, they argue, could be a sufficient (though not a necessary) basis of en-hanced fluency.

[8] A study by Brown, Zimmermann, Linville, and Hegmann (1990) also failed to provide evidence of unusual variability in the jaw onset-offset duration during the production of "ah" by 10 stutterers when compared with 10 nonstutterers. While the abstract states that "the stutterers . . . were less variable than nonstut-terers," the data analyses (see p. 319) actually failed to find significant differ-ences between the groups.

Are "Oscillations" Also Shaky?

Finally, there is the issue of orofacial muscle oscillations. This AD model cornerstone has been studied most by Anne Smith and her students. The promise of their research program rested on earlier evidence of abnormal muscle activity in the laryngeal region during stuttering (Conture, McCall, & Brewer, 1977; Conture, Schwartz, & Brewer, 1985; Fibiger, 1971; Freeman & Ushijima, 1978; Platt & Basili, 1973; Shapiro, 1980). Most of the recent studies have been focused on allegedly "abnormal" (see, for example, Kelly, Smith, & Goffman, 1995, p. 1025) 5–15 Hz orofacial muscle oscillations during stuttering. Why? Because, to quote Smith and colleagues, the "patterns of muscle contraction necessary for normally coordinated speech movements would be disrupted by the synchronized firing of groups of motor units at 5–15 Hz" (Smith et al., 1993, p. 1309). However, no clear evidence has emerged to justify this claim. Furthermore, while 5–15 Hz oscillations often do have a pathological origin (e.g., Parkinsonism), quite often they do not (see Freund & Dietz, 1978). In fact, they often occur among the orofacial muscles of normal speakers (McFarland, Smith, Moore, & Weber, 1986; Palla & Ash, 1979). Not surprisingly, this makes it extremely difficult to relate these oscillations to stuttering. An equally difficult problem for readers of this research is that the mere appearance of a 5–15 Hz oscillation with stuttering often appears to merit far more significance than the nonappearance of these oscillations during stuttering.

So what have these studies shown? Answer: At best a pattern of inconsistent positive findings that are not always decisively associated with stuttering. These 5–15 Hz oscillations have been observed during the stuttered speech of 24/45 (53%) stutterers studied in this research (Denny & Smith, 1992; Kelly et al., 1995; McClean, Goldsmith, & Cerf, 1984; Smith, 1989; Smith et al., 1993). However, they have also appeared among normally fluent controls and during stutterers' fluent speech (Denny & Smith, 1992; Kelly et al., 1995). Small wonder that Denny and Smith (1992) were forced to conclude from their review that:

> The present results clearly indicate that *none of the elements of the oscillatory pattern are necessary concomitants of disfluency.* Stuttering can and does occur in the absence of tremorlike oscillations or high levels of activation in muscles consistently recruited for speech. (Denny & Smith, 1992, p. 1226; emphasis added)[9]

---

[9] However, that has not diminished their importance for these researchers. Most recently Denny and Smith (1997, p. 138) have argued that one reason why these oscillations are not consistently observed is because they might be prompted by different levels of sympathetic arousal. Their claim relied on a study by Weber and Smith (1990), which supplies remarkably frail support for any hypothesized association between sympathetic arousal and stuttering. Weber and Smith's highest reported correlation between autonomic system measures and "disfluent" events was 0.33 during oral reading, which would account for little more than 10% of variance. During more customary speech, a spontaneous speaking task, the correlation was only 0.12, which would account for a meager 1% of variance.

Surely this is sufficient reason to suggest that tremor-like oscillations are not likely to be a powerful distinguishing or functionally important speech motor variable. Furthermore, literally no evidence has been presented to show that 5–15 Hz oscillations have any greater claim to importance in understanding (let alone treating) stuttering than, say, head movements or any bodily movements that occur in conjunction with stuttering.[10]

Ironically, the search for muscle oscillation has actually produced one very important clinical implication: It has finally confirmed that Botox is not a very sensible treatment for stuttering. During the early 1980s, studies by Freeman and Ushijima (1978) and Shapiro (1980) were used to argue that the source of stuttering may reside in the larynx (Freeman, 1979). These studies were obviously flawed, a point also made by Smith et al. (1996). They were also undercut, as it were, by compelling evidence that stuttering may continue after a laryngectomy (see Ingham, 1984, Chapter 10). Nevertheless, this flawed research was used to justify risky Botox injections in the vocal folds as a treatment for stuttering. It should be no surprise that those treatments appear to have completely failed (Brin, Stewart, Blitzer, & Diamond, 1994; Stager & Ludlow, 1994). Smith et al. (1996) also reported that excess electromyographic-recorded laryngeal muscle activation is not a necessary concomitant of stuttering, which then led to a rather belated conclusion that Botox injections might not be a good idea after all.

---

[10]There is an interesting sidelight to this research. Its conclusions clearly derive from studies that have compared judgments of stuttered and nonstuttered segments of speech, yet Smith and Kelly (1997) have recently derided such judgments as "fictive in time and space." This creates some logical and scientific complications. For instance, within the same chapter, Smith and Kelly stated that, "Stuttering emerges in individuals . . . (who) . . . produce failures in fluency that the individuals and their culture judge to be aberrant" (1997, p. 210).

The fact is that individuals and researchers are obliged to judge when that aberrant behavior is present or absent if they are ever going to be able to relate stuttering to clinically or theoretically relevant variables. This is precisely what Smith and colleagues did in order to test their hypothesis that 5–15 Hz oscillations might be associated with stuttering. On the other hand, the claim that these oscillations are associated with "fictive" events does enable Smith and colleagues to maintain the relevance of 5–15 Hz oscillations to the problem of stuttering. The mounting evidence that these oscillations do not consistently occur during stuttering, let alone in conjunction with all stuttering events, can be simply ignored by these researchers as long as they insist that stuttering events have no reality.

SMC SANS AD MODEL

Perhaps There Is Some Gold

None of the foregoing is meant to suggest that there may not be fundamentally important differences between stutterers and normals with respect to their sequencing and timing skills, differences that may have neurophysiological origins. The most replicable findings appear to relate to finger tapping or, more specifically, the sequencing of finger tapping. A range of studies by Webster and colleagues (see Webster, 1993) and, more recently, Jäncke, Hefter, and Kalveram (1995), make clear that stutterers do indeed display poorer skills in handling the sequencing or timing of finger tapping. This effect may also be related to their relatively poorer ability to time (independently of speaking) the duration of utterance intervals (Cooper & Allen, 1977), a skill, incidentally, that appears to be retrieved after treatment. The origin of those differences may reside far beyond articulatory dynamics. This effect may also be related to a large body of research that suggested, in some relatively nonspecific fashion, that stutterers exhibit unusual levels of right hemisphere activity during speech related tasks (see Moore, 1990). The ability to prepare and rapidly produce sequences of motor behaviors, for instance, seems at the neurophysiological level to depend on Supplementary Motor Area's (SMA) executive functions (Marsden et al., 1996). However, SMA's executive functions are not necessarily reflected among the regions related to Mouth (M1), a region that seems to be neurologically organized to most directly influence articulatory dynamics.

Of course, what has still remained unresolved in the midst of abundant evidence of differences between stutterers and nonstutterers is whether these differences are simply benign ephemera. Many almost certainly are, given their notable absence among young children who stutter. For instance, in 1991 Ed Conture reviewed research on the respiratory, laryngeal, and articulatory systems in stuttering and nonstuttering children, including his own group's research (Caruso, Conture, & Colton, 1988; Conture, Colton, & Gleason, 1988; Conture, Rothenberg, & Molitor, 1986; Schwartz, 1987). He then reached this rather decisive conclusion:

> it seems about time that we talk about the emperor's lack of new clothes. Despite all good intentions, no one has been able to show that young stutterers' speech production abilities and behaviors are useful, objective or observer-independent criteria for distinguishing between (1) children's stuttered and nonstuttered disfluencies, (2) children who are or are not stutterers and (3) those young stutterers who will or will not continue to stutter as adults . . . . (Conture, 1991, p. 378)

There is also evidence that some motoric differences, acoustic and kinematic (Mallard & Westbrook, 1985; Metz, Onufrak, & Ogburn, 1979; Samar, Metz, & Sacco, 1986; Story, Alfonso, & Harris, 1996), might not only change as a result of stuttering treatment, but might also reflect specific motor targets taught in treatment. On the other hand, more significance might be attached to changes in hemispheric processing that occur in conjunction with treatment. Superficially at least, these changes do seem to be toward the normalizing of hemispheric processing (Boberg, Yeudall, Schopflocher, & Bo-Lassen, 1983; Moore, 1984).

However, before we conclude that SMC may not offer anything to the treatment of stuttering, it is worth considering three peripheral but clinically profitable research areas that appear to have been largely bypassed because of SMC's orientation. These developments pertain to an understanding of (1) the motor variables that may be responsible for the prolonged speech effect, (2) the role of respiration, and (3) the place of auditory factors in treatment. All appear to have the potential of locating powerful and clinically meaningful effects.

Wither Not Prolonged Speech

There are some experimental investigations that have started to tease apart the motor variables that might be most functional within *prolonged speech*, surely the most widely used and least researched stuttering treatment procedure. The descriptions of this speech pattern (generally, increased durations of phonation, gradual voice onsets, reduced articulatory contrasts) seem to be tantalizingly amenable to empirical study, but for some reason that has not occurred. Some investigations from the author's lab (Gow & Ingham, 1992; Ingham, Montgomery, & Ulliana, 1983) have shown that systematically manipulating the frequency of relatively short phonated intervals (via EGG or accelerometers) will exert decisive control over stuttering frequency. It is not clear, though, to what extent these effects are related to alterations in the gradients of voice onsets. The importance of abrupt onsets seems evident in data from Peters and Boves (1988). They found that even in adult stutterers' fluent speech there was a disproportionate number of EGG-recorded abrupt onsets, while Bakker, Ingham, and Netsell (1997) reported that speakers showed reasonable accuracy in self-judging the level of abruptness in the initial acoustic signal of a production. Taken together, these findings almost scream out for conversion to investigations of the effect of onset abruptness on stuttering.[11] It would also be

---

[11] Of course, this also touches the thorny issue of the reliability with which judges, including the speaker, are able to discriminate between abrupt and gentle voice onsets. That same issue applies to any attempts to measure the parameters of soft and hard articulatory contacts.

research directed at one of the most powerful procedures available for stuttering treatment, yet we do not know how to measure its features reliably, nor why it works.

Could It Be Bad Breath?

The AD model's influence may have also diminished interest in respiration, even though breathstream management seems to have clinical relevance. A number of studies have reported unusual respiration patterns in adult stutterers (Baken, McManus, & Cavallo, 1983; Peters & Boves, 1988), but two recent studies deserve much more attention because of their clinical significance. Zocchi et al. (1990) measured the subglottic pressure of 10 adult stutterers during speech and showed that Psg during stuttering "varied substantially and sometimes chaotically from too high to too low, rendering normal speech impossible. During periods of fluency, Psg was much better controlled" (Zocchi et al., 1990, p. 1510). Their data show that unlike the controls, the stutterers' (n = 10) Psg was never kept at a relatively constant level. This finding is also consistent with data from four adult stutterers and controls presented by Johnston, Watkin, and Macklem (1993). At the very least these studies confirm that subglottic air pressure does behave aberrantly in stutterers, thereby inviting the possibility that feedback signaling departures from a normal pressure range might functionally control stuttering. Why are these findings especially interesting? Because they are replicated and report unambiguous differences between *all* stutterers and nonstutterers.

Shouldn't We Peer More Closely at the Ear?

Arguably, another casualty of SMC has been the minimal interest in the role of auditory factors in stuttering, although that has been partly redressed by the surprising interest in the ameliorative effects of frequency-altered feedback (Howell, El-Yaniv, & Powell, 1987; Kalinowski, Armson, Roland-Mieszkowski, Stuart, & Gracco, 1993). This procedure which, incidentally, does not produce consistent clinically significant effects (Ingham, Moglia, Frank, Ingham, & Cordes, 1997), may have restored attention to the poorly understood relationship between auditory processing and stuttering. Numerous studies have suggested that stutterers do display unusual central auditory processing. These include findings of central auditory problems (Hall & Jerger, 1978; Rosenfield & Jerger, 1984; Tosher & Rupp, 1978) and nonnormal processing and matching of acoustic stimuli by stutterers (Nudelman, Herbrich, Hess, Hoyt, & Rosenfield, 1992; Stromsta, 1972). But it is the powerful and dramatic reductions in stuttering produced by some auditory stimulation procedures (e.g., chorus reading) that leads to the suspicion that the origin of these changes resides at a neurologic rather than motoric level. Some changes may be attributable to motor variables (Stager & Ludlow, 1991), but that seems increasingly unlikely. Why, for instance, should auditory masking during *nonspeech intervals* also reduce stuttering (Sutton & Chase, 1961; Webster & Dorman, 1970); or why should stuttering be reduced during amplified sidetone conditions, but only when those conditions are preceded by speech during auditory masking rather than rhythmic stimulation (Martin, Johnson, Siegel, & Haroldson, 1985; Martin, Siegel, Johnson, & Haroldson, 1984)? It seems reasonably likely that auditory masking produces some temporary alteration or even activation within an unusual auditory system, an activation that might be responsible for these changes. And that possibility may be somewhat more probable as the findings of the first brain imaging studies on stutterers have begun to appear.

THE RUSH TO THE BRAIN

This section will offer one perspective on an emerging neuroscience orientation to stuttering research. Perhaps it is worth mentioning, prefatorily, that the new brain imaging technologies are also perfectly designed for yet more aimless searching for differences between stutterers and nonstutterers, albeit at the level of cerebral blood flow analyses. Indeed, their growing use could confirm Quesal's (1989) claim that stuttering research is more often driven by technology than theory, or simply the opportunity to try something different. Dick Curlee has made a much more telling point in personal communications with this author: He suggests that it would be surprising indeed if brain imaging actually *failed* to locate differences in the neural processing systems used by stutterers and nonstutterers. Therefore, this section will briefly review the background to this emerging neuroscience orientation and then try to show how this author and colleagues at the University of Texas Health Science Center in San Antonio have been endeavoring to use this technology rather more purposefully.

A number of cerebral blood flow (CBF) technologies are now generally accepted methods for mapping and monitoring the neural systems that subserve or control behavior. Thanks to the popular press, the reigning CBF brain mapping procedures are now reasonably well known, as is their suitability for investigating neural areas associated with behavior and behavior change (see Posner & Raichle, 1994). F-18 deoxyglucose (FDG) PET actually records metabolic activity in the brain by recording glucose uptake while behavior is occurring. The scanning period is about 45 minutes and whatever behavior activations occur during that time are assumed to be reflected in the altered CBF state. $H_2{}^{15}O$ PET, in conjunction with magnetic resonance imaging (MRI), has become one of the most widely used means for tracing CBF activity throughout the whole brain during different conditions. The scanning period is only 40 seconds, but, like FDG, all behavioral activations and deactivations during that period are reflected in the scan record. Functional MRI (fMRI) records neural activation with much more temporal specificity than PET by recording blood oxygenation at 1–3 second interval resolution. However, fMRI is still problematic for stuttering research because it requires an extremely noisy imaging environment, one that could suppress stuttering and diminish recording quality. Another procedure, SPECT (or single photon emission computerized tomography), provides *single* plane ("slices") images of the brain, but without the resolution of PET. More recently, these procedures have been joined by transcranial magnetic stimulation, or TMS, which may provide an alternative brain mapping procedure as well as a relatively noninvasive method of stimulating and altering the levels of activation in focal regions of the brain.

   The first blood-flow brain maps of the speech motor system appeared in the late 1980s. They were derived from single-word production (verb generation) tasks (e.g., Peterson, Fox, Posner, Mintun, & Raichle, 1989) using $H_2{}^{15}O$ PET. These studies clearly showed that SMA, M1 (mouth), Broca's area, temporal lobe, and cerebellum were reliably activated during speech. Since that time the developments in PET technology have made it possible to obtain a better understanding of the various interactions among these regions as well as others, especially those in the basal ganglia region. Those same developments now permit very high resolution images that not only identify these regions of activation and deactivation from within group studies, but now make it possible to locate these regional activations within individual subjects. Indeed, many of these developments have literally occurred during the lifetime of this 4-year-old research program. They permit increasingly sophisticated analyses, even from this program's original data, some of which are described below.

The Short History of Brain Imaging and Stuttering

At the time of this writing there have been five published accounts of CBF brain imaging studies on stuttering. Three are functional activation studies (Fox et al., 1996; Wood, Stump, McKeehan, Sheldon, & Proctor,

1980; Wu et al., 1995) in which scans were obtained during a speech task when stuttering is present and others when stuttering is absent in order to isolate neural activations related to stuttering. If scans are also obtained during a rest or nonspeech condition, then nonspeech related activations can be removed from the image analysis; that control condition also makes it possible to identify neural *de*activations as well as activations. There have also been two functional lesion studies (Ingham et al., 1996; Pool, Devous, Freeman, Watson, & Finitzo, 1991). These studies record brain blood flow at rest and are designed to identify the presence of neural lesions or disease-related activations, largely by comparing rest-state neural activations in, say, stutterers and nonstutterers. Two other research groups have described $H_2^{15}O$ PET activation studies at conferences (Braun, Ludlow, Varga, Shulz, & Stager, 1994; De Nil, Kroll, Kapur, & Houle, 1995), but only cursory accounts of their findings are available. Of course, it would be helpful if the findings from within both groups of studies could be directly compared, but, as will be explained, there are some reasons why that is not immediately possible.

The first published activation study was by Wood et al. (1980) and employed a then modern, but now relatively insensitive, scanning system (a single-photon system which could only record activations near cortex surface) with two right-handed adult stutterers. Unfortunately, the technical limitations of this system make it difficult to relate their activations to known regions within the brain, or to later imaging studies.

In 1995 a FDG PET activation study was reported by Wu et al. Their study involved four adult stutterers and four controls (three males and one female in each group). The scan conditions were reading aloud and chorus reading, but there was no rest condition and not all of the brain was scanned (for instance, the SMA region was omitted). Their principal finding was that the stutterers' left caudate was hypometabolized during all conditions and may, therefore, be a "trait marker for stuttering." However, there are some serious methodological concerns that may have affected the interpretation of the data in this study (see Ingham et al., 1996, p. 1224). Furthermore, three PET $H_2^{15}O$ activation studies with adult stutterers (Braun et al., 1994; De Nil et al., 1995; Fox et al., 1996) have all failed to identify a caudate abnormality. Thus, Wu and associates' (1995) findings must await replication.

The two unpublished PET $H_2^{15}O$ activation studies with adult stutterers have, unfortunately, not provided either regional activation (Braun et al., 1994) or speech performance (De Nil et al., 1995) data. Nevertheless, both studies do report that during speech tasks their stutterers displayed either indistinct lateralization or unusual right hemisphere activation when compared with controls.

Perhaps the most controversial study is the 1991 functional lesion study by Pool et al. They used SPECT to record rCBF values in 22 regions of interest from 20 adult stutterers and 78 age-matched controls during rest state conditions. The blood flow data for this study were derived from only one horizontal "slice" (1.7–1.9 cm) of the brain. They reported finding "preliminary evidence for cortical dysfunction in stutterers related to reduced and asymmetric left frontal and temporal perfusion" (1991, p. 512), but there are reasons to doubt the validity of that finding. For instance, they made the rather questionable claim that the whole-brain blood flow level of their stutterers was, on average, 20% below that of their controls.[12] Whole brain PET analyses conducted by the San Antonio group (see below) and by Alan Braun (personal communication, 1996) at NIH have failed to find *any* neural differences between matched stutterers and controls at rest. Suffice to say that the Pool et al. findings await replication.

The foregoing gives some reasons why there are still too few replicated findings across these studies. Nonetheless, it is reasonably clear that unusual right hemisphere activation *does occur* during stuttering and that these activations *do* tend to normalize when stuttering is reduced. It is also highly unlikely that stutterers display unusual activations during nonspeaking conditions.

The San Antonio Studies

These studies are part of a research program that is being conducted by the author and colleagues for the purpose of identifying and then, if at all possible, rectifying the neural systems that characterize stuttering. It has been built on two assumptions. The first is that environmental stimuli and motor behavior changes (among other factors) are powerful modifiers of neural systems. There is certainly considerable evidence that behavior change (i.e., therapy or fluency induction) may produce

---

[12] Fox, Lancaster, and Ingham (1993) have pointed out that this largely ignored finding in the study of Pool et al. (1991) implies that stutterers exhibit whole-brain dysfunction of a magnitude equivalent to that found in the later stages of Alzheimer's disease.

lasting neural reorganization.[13] The second assumption, and the one occupying the most attention in this program, is that the source of functional control over stuttering may reside in neural processes that can be directly modified. The result has been a program that is designed to try to isolate those neural processes that might be "switched" on and off when stuttering is present and absent within an individual. That program began by (1) exploiting different fluency-inducing procedures in order to identify potentially "switchable" neural processes. It will then (2) use a recently developed noninvasive procedure in order to demonstrate their functional control over stuttering, and finally (3) it will use that control as a treatment if the effects appear to be clinically significant.

This program began with a recently reported $H_2^{15}O$ PET functional activation study (Fox et al., 1996). CBF imaging scans were collected from 10 adult right-handed male stutterers and 10 matched controls dur-

---

[13] An important clinical issue in much of the recent interest in neural structures and systems that might be associated with stuttering is the extent to which such systems can be modified or reorganized, even in adults. Pioneering studies demonstrated that cortical reorganization readily occurs after, say, finger amputations (Kass, Merzenich, & Killachey, 1983; Merzenich, Recanzone, Jenkins, Allard, & Judo, 1988), which suggested that neural plasticity is driven by a self-organizing principle, rather than being genetically "hard-coded" (Stryker, 1988). Other principles or models emerged with later studies. Rakic, Suner, and Williams (1991), for example, showed that early occular ennucleation results in an aberrant cortical organization. Even more dramatic, following prenatal transposition of auditory and visual cortex (Kass, 1988; Sur & Garraghty, 1986), transposed cortex assumed the functional properties appropriate to its new location. This has suggested that both thalamo-cortical and cortico-cortical connectivity controls the functionality of neural regions. As cortical projections are regionally broad, overlapping and, in part, redundant, this provides a neuroanatomic mechanism for adaptive reorganization that may persist into adult life.

Some recent PET studies of aphasic patients have also been informative regarding neural reorganization (Weiller, Chollet, Friston, Wise, & Frackowiak, 1992; Weiller et al., 1995). They include suggestions that some regional reorganization may even impede recovery. A recent PET study by Belin et al. (1996) evaluated the effects of Melodic Intonation Therapy (MIT) among seven nonfluent recovered aphasic patients—all with left sided lesions and four out of seven with infarcts recorded in Broca's area. The group displayed abnormally activated right hemisphere regions (corresponding to those activated in the left hemisphere for normal subjects) and deactivated left hemisphere language related regions during speech. During MIT, however, Broca's area and the left prefrontal cortex were significantly activated (unclear whether that was true for all patients) while the right hemisphere counterpart of Wernicke's area was deactivated. In other words, their findings suggest that a previously damaged

ing three conditions: during eyes-closed rest, while orally reading paragraphs (*Solo* reading), and while *Chorus* reading to an audio recording of the same paragraphs at a subject-selected rate. A subtraction analysis was then used to identify neural activations that were present during stuttering in comparison to those that were present when stuttering was absent.

The speech performance data were the number of 4-second intervals during 40-second scanning periods that were judged to contain stuttering (i.e., the number out of 10) (Ingham, Cordes, & Finn, 1993), the number of syllables per 40 second, and the mean 1–9 speech naturalness rating (Martin, Haroldson, & Triden, 1984) per 40-second scan. The results showed that during *Solo* reading all stutterers produced stuttering and spoke more slowly than the controls. During *Chorus* reading, by contrast, there was no stuttering and the stutterers and the controls

and deactivated region could be activated by MIT and that abnormally activated regions could be deactivated. This suggests that perhaps neural reorganization without intervention may actually impede recovery.

Two neuroimaging studies of training-induced plasticity in normal subjects also provide suggestive data for stuttering treatment. Raichle et al. (1994) reported that an initial verb-generation task activated well-established regions for this task (anterior cingulate, left prefrontal and left posterior temporal cortices, and right cerebellum) but these activations essentially normalized with practice on this task. They may also become more extensive with practice. Karni et al. (1995) imaged normal subjects during an initial complex, finger tapping task, and then again after several weeks of training. After training, the extent of primary and periprimary motor cortex activated during task performance was significantly increased. This increase, however, was found only during performance of the overlearned task. It was not seen during performance of other complex, motor tasks that had not been overlearned. This "plasticity" then, is now being regarded more as a learning mechanism, rather than plastic reorganization. That has been verified in a TMS investigation by Pascual-Leone and Torres (1993). They reported that proficient right handed Braille readers displayed sensorimotor evoked potentials (they were elicited by TMS over the M1/S1 region) that were substantially larger and more extensive for their right hand when compared with a control group's right hand, and also relative to the left hand in both groups.

The effect of behavior change on neural reorganization has also been demonstrated. Baxter et al. (1992), using PET (FDG at rest), showed that successful responders to treatment for obsessive-compulsive disorder by either behavioral or drug therapy showed identical increased activations in right caudate (part of basil ganglia) relative to left, while all other regions scanned showed no significant change. The important feature of this study was that specific regional activation changes were evident as a result of a strictly behavioral treatment.

produced similar speech rates and similar speech naturalness ratings. There is one important feature of this study that needs to be underscored: this was a restricted population of adult stutterers and may have been unusual. They were all adult right-handed males and preliminary and experimental findings showed that they were definite responders to Chorus reading.

So what was the result? In summary, the stutterers displayed distinguishing and significant activations in SMA, superior lateral premotor cortex (SLPrM) on the *right* (a previously unreported region of activation during speech), a right lateralized M1 (relative to the controls), and Broca's area that was substantially more right lateralized than it was in the controls. The cerebellar activations were remarkably prominent; they were more than double the size found in the controls. (There were other motor system activations, especially in basal ganglia, that were not seen in the controls.) However, the most surprising finding was that the primary auditory area (left and right superior temporal cortex) activations, so prominent in the controls, was literally *nonactivated* during stuttering, while the associated auditory area (BA 22) was actually deactivated, mainly on the right. In many respects the latter finding is especially interesting because it might mean that stutterers simply do not self-monitor their speech to the same extent as nonstutterers during oral reading. That finding is also of added interest because it seems to be in conflict with theories that claim that stutterers monitor their speech excessively (e.g., Postma & Kolk, 1993).

Chorus reading reduced many differences between the stutterers and the controls. The prominent SMA activations and the right activations in SLPrM and Broca's were either reduced or normalized, although the stutterers still displayed exceedingly large cerebellum activations. The auditory region activations were restored, although this was expected because of the presence of the *Chorus* reading stimulus which was delivered in the left ear.

Another very significant finding was that the regional activations and deactivations observed during stuttering also showed high intersubject agreement. The most prominent were present in 70–100% of subjects. Such high intersubject agreement carries added interest because the subjects ranged from very mild to very severe stutterers.

As mentioned above, the author and colleagues also conducted a functional-lesion study (Ingham et al., 1996) on the rest-state condition data from the preceding study. The controls were augmented by subjects who had participated in a related study that also required an eyes-closed rest condition. The purpose was to determine whether the stutterers in the Fox et al. (1996) study also displayed physiological abnormalities that are independent of speech production abnormalities. To test this hypothesis, 74 regions of interest throughout the brain were sampled, including areas referred to in the Pool et al. (1991) study. The results showed that there were literally *no* significant differences between the stutterers and controls ($n = 19$) for any of the regional CBF values.

Can Correlation Point to Cause?

From one perspective, of course, all that was really learned from the Fox et al. (1996) study was that during oral reading certain activations *did occur* when stuttering was present and *did not occur* when stuttering was absent, and that they also *did not occur* when normally fluent speakers read aloud. That finding provides no information about the source of those differences; arguably, they may be little more than the consequences of speaking with a stuttering problem. As a result, attempts are now being made to address the "cause or consequence issue," albeit via two very different approaches.

The first approach has been to evaluate the level of correlation between the rate of behavior and the regional activations. The purpose has been to learn if the significant activations in these regions are correlates of stuttering and not simply correlates of the rate of syllable production. This is an important question because the stutterers in the Fox et al. (1996) study did speak more slowly at the same time that they stuttered more frequently, and so some of the differences might have reflected differences in the rate of syllable production. To that end, correlation analyses were conducted in order to test whether some regions activate unusually (i.e., relative to controls) in conjunction with the amount of stuttering, while others might activate unusually in conjunction with the amount of speaking. If that were the case then, it was speculated, this might also help to narrow the search for the most functional regions.

Table 4–1 summarizes the findings of these correlation analyses. Incidentally, the magnitude of these analyses was considerable; for instance, each correlation analysis (e.g., the frequency of stuttered intervals × activations in all scanning conditions) produced 132,812 correlation coefficients. This permitted the identification of the clusters of significantly correlated voxels ($2 \times 2 \times 2$ mm areas) and then related the resulting clusters to regions within the Talairach brain atlas (Talairach & Tournoux, 1988). These regions were then related to the activation regions that were identified in the Fox et al. (1996) PET study.

The Fox et al. PET study suggested that SMA (actually an unusually superior SMA), SLPrM, M1 (mouth), Broca's, temporal lobe (auditory region), insula (basal ganglia), and cerebellum were functionally related to stuttering. These regions mainly activated on the right. The important exception was A2 which mainly deactivated on the right.

In Table 4–1 those regions of interest (ROIs) are shown in Column 1, with the hemisphere in which they were located in Column 2. Reduced to their simplest form, the findings show that the correlations between

TABLE 4–1. Neural Regions Identified in the Fox et al. (1996) PET Study and the Neural Region CBF Correlations with Stuttering and Syllables Spoken.*

Column 1 shows the neural regions (plus hemisphere location in *Column 2*) that were identified as unusual among the 10 stutterers in the Fox et al. (1996) study. *Column 3* shows regions where there were voxel clusters that showed significant correlations between CBF and Stuttering (stuttered intervals). *Column 4* shows the regions where there were significant correlations between CBF and Syllables spoken for Stutterers (n = 10). *Column 5* shows the regions where there were significant correlations between CBF and Syllables spoken for the Controls (*n* = 10).

Columns 4 and 5 show that the CBF activations for stutterers and controls produced virtually identical correlations with the rate of syllable production. The stuttering correlations (displayed in Column 3) appeared to relate to different regions.

			Behavioral Correlation Data (regional activations × stuttering [stuttered intervals] or syllables spoken)	
			Stutterers	Controls
1	**2**	**3**	**4**	**5**
Region	**Stuttering**	**Stuttering**	**Syllables**	**Syllables**
SMA	Bilateral	**Bilateral**	Medial	Medial
SLPrM	Right			
M1	Left		Bilateral	Bilateral
BROCA'S	Right	**Right**	Bilateral	Bilateral
AUD	-Right	**-Right**		
Insula	Bilateral			
Cerebellum	Bilateral	**Bilateral**	Medial	Medial

*Regions were identified from the Talairach and Tournoux (1988) coordinates and the correlations were those significant with a z-score > 1.96. The 2 × 2 × 2 mm voxel cluster sizes ranged from 15 to 106.

the number of syllables spoken and areas of prominent activation were virtually identical for the stutterers and for the controls. In other words, the stutterers' and nonstutterers' speech production systems appear to be subserved by the same neural regions (SMA, M1, Broca's, and cerebellum)—virtually textbook areas associated with speech production. However, stuttering (actually stuttered intervals) appears to correlate reasonably well with only a subset of these regions (shown in bold), and in slightly different ways. The most obvious is SMA, which emerged as being strongly bilateral and distinctively different to the syllable rate correlations for the stutterers and the controls. M1 (mouth) *was not* correlated with stuttering, but Broca's on the right (not bilaterally) *was* correlated with stuttering. The temporal lobe region was again definitely deactivated and negatively correlated with stuttering, a feature unrelated to syllable production. Finally, there was still evidence of considerable cerebellum involvement, a finding that probably carries immense significance. However, in view of current controversies over the function of cerebellum (see *Behavioral and Brain Sciences*, December 1996), the nature of that significance is difficult to judge.

TMS: Not Yet Time to Worry About What's Flying Over the Cuckoo's Nest

Actually, the San Antonio group's plans regarding a second approach to the "cause or consequence" issue have been rather publicly and perhaps overdramatically advertised in a recent article in *New Scientist* (Motluk, 1997). Contrary to article claims, the purpose is *not* to perform neurosurgery; it is to use a noninvasive procedure called repeated transcranial magnetic stimulation (rTMS) in order to try to deactivate some of these abnormally activated regions (George, Wassermann, & Post, 1996). rTMS uses the principle of induction to transfer electrical energy across the scalp and skull and into the brain. A brief electrical pulse through a wire coil placed on the scalp provides a magnetic field. The field passes unimpeded through the tissues of the head and induces an electrical current in the brain. The strength and frequency of the charge influences the level and extent of depolarization of neurons. This is also a function of the shape of the coil: a butterfly (figure 8) shape coil produces fairly focal stimulation. The current stimulators develop about 1.5 to 2 Tesla at the face of the coil and are able to activate neurons 1.5 to 2 cm from the surface of the coil in the cortex (Epstein, Schwartzberg, Davey, & Sudderth, 1990).

Recent developments with TMS have suggested that it may also be possible to either stimulate or "quench" (i.e., deactivate) neural activations in relatively focal areas (see Fox et al., 1996). TMS also appears to be a very safe procedure for creating temporary deactivations and activations in order to map functional regions of the brain.[14] Peter Fox (see

---

[14] Of course, this is precisely what Penfield and Roberts (1959) attempted to do by electrostimulating certain sites in the exposed cortex. That type of "fortuitous" research is still being conducted with different patients (e.g., Weber & Ojemann, 1995), but it depends on the study of essentially nonnormal or lesioned patients. Rather similar procedures were reported by Bhatnager and Andy (1989) to produce electrical stimulation of the thalamic region of some persons who stutter. However, this is an extremely hazardous invasive procedure that may only be suitable in rare cases of stuttering where the brain is exposed for some other health reason.

Motluk, 1997) has also recently suggested that this procedure may make it possible to conduct "systems neurosurgey," a method for directly altering the action of those disorders that appear to be associated with, or subserved by, unusual regions of activation and deactivation. Such regional intervention may actually make it possible to "turn a disorder on and off." It is at least possible that stuttering may also fall into that class of disorder.

Even more interesting is the implication of studies that have shown that daily periods of approximately 30 minutes of low frequency (1 Hz) TMS will not only interrupt aberrant neural activity, but may succeed in producing sustained low levels of activity (George, Wassermann, & Post, 1996). Of course, a host of unknowns could occur in conjunction with this procedure. For instance, it is possible that TMS might produce a neural reorganization that "rejects" such alterations, or perhaps it will produce other abnormal activations and behavior. However, recent studies do not appear to have produced these untoward effects (see Wassermann, 1997).

Most of the evidence about the effect of rTMS have derived from studies of the motor cortex. However, there have now been investigations of the effects of extensive low frequency rTMS with Parkinsonism and depressed patients. They have shown that focal stimulation of specific regions may induce sustained changes in behavior and in activation areas (George, Wassermann, & Post, 1996; Stallings, Speer, Spicer, Cheng, & George, 1997). Among the more interesting recent studies is one by Karp and colleagues (Karp, Wassermann, Porter, & Hallett, 1997) at the NIH on Tourette's syndrome (TS), a disorder that some have suggested is related to stuttering (Comings & Comings, 1994; Ingham, 1984). In this particular study, six TS subjects received initially 1 Hz rTMS (30 seconds on/15 s off) over various sites (including sham stimulation) and showed a 44% decrease in motor tics during stimulation to contralateral M1 and a 37% decrease during stimulation to SMA (sham stimulation produced a 2% decrease). The sites selected for stimulation in these subjects were not based on the systematic identification of abnormal regions of activation. Nevertheless, the evidence from Karp et al. (1997) is particularly interesting and appears to offer some additional justification for testing the effects of sustained low frequency rTMS on stuttering.

Initial research using rTMS will be directed toward isolating the functional role of SMA and SLPrM on stuttering. A series of single subject experiments have been planned in order to investigate the effects of brief "trains" of high frequency (20 Hz) rTMS delivered to both of these sites during oral reading trials. These studies will be conducted with some of the 10 adult stutterers who were subjects in the Fox et al. (1996) PET study. In all likelihood, the effect of rTMS on all sites will be evaluated, depending on the results of some studies that we are currently conducting in San Antonio, some literally on the researchers (e.g., Fox et al., 1997). One purpose of these studies, incidentally, is to carefully document the effects of TMS on CBF. Thus far it seems that that there is every reason to expect that these effects should be readily detected in the CBF data required for this research. The primary purpose of these studies with stutterers, therefore, will be to assess the effects on stuttering of reducing the level of rCBF activation in SMA and SLPrM during oral reading. In the event that it is found that rTMS does reduce stuttering, assessment of the effects of extended low frequency (1 Hz) rTMS on stuttering during speech across time and over a variety of speaking situations is planned. Hopefully, this will produce some useful therapeutic consequences; at the very least it should determine the contribution of these regional activations to stuttering.

CONCLUSIONS

The recent emergence of a neuroscience orientation within stuttering research certainly appears to have a lot of promise and a lot of pitfalls. The promising feature of this orientation is that it does offer the possibility of achieving more than the simple mapping of neural regions associated with stuttering; it is beginning to appear that it will also be possible to identify powerful and pivotal variables that have clinical promise. Of course, many of the new directions may turn out to do little more than cancel out hypothetically promising avenues, and that will still be a considerable contribution to stuttering research. However, this new orientation has emerged in conjunction with new technologies that have the capability of identifying functional variables that may become important treatment agents. Arguably, it is this feature, above most others, that may ultimately help to separate this orientation from much of the recent and clinically uninspiring history of stuttering research.

ACKNOWLEDGMENT: Paper read to the conference "Toward Treatment Efficacy for Stuttering" held at The University of Georgia, Athens, Georgia, March 20, 1997.

REFERENCES

Adams, M. R. (1987). Voice onsets and segment durations of normal speakers and beginning stutterers. *Journal of Fluency Disorders, 12,* 133–139.

Adams, M. R. (1990). The demands and capacities model I: Theoretical elaboration. *Journal of Fluency Disorders, 15*, 135–141.

Adams, M. R., & Hayden, P. (1976). The ability of stutterers and nonstutterers to initiate and terminate phonation during production of an isolated vowel. *Journal of Speech and Hearing Research, 19*, 290–296.

Agnello, J. G. (1975). Voice onset and voice termination features of stutterers. In L. M. Webster & L. C. Furst (Eds.), *Proceedings of the First Annual Hayes Martin Conference on Vocal Tract Dynamics*. New York: New York Speech and Hearing Institute.

Alfonso, P. J. (1991). Implications of the concepts underlying task-dynamic modeling on kinematic studies of stuttering. In H. F. M. Peters, W. Hulstjin, & W. Starkweather (Eds.), *Speech motor control and stuttering* (pp. 79–100). Amsterdam: Excerpta Medica.

Andrews, G., Craig, A., Feyer, A-M., Hoddinott, S., Howie, P., & Neilson, M. (1983). Stuttering: A review of research findings and theories circa 1982. *Journal of Speech and Hearing Disorders, 48*, 226–246.

Armson, J., & Kalinowski, J. (1994). Interpreting results of the fluent speech paradigm in stuttering research: Difficulties in separating cause from effect. *Journal of Speech and Hearing Research, 37*, 69–82.

Baken, R., McManus, D. A., & Cavallo, S. A. (1983). Prephonatory chest wall posturing in stutterers. *Journal of Speech and Hearing Research, 26*, 444–450.

Bakker, K., & Brutten, G. J. (1990). Speech-related reaction times of stutterers and nonstutterers: Diagnostic implications. *Journal of Speech and Hearing Disorders, 55*, 295–299.

Bakker, K., Ingham, R. J., & Netsell, R. (1997). The measurement of voice onset abruptness via acoustic, accelerometric, and aerodynamic signal analysis. In W. Hulstjin, H. F. M. Peters, & P. H. H. M. van Lieshout (Eds.), *Speech motor production: Motor control, brain research and fluency disorders* (pp. 405–412). Amsterdam: Elsevier.

Baxter, L. R., Schwartz, J. M., Bergman, K. S., Szuba, M. P., Guze, B. H., Mazziotta, J. C., Alazaraki, A., Selin, C. E., Ferng, H-K., Munford, P., & Phelps, M. (1992). Caudate glucose metabolic rate changes with both drug and behavior therapy for obsessive-compulsive disorder. *Archives of General Psychiatry, 49*, 681–689.

Belin, P., Van Eeckhout, P., Zilbovicius, M., Remy, P., François, C., Guillaume, S., Chain, F., Rancurel, G., & Samson, Y. (1996). Recovery from nonfluent aphasia after melodic intonation therapy: A PET study. *Neurology, 47*, 1504–1511.

Bennett, S. (1981). Vowel formant frequency characteristics of preadolescent males and females. *Journal of the Acoustical Society of America, 69*, 231–238.

Bhatnagar, S. C., & Andy, O. J. (1989). Alleviation of acquired stuttering with human centermedian thalamic stimulation. *Journal of Neurology, Neurosurgery, and Psychiatry, 52*, 1182–1184.

Bloodstein, O. (1995). *A handbook on stuttering* (5th ed.). San Diego, CA: Singular Publishing Group.

Boberg, E., Yeudall, L. T., Schopflocher, D., & Bo-Lassen, P. (1983). The effect of an intensive behavioral program on the distribution of EEG alpha power in stutterers during the processing of verbal and visuospatial information. *Journal of Fluency Disorders, 8*, 245–263.

Borden, G. J. (1983). Initiation versus execution time during manual and oral counting by stutterers. *Journal of Speech and Hearing Research, 26,* 389–396.

Braun, A. R., Ludlow, C. L., Varga, M., Shulz, G. M., & Stager, S. (1994). Central correlates of speech motor control in stuttering: An $H_2{}^{15}O$ PET study. *Neurology, 44*(Suppl. 2), A261.

Brin, M. F., Stewart, C., Blitzer, A., & Diamond, B. (1994). Laryngeal botulinum toxin injections for disabling stuttering in adults. *Neurology, 44,* 2262–2268.

Brown, C. J., Zimmermann, G. N., Linville, R. N., & Hegmann, J. P. (1990). Variations in self-paced behaviors in stutterers and nonstutterers. *Journal of Speech and Hearing Research, 33,* 317–323.

Caruso, A. J., Abbs, J. H., & Gracco, V. L. (1988). Kinematic analysis of multiple movement coordination during speech in stutterers. *Brain, 111,* 439–455.

Caruso, A. J., Conture, E. G., & Colton, R. H. (1988). Selected temporal parameters of coordination associated with stuttering in children. *Journal of Fluency Disorders, 13,* 57–82.

Colcord, R. D., & Adams, M. R. (1979). Voicing duration and vocal SPL changes associated with stuttering reduction during singing. *Journal of Speech and Hearing Research, 22,* 468–479.

Comings, D. E., & Comings, B. G. (1994). TS, learning, and speech problems. *Journal of the American Academy of Child and Adolescent Psychiatry, 33,* 429–430.

Conture, E. G. (1991). Young stutterers' speech production: A critical perspective. In H. F. M. Peters, W. Hulstjin, & W. Starkweather (Eds.), *Speech motor control and stuttering* (pp. 365–384). Amsterdam: Springer-Verlag.

Conture, E. G., Colton, R. H., & Gleason, J. R. (1988). Selected temporal aspects of coordination during fluent speech of young stutterers. *Journal of Speech and Hearing Research, 31,* 640–653.

Conture, E. G., McCall, G. N., & Brewer, D. W. (1977). Laryngeal behavior during stuttering. *Journal of Speech and Hearing Research, 20,* 661–668.

Conture, E. G., Rothenberg, M., & Molitor, R. D. (1986). Electroglottographic observations of young stutterers' fluency. *Journal of Speech and Hearing Research, 29,* 384–393.

Conture, E. G., Schwartz, H. D., & Brewer, D. (1985). Laryngeal behavior during stuttering: A further study. *Journal of Speech and Hearing Research, 28,* 233–240.

Cooper, M. H., & Allen, G. D. (1977). Timing control accuracy in normal speakers and stutterers. *Journal of Speech and Hearing Research, 20,* 55–71.

Cullinan, W. L., & Springer, M. T. (1980). Voice initiation and termination times in stuttering and nonstuttering children. *Journal of Speech and Hearing Research, 23,* 344–360.

Curlee, R. F. (1993). Neuropsychological aspects of stuttering. Implications for diagnosis. In E. Boberg (Ed.), *Neuropsychology of stuttering* (pp. 165–175). Edmonton: The University of Alberta Press.

Curlee, R. F., & Siegel, G. M. (1997). *Nature and treatment of stuttering: New directions* (2nd ed.), Boston: Allyn & Bacon.

De Nil, L. F., Kroll, R. M., Kapur, S., & Houle, S. (1995, December). *Silent and oral reading in stuttering and nonstuttering adults: A positron emission tomography study.* Paper read at the annual meeting of the American Speech-Language-Hearing Association, Orlando, FL.

Denny, M., & Smith, A. (1992). Gradations in a pattern of neuromuscular activity associated with stuttering. *Journal of Speech and Hearing Research, 35,* 1216–1229.

Denny, M., & Smith, A. (1997). Respiratory and laryngeal control in stuttering. In R. F. Curlee & G. M. Siegel (Eds.), *Nature and treatment of stuttering: New directions* (2nd ed., pp. 128–142). Boston: Allyn and Bacon.

Di Simoni, F. G. (1974). Preliminary study of certain timing relationships in the speech of stutterers. *Journal of the Acoustical Society of America, 56,* 695–696.

Epstein, C. M., Schwartzberg, D. G., Davey, K. R., & Sudderth, D. B. (1990). Localizing the site of magnetic brain stimulation in humans. *Neurology, 40,* 666–670.

Fant, G. (1966). A note on vocal tract size factors and nonuniform F-pattern scalings. *Speech Transmission Laboratory: Quarterly Report (Stockholm Royal Institute of Technology), 4,* 22–30.

Fibiger, S. (1971). Stuttering explained as a physiological tremor. *Speech Transmission Laboratory—Quarterly Progress and Status Report, 2–3,* 1–24.

Fox, P. T., Ingham, R. J., George, M. S., Mayberg, H., Ingham, J., Roby, J., Martin, C., & Jerabek, P. (1997). Imaging human intra-cerebral connectivity by PET during TMS. *Neuroreport, 8,* 2787–2791.

Fox, P. T., Ingham, R. J., Ingham, J. C., Hirsch, T., Downs, J. H., Martin, C., Jerabek, P., Glass, T., & Lancaster, J. L. (1996). A PET study of the neural systems of stuttering. *Nature, 382,* 158–162.

Fox, P. T., Lancaster, J. L., & Ingham, R. J. (1993). On stuttering and global ischemia. *Archives of Neurology, 50,* 1287–1288.

Freeman, F. J. (1979). Phonation in stuttering: A review of current research. *Journal of Fluency Disorders, 4,* 79–89.

Freeman, F., & Ushijima, T. (1978). Laryngeal muscle activity during stuttering. *Journal of Speech and Hearing Research, 21,* 538–562.

Freund, H. J., & Dietz, V. (1978). The relationship between physiological and pathological tremor. In J. E. Desmedt (Ed.), *Physiological tremor, pathological tremors and clonus* (pp. 66–89). Basel, Switzerland: Karger.

George, M. S., Wassermann, E. M., & Post, R. M. (1996). Transcranial magnetic stimulation: A neuropsychiatric tool for the 21st century. *Journal of Neuropsychiatry and Clinical Neuroscience, 8,* 373–382.

Goldberger, A. L., Rigney, D. R., Mietus, J., Antman, E. M., & Greenwald, S. (1988). Nonlinear dynamics in sudden cardiac death syndrome: Heartrate oscillations and bifurcations. *Experientia, 44,* 983–987.

Goldsmith, H. (1983). Some comments on "Articulatory dynamics of fluent utterances of stutterers and nonstutterers." *Journal of Speech and Hearing Research, 26,* 319–320.

Gow, M. L., & Ingham, R. J. (1992). Modifying electroglottograph-identified intervals of phonation: The effect on stuttering. *Journal of Speech and Hearing Research, 35,* 495–511.

Hall, J., & Jerger, J. (1978). Central auditory function in stutterers. *Journal of Speech and Hearing Research, 21,* 324–337.

Healey, E. C., & Gutkin, B. (1984). Analysis of stutterers' voice onset times and fundamental frequency contours during fluency. *Journal of Speech and Hearing Research, 27*, 219–225.

Hillman, R. E., & Gilbert, H. R. (1977). Voice onset time for voiceless stop consonants in the fluent reading of stutterers and nonstutterers. *Journal of the Acoustical Society of America, 61*, 610–611.

Howell, P., El-Yaniv, N., & Powell, D. J. (1987). Factors affecting fluency in stutterers when speaking under altered auditory feedback. In H. F. M. Peters & W. Hulstijn (Eds.), *Speech motor dynamics in stuttering* (pp. 361–369). New York: Springer-Verlag.

Hulstijn, W., Starkweather, C. W., & Peters, H. F. M. (1991). Speech motor control and stuttering: An introduction. In H. F. M. Peters, W. Hulstijn, & W. Starkweather (Eds.), *Speech motor control and stuttering.* (pp. xvii–xxiii). New York: Springer-Verlag.

Ingham, R. J. (1984). *Stuttering and behavior therapy: Current status and experimental foundations.* San Diego: College-Hill Press.

Ingham, R. J. (1993). The neuropsychology of stuttering: Are there implications for clinical management? In E. Boberg (Ed.), *Neuropsychology of stuttering* (pp. 177–198). Edmonton, Alberta: The University of Alberta Press.

Ingham, R. J., & Cordes, A. K. (1997). Self-measurement and evaluating treatment efficacy. In R. F. Curlee & G. M. Siegel (Eds.), *Nature and treatment of stuttering: New directions* (2nd ed., pp. 413–438). Boston: Allyn & Bacon.

Ingham, R. J., Cordes, A. K., & Finn, P. (1993). Time-interval measurement of stuttering: Systematic replication of Ingham, Cordes, and Gow (1993). *Journal of Speech and Hearing Research, 36*, 1168–1176.

Ingham, R. J., Fox, P. T., Ingham, J. C., Zamarripa, F., Jerabek, P., & Cotton, J. (1996). A functional lesion investigation of developmental stuttering using positron emission tomography. *Journal of Speech and Hearing Research, 39*, 1208–1227.

Ingham, R. J., Moglia, R. A., Frank, P., Ingham, J. C., & Cordes, A. K. (1997). Experimental investigation of the effects of frequency-altered auditory feedback on the speech of adults who stutter. *Journal of Speech, Language, and Hearing Research, 40*, 349–360.

Ingham, R. J., Montgomery, J., & Ulliana, L. (1993). The effect of manipulating phonation duration on stuttering. *Journal of Speech and Hearing Research, 26*, 579–587.

Jäncke, L., Hefter, H., & Kalveram, K. T. (1995). Fast finger extensions are slower in stutterers than in nonstutterers. *Perceptual and Motor Skills, 80*, 1103–1107.

Jäncke, L., Kaiser, P., Bauer, A., & Kalveram, K. T. (1995). Upper lip, lower lip, and jaw peak velocity sequence during bilabial closures: No differences between stutterers and nonstutterers. *Journal of the Acoustical Society of America, 97*, 3900–3903.

Janssen, P., & Wieneke, P. (1987). The effects of fluency-inducing conditions on the variability in the duration of laryngeal movements during stutterers' fluent speech. In H. F. M. Peters & W. Hulstijn (Eds.), *Speech motor dynamics in stuttering* (pp. 337–344). New York: Springer-Verlag.

Johnston, S. J., Watkin, K. L., & Macklem, P. T. (1993). Lung volume changes during relatively fluent speech in stutterers. *Journal of Applied Physiology*, *75*, 696–703.

Kalinowski, J., Armson, J., Roland-Mieszkowski, M., Stuart, A., & Gracco, V. (1993). Effects of alterations in auditory feedback and speech rate on stuttering frequency. *Language and Speech*, *36*, 1–16.

Karni, A., Meyer, G., Jezzard, P., Adams, M. M., Turner, R., & Ungerleider, L. G. (1995). Functional MRI evidence for adult motor cortex plasticity during motor skill learning. *Nature*, *377*, 155–158.

Karp, B. I., Wassermann, E. M., Porter, S., & Hallett, M. (1997). Transcranial magnetic stimulation acutely decreases motor tics. *Neurology*, *48*, A397–398.

Kass, J. H. (1988). Development of cortical sensory maps. In P. Rakic & W. Singer (Eds.), *Neurobiology of neocortex* (pp. 41–67). New York: John Wiley.

Kass, J., Merzenich, M., & Killachey, H. (1983). The reorganization of somatosensory cortex following peripheral nerve damage in adult and developing mammals. *Annual Review of Neuroscience*, *6*, 325–356.

Kelly, M., Smith, A., & Goffman, L. (1995). Orofacial muscle activity of children who stutter: A preliminary study. *Journal of Speech and Hearing Research*, *38*, 1025–1036.

Love, L. R., & Jeffress, L. A. (1971). Identification of brief pauses in the fluent speech of stutterers and nonstutterers. *Journal of Speech and Hearing Research*, *14*, 229–240.

Mallard, A. R., & Westbrook, J. B. (1985). Vowel duration in stutterers participating in Precision Fluency Shaping. *Journal of Fluency Disorders*, *10*, 221–228.

Marsden, C. D., Deecke, L., Freund, H-J., Hallett, M., Passingham, R. E., Shibasaki, H., Tanji, J., & Wiesendanger, M. (1996). The functions of the supplementary motor area. *Advances in Neurology*, *70*, 477–487.

Martin, R. R., Haroldson, S. K., & Triden, K. A. (1984). Stuttering and speech naturalness. *Journal of Speech and Hearing Disorders*, *49*, 53–58.

Martin, R. R., Johnson, L. J., Siegel, G. M., & Haroldson, S. K. (1985). Auditory stimulation, rhythm, and stuttering. *Journal of Speech and Hearing Research*, *28*, 487–495.

Martin, R. R., Siegel, G. M., Johnson, L. J., & Haroldson, S. K. (1984). Sidetone amplification, noise, and stuttering. *Journal of Speech and Hearing Research*, *27*, 518–527.

McClean, M., Goldsmith, H., & Cerf, A. (1984). Lower-lip EMG and displacement during bilabial disfluencies in adult stutterers. *Journal of Speech and Hearing Research*, *27*, 342–349.

McClean, M. D., Kroll, R. M., & Loftus, N. S. (1990). Kinematic analysis of lipclosure in stutterers' fluent speech. *Journal of Speech and Hearing Research*, *35*, 755–760.

McClean, M. D., Levandowski, D. R., & Cord, M. T. (1994). Intersyllabic movement timing in the fluent speech of stutterers with different disfluency levels. *Journal of Speech and Hearing Research*, *37*, 1060–1066.

McFarland, D., Smith, A., Moore, C. A., & Weber, C. M. (1986). Relationship between amplitude of tremor and reflex responses of the human jaw-closing system. *Brain Research*, *366*, 272–278.

Merzenich, M. M., Recanzone, G., Jenkins, W. M., Allard, T. T., & Judo, R. J. (1988). Cortical representational plasticity. In P. Rakic & W. Singer (Eds.), *Neurobiology of Neocortex* (pp. 41–67). New York: John Wiley.

Metz, D. E., Onufrak, J. A., & Ogburn, R. S. (1979). An acoustical analysis of stutterers' speech prior to and at the termination of speech therapy. *Journal of Fluency Disorders, 4*, 249–254.

Moore, W. H., Jr. (1984). Hemispheric alpha asymmetries during an electromyographic biofeedback procedure for stuttering. *Journal of Fluency Disorders, 17*, 143–162.

Moore, W. H., Jr. (1990). Pathophysiology of stuttering: Cerebral activation differences in stutterers vs. nonstutterers. *ASHA Reports, 18*, 72–80.

Moore, W. H., Jr., & Haynes, W. O. (1980). Alpha hemispheric asymmetry and stuttering: Some support for segmentation dysfunction hypothesis. *Journal of Speech and Hearing Research, 23*, 229–247.

Motluk, A. (1997, February 1). Cutting out stuttering. *New Scientist*, 32–35.

Nudelman, H. B., Herbrich, K. E., Hess, K. R., Hoyt, B. D., & Rosenfield, D. B. (1992). A model of the phonatory response time of stutterers and fluent speakers to frequency-modulated tones. *Journal of the Acoustical Society of America, 92*, 1882–1888.

Onslow, M., Packman, A., Stocker, S., van Doorn, J., & Siegel, G. M. (1997). Control of children's stuttering with response-contingent time-out: Behavioral, perceptual, and acoustic data. *Journal of Speech, Language, and Hearing Research, 40*, 121–133.

Onslow, M., van Doorn, J., & Newman, D. (1992). Variability of acoustic segment durations after prolonged-speech treatment for stuttering. *Journal of Speech and Hearing Research, 35*, 529–536.

Packman, A., Onslow, M., Richards, F., & van Doorn, J. (1996). Syllabic stress and variability: A model of stuttering. *Clinical Linguistics and Phonetics, 10*, 235–263.

Packman, A., Onslow, M., & van Doorn, J. (1994). Prolonged speech and modification of stuttering: Perceptual, acoustic, and electroglottographic data. *Journal of Speech and Hearing Research, 37*, 724–737.

Palla, S., & Ash, M. M. (1979). Frequency analysis of human jaw tremor at rest. *Archives of Oral Biology, 24*, 709–718.

Pascual-Leone, A., & Torres, F. (1993). Plasticity of the sensorimotor cortex representation of the reading finger in Braille readers. *Brain, 116*, 39–52.

Penfield, W., & Roberts, L. (1959). *Speech and brain-mechanisms.* Princeton, NJ: Princeton University Press.

Perkins, W. H. (1997). Stuttering: Why science hasn't solved it. In R. F. Curlee & G. M. Siegel (Eds.), *Nature and treatment of stuttering: New directions* (2nd ed., pp. 218–235). Boston: Allyn & Bacon.

Peters, H. F. M., & Boves, L. (1988). Coordination of aerodynamic and phonatory processes in fluent speech utterances of stutterers. *Journal of Speech and Hearing Research, 31*, 352–361.

Peters, H. F. M., & Hulstijn, W. (1987). *Speech motor dynamics in stuttering.* New York: Springer-Verlag.

Peters, H. F. M., Hulstijn, W., & Starkweather, C. W. (1989). Acoustic and physiologic reaction times of stutterers and nonstutterers. *Journal of Speech and Hearing Research, 32*, 668–680.

Peters, H. F. M., Hulstijn, W., & Starkweather, C. W. (1991). *Speech motor control and stuttering.* Amsterdam: Exerpta Medica.

Petersen, S. E., Fox, P. T., Posner, M. I., Mintun, M., & Raichle, M. E. (1989). Positron emission tomographic studies of the processing of single words. *Journal of Cognitive Neuroscience, 1*, 153–170.

Platt, L. J., & Basili, A. (1973). Jaw tremor during stuttering block. *Journal of Communication Disorders, 6*, 102–109.

Pool, K. D., Devous, M. D., Sr., Freeman, F. J., Watson, B. C., & Finitzo, T. (1991). Regional cerebral blood flow in developmental stutterers. *Archives of Neurology, 48*, 509–512.

Posner, M. I., & Raichle, M. E. (1994). *Images of mind.* New York: Scientific American Library.

Postma, A., & Kolk, H. H. J. (1993). The covert repair hypothesis: Prearticulatory repair processes in normal and stuttered disfluencies. *Journal of Speech and Hearing Research, 36*, 472–487.

Prosek, R. A., & Runyan, G. M. (1982). Temporal characteristics related to the discrimination of stutterers' and nonstutterers' speech samples. *Journal of Speech and Hearing Research, 25*, 29–33.

Prosek, R. A., & Runyan, G. M. (1983). Effects of segment and pause manipulations on the identification of treated stutterers. *Journal of Speech and Hearing Research, 26*, 510–516.

Quesal, R. W. (1989). Stuttering research: Have we forgotten the stutterer? *Journal of Fluency Disorders, 14*, 153–164.

Raichle, M. E., Fiez, J. A., Videen, T. O., MacLeod, A. M., Pardo, J. V., Fox, P. T., & Petersen, S. E. (1994). Practice-related changes in human brain functional anatomy during nonmotor learning. *Cerebral Cortex, 4*, 8–26.

Rakic, P., Suner, I., & Williams, R. W. (1991). A novel cytoarchitectonic area induced experimentally within the primary visual cortex. *Proceedings of the National Academy of Sciences of the United States of America, 88*, 2083–2087.

Ramig, P. R., Krieger, S. M., & Adams, M. R. (1982). Vocal changes in stutterers and nonstutterers when speaking to children. *Journal of Fluency Disorders, 7*, 369–384.

Rosenfield, D. B., & Jerger, J. (1984). Stuttering and auditory function. In R. F. Curlee & W. H. Perkins (Eds.), *Nature and treatment of stuttering: New directions* (pp. 73–87). San Diego: College-Hill Press.

Samar, V. J., Metz, D. E., & Sacco, P. R. (1986). Changes in aerodynamic characteristics of stutterers' fluent speech associated with therapy. *Journal of Speech and Hearing Research, 29*, 106–113.

Schwartz, H. D. (1987). Subgrouping young stutterers: A physiological perspective. In H. F. M. Peters & W. Hulstijn (Eds.), *Speech motor dynamics in stuttering* (pp. 215–227). New York: Springer-Verlag.

Shapiro, A. I. (1980). An electromyographic analysis of the fluent and dysfluent utterances of several types of stutterers. *Journal of Fluency Disorders, 5*, 203–231.

Smith, A. (1989). Neural drive to muscles in stuttering. *Journal of Speech and Hearing Research, 32,* 252–264.

Smith, A., Denny, M., Shaffer, L. A., Kelly, E. M., & Hirano, M. (1996). Activity of intrinsic laryngeal muscles in fluent and disfluent speech. *Journal of Speech and Hearing Research, 39,* 329–348.

Smith, A., Denny, M., & Wood, J. L. (1991). Instability in speech muscle systems in stuttering. In H. F. M. Peters, W. Hulstijn, & W. Starkweather (Eds.), *Speech motor control and stuttering* (pp. 231–242). Amsterdam: Excerpta Medica.

Smith, A., & Kelly, E. (1997). Stuttering: A dynamic, multifactorial model. In R. F. Curlee & G. M. Siegel (Eds.), *Nature and treatment of stuttering: New directions* (2nd ed., pp. 204–217). Boston: Allyn & Bacon.

Smith, A., Luschei, E., Denny, M., Wood, J. L., Hirano, M., & Badylak, S. (1993). Spectral analyses of activity of laryngeal and orofacial muscles in stutterers. *Journal of Neurology, Neurosurgery, and Psychiatry, 56,* 1303–1311.

Stager, S. V., & Ludlow, C. L. (1991). Do fluency-evoking conditions elicit continuous voicing in normal speakers? In H. F. M. Peters, W. Hulstijn, & C. W. Starkweather (Eds.), *Speech motor control and stuttering* (pp. 355–362). Amsterdam: Excerpta Medica.

Stager, S. V., & Ludlow, C. L. (1994). Responses of stutterers and vocal tremor patients of treatment with botulinum toxin. In J. Jankovic, & M. Hallett (Eds.), *Therapy with botulinum toxin* (pp. 481–490). New York: Marcel Dekker.

Stallings, L. E., Speer, A. M., Spicer, K. M., Cheng, M. S., & George, M. S. (1997, May). *Combining SPECT and repetitive transcranial magnetic stimulation (rTMS) - Left prefrontal stimulation decreases relative perfusion locally in a dose-dependent manner.* Paper read to 3rd International Conference on Functional Mapping of the Human Brain, Copenhagen, Denmark.

Starkweather, C. W. (1987). *Fluency and stuttering.* Englewood Cliffs, NJ: Prentice Hall.

Starkweather, C. W., & Myers, M. (1979). Duration of subsegments within the intervocalic intervals in stutterers and nonstutterers. *Journal of Fluency Disorders, 4,* 205–214.

Story, R. S., Alfonso, P. J., & Harris, K. S. (1996). Pre- and posttreatment comparison of the kinematics of the fluent speech of persons who stutter. *Journal of Speech and Hearing Research, 39,* 991–1005.

Stromsta, C. (1972). Interaural phase disparity of stutterers and nonstutterers. *Journal of Speech and Hearing Research, 15,* 771–780.

Stryker, M. P. (1988). Principles of cortical self-organization. In P. Rakic & W. Singer (Eds.), *Neurobiology of neocortex* (pp. 115–136). New York: John Wiley.

Sur, M., & Garraghty, P. (1986). Experimentally induced visual responses from auditory thalamus and cortex. *Society for the Neurosciences Abstracts, 12,* 592.

Sutton, S., & Chase, R. A. (1961). White noise and stuttering. *Journal of Speech and Hearing Research, 4,* 72.

Talairach, J., & Tournoux, P. (1988). *Co-planar stereotaxic atlas of the human brain.* Verlag: Thieme.

Tosher, M., & Rupp, R. (1978). A study of the central auditory processes in stutterers using the synthetic sentence identification (SSI) test battery. *Journal of Speech and Hearing Research, 21*, 779–792.

Travis, L. E. (1934). Dissociation of the homologous muscle function in stuttering. *Archives of Neurology and Psychiatry, 31*, 127–133.

Wassermann, E. M. (1997). Repetitive transcranial magnetic stimulation: An introduction and overview. *CNS Spectrums, 2*, 21–25.

Watson, B. C., & Alfonso, P. J. (1983). Foreperiod and stuttering severity effects on acoustic laryngeal reaction time. *Journal of Fluency Disorders, 8*, 183–205.

Watson, B. C., & Alfonso, P. J. (1987). Physiological bases of acoustic LRT in nonstutterers, mild stutterers and severe stutterers. *Journal of Speech and Hearing Research, 30*, 434–437.

Weber, C. M., & Smith, A. (1990). Autonomic correlates of stuttering and speech assessed in a range of experimental tasks. *Journal of Speech and Hearing Research, 33*, 690–706.

Weber, P. B., & Ojemann, G. A. (1995). Neuronal recordings in human lateral temporal lobe during verbal paired associate learning. *Neuroreport, 6*, 685–689.

Webster, R. L., & Dorman, M. T. (1970). Decreases in stuttering frequency as a function of continuous and contingent forms of auditory masking. *Journal of Speech and Hearing Research, 13*, 82–86.

Webster, W. G. (1993). Hurried hands and tangled tongues. Implications of current research for the management of stuttering. In E. Boberg (Ed.), *Neuropsychology of stuttering* (pp. 73–127). Edmonton: The University of Alberta Press.

Weiller, C., Chollet, F., Friston, K. J., Wise, R. J. S., & Frackowiak, R. S. J. (1992). Functional reorganization of the brain in recovery from striatocapsular infarction in man. *Annals of Neurology 32*, 463–472.

Weiller, C., Isensee, C., Rijntjes, M., Huber, W., Müller, S., Bier, D., Dutschka, K., Woods, R. P., Noth, J., & Diener, H. C. (1995). Recovery from Wernicke's aphasia: A positron emission tomographic study. *Annals of Neurology, 37*, 723–732.

Wieneke, G., & Janssen, P. (1987). Duration variations in the fluent speech of stutterers and nonstutterers. In H. F. M. Peters & W. Hulstijn (Eds.), *Speech motor dynamics in stuttering* (pp. 345–352). New York: Springer-Verlag.

Wieneke, G., & Janssen, P. (1991). Effect of speaking rate on speech timing variability. In H. F. M. Peters, W. Hulstijn, & W. Starkweather (Eds.), *Speech motor control and stuttering* (pp. 325–331). Amsterdam: Excerpta Medica.

Wingate, M. E. (1969). Sound and pattern in "artificial" fluency. *Journal of Speech and Hearing Research, 12*, 677–686.

Wingate, M. E. (1970). Effect on stuttering of changes in audition. *Journal of Speech and Hearing Research, 13*, 861–873.

Wood, F., Stump, D., McKeehan, A., Sheldon, S., & Proctor, J. (1980). Patterns of regional cerebral blood flow during attempted reading aloud by stutterers both on and off haloperidol medication: Evidence for inadequate left frontal activation during stuttering. *Brain and Language, 9*, 141–144.

Wu, J. C., Maguire, G., Riley, G., Fallon, J., LaCase, L., Chin, S., Klein, E., Tang, C., Cadwell, S., & Lottenberg, S. (1995). A positron emission tomography

(F-18) deoxyglucose study of developmental stuttering. *Neuroreport, 6,* 501–505.

Young, M. A. (1994). Evaluating differences between stuttering and nonstuttering speakers: The group difference design. *Journal of Speech and Hearing Research, 37,* 522–534.

Zimmermann, G. (1980a). Articulatory behaviors associated with stuttering: A cinefluorographic analysis. *Journal of Speech and Hearing Research, 23,* 108–121.

Zimmermann, G. (1980b). Articulatory dynamics of fluent utterances of stutterers and nonstutterers. *Journal of Speech and Hearing Research, 23,* 95–107.

Zimmermann, G. (1980c). Stuttering: A disorder of movement. *Journal of Speech and Hearing Research, 23,* 122–136.

Zimmermann, G. (1983). In agreement with Goldsmith. *Journal of Speech and Hearing Research, 26,* 320.

Zimmermann, G., & Hanley, J. M. (1983). A cinefluorographic investigation of repeated fluent productions of stutterers in an adaptation procedure. *Journal of Speech and Hearing Research, 26,* 35–42.

Zimmermann, G. N., Smith, A., & Hanley, J. M. (1981). Stuttering: In need of a unifying conceptual framework. *Journal of Speech and Hearing Research, 24,* 25-31.

Zocchi, L., Estenne, M., Johnston, S., Del Ferro, L., Ward, M. E., & Macklem, P. T. (1990). Respiratory muscle incoordination in stuttering speech. *American Review of Respiratory Disease, 141,* 1510–1515.

CHAPTER

Stuttering: Theory, Research, and Therapy

GERALD M. SIEGEL, Ph.D.

The current chapter expands on a theme first explored several years ago as part of a conference on cognitive science (Siegel, 1992). The main thesis of the 1992 conference paper was that in applied fields such as speech-language pathology, theories have practical and immediate consequences for the people served. These consequences are not simply academic. They affect the lives and welfare of clients. In the area of stuttering, for example, the development of a new theory of stuttering has periodically liberated clinical practice and opened up approaches that previously seemed hardly possible. At other times, stuttering theories have had a constraining influence. Those who do research in applied areas are constantly confronted with the tension between the liberating and constraining aspects of theory.

The current chapter revisits this general topic, recognizing full well that these issues crop up during periods when there is uncertainty about how research efforts should be directed (e.g., Johnston, 1983; Kent & Fair, 1985; Perkins, 1986; Ringel, Trachtman, & Prutting, 1984; Siegel, 1987; Siegel & Ingham, 1987). The first part of the chapter will draw on familiar examples from the history of stuttering, briefly examining the cerebral dominance, diagnosogenic, and operant theories of stuttering. It will then be argued that, unlike past eras, there currently is no truly dominant theory or approach to the disorder. Finally, possible reasons for this change, and its implications, will be explored.

THE CEREBRAL DOMINANCE THEORY

The first approximation to a formal theory of stuttering was undoubtedly the Orton and Travis cerebral dominance theory, elaborated by Travis in 1931. Travis (1931, p. 95) regarded stuttering as "a deep-seated neurophysiological disturbance" caused by a failure in cerebral dominance, often related to ambiguous or changed handedness. The cerebral dominance theory highlighted the absurdity of some of the bizarre treatments for stuttering practiced earlier, including incision of parts of the tongue. It led to the development of ingenious measurement tools and generated a great deal of physiological research. It offered an explanation for what appeared to be some curious "facts" about stuttering and handedness, and, perhaps more importantly, it provided a motivation to study them (Bloodstein, 1995). Consistent with the theory, a great deal of attention was devoted to training stutterers to use their preferred hand. And although Travis later acknowledged that this form of therapy was ineffectual, at the very least it discouraged the foolish practice in the schools of forcibly changing the handedness of left-handed children.

An unexpected byproduct of the cerebral dominance theory was a concern for personal adjustment. In the very first publication of his *Handbook on Stuttering*, Bloodstein (1959) observed that, "It is a curious feature of an essentially neurophysiological or other type of breakdown theory that it permits considerable emphasis in therapy on the stutterer's attitudes and adjustments" (p. 71) to help persons who stutter cope with the strong emotional reactions which may precipitate breakdowns of their vulnerable neuromuscular organization.

As the first major, systematic theory of stuttering, Travis's contributions were extremely influential and though certainly no longer central, allusions to the theory appear in very modern investigations of brain mechanisms in stutterers (e.g., Fox et al., 1996; Watson & Freeman, 1997).

The cerebral dominance theory also had unfortunate consequences. For example, children were discouraged from participating in sports or musical activities that involved both hands. Under the influence of the theory, Van Riper (1958) reported that "one male, an excellent flute and piano player, was shifted to the trumpet" (p. 279). Furthermore, the theory encouraged the belief that the person who stutters is neurologically fragile and organically defective, labels that Wendell Johnson, one of Travis's students and a stutterer himself, ultimately rejected. In its place, of course, Johnson developed the "diagnosogenic theory," discussed in the next section.

THE DIAGNOSOGENIC THEORY

Johnson (Johnson, 1956a, 1959; Johnson & Leutenegger, 1955) insisted that stutterers are normal individuals with normal nervous systems who struggle with phantoms when all they need to do is to talk, to stumble occasionally, but simply to go on talking. His theory was enormously appealing against the backdrop of Travis's views. Johnson's formulation led to the logical and optimistic conclusion that stuttering is never inevitable, that it is not written into the genes, and that with proper education it can be eradicated as surely as polio or diphtheria. The theory shifted the emphasis from the search for an underlying pathology to a focus on the variability of stuttering behavior, and led to the explication of the adaptation, consistency, and expectancy effects. Within the framework of diagnosogenic theory, young basketball players who stuttered were permitted to dribble and shoot with both hands, and aspiring musicians might play the piano or the flute, as well as the trumpet, despite their stuttering. The theory emphasized the ways in which persons who stutter are similar to others, rather than their organic differences.

Diagnosogenic theory also imposed heavy burdens on the stuttering child's family and limited the universe of possibilities for therapists and researchers. As part of the public education plan that was to eradicate stuttering, Johnson, in his famous "Open letter" (1956b, p. 565), advised parents, "Do nothing at any time, by word or deed or posture or facial expression, that would serve to call Fred's attention to the interruptions in his speech." The point of therapy for young children was to modify the evaluations and the responses of the significant persons in the child's environment rather than to treat the child's stuttering behaviors directly (Johnson, 1956a). If the stuttering had progressed beyond such indirect approaches, the focus in therapy would not be on eliminating stuttering, because that, in Johnson's view, would only strengthen avoidance tendencies, but rather would be to teach the child to stutter without associated mannerisms.

The case against punishment or disapproval of stuttering responses was made very unequivocally:

> One word of caution is absolutely essential. The child must never get the impression that he is being disapproved for stuttering. That would intensify his fear of stuttering and result in greater tension and generally more severe blocking. He is to be given every assurance that he may stutter as much as he likes. (Johnson, 1956a, p. 290)

The preoccupation with stuttering as a fear-motivated avoidance response discouraged the experimental use of punishment and reinforcement. This attitude was captured in a presentation by Sheehan

(1970) that was very critical of the burgeoning research based on operant conditioning methods:

> Johnson and others showed many years ago that most stutterers speak most of their words fluently . . . It is our view that stuttering is learned in response to punishment and is perpetuated in most stutterers by the anticipation of further punishment. Therefore, the stutterer does not need reinforcement for fluent words. . . . Any plea for the use of punishment as a therapeutic technique must be viewed as a step backward. . . . Obviously, stuttering is punished more than it is rewarded . . . We have never encountered stutterers whose case histories lacked an abundance of punishment. (p. 132)

Against this backdrop, it took a major reconceptualization to recognize and break through the constraints imposed by Johnson's views of stuttering as fear-motivated behavior. Interestingly, the impetus came from an outsider to the field, Israel Goldiamond, an experimental psychologist who had little experience with stuttering research but was well versed in operant conditioning and behavior modification. Undeterred by stuttering lore, Goldiamond experimented with the application of punishment to stuttering behaviors. Though he contributed only a handful of papers, he ushered in an approach that dominated stuttering research and theory for nearly the next two decades.

THE OPERANT BEHAVIOR APPROACH

Although he had little to say about the basic cause of stuttering, Goldiamond (1965) claimed that it could be eliminated in adults by the application of operant methods of behavior analysis. At first glance, Goldiamond's ideas seemed to have much in common with Johnson's. Both eschewed organic variables and both treated stuttering as learned, but they defined learning in vastly different ways. Johnson was concerned with learned cognitions—the anticipation and fear that presumably led to hypertonic avoidance behaviors. In his version of learning, penalty for stuttering is pernicious because it increases the tendency to avoid, and thus exacerbates the stuttering itself. Goldiamond applied his learning principles to the external behaviors and assumed that the maladaptive cognitions need not be treated directly; they would disappear along with the stuttering. From Goldiamond's perspective, stuttering could be managed like any other operant behavior and, like most other behaviors, should decrease when punished.

The two theories make different predictions concerning the effects of punishment, but the conflict was not apparent until operant theory, which had been around for several decades, was finally applied to stuttering. Furthermore, experiments to resolve the conflict could not be conceived of until the new theory provided a framework that highlighted the very different ways in which punishment was defined in the two approaches. Once again a new theory encouraged modes of experimentation, and eventually of therapy, that were previously unimaginable.

The operant approach made at least two fundamental contributions to the understanding of stuttering. The first was to provide data, and a theoretical framework, that liberated clinicians and researchers from the fear that manipulating stuttering moments will necessarily have catastrophic consequences for the stutterer. The second contribution was to insist that the collection of objective, verifiable data should be part of every clinical encounter (J. C. Ingham, 1993).

PARADIGMS LOST

Much like the preceding theories, the operant approach eventually fell out of favor and no longer dominates stuttering research or therapy, as reflected in the title of a recent article by Kuhr (1994): "Rise and fall of operant programs for the treatment of stammering." Although there are exceptions, especially in the work of Onslow and colleagues (Lincoln, Onslow, Lewis, & Wilson, 1996; Onslow, Andrews, & Lincoln, 1994; Onslow, Costa, & Rue, 1990; Onslow, Packman, Stocker, van Doorn, & Siegel, 1997), operant theory is no longer a significant influence in stuttering research. Curlee (1993) has remarked that even when methods that grew directly from operant research are used, the origins are seldom recognized. Similar observations have been made by Martin (1993) and J. C. Ingham (1993).

There are several possible reasons why interest in the operant approach waned. One possibility is that the punishment effects typically didn't generalize beyond the laboratory, especially in adults, a common problem in almost all therapy regimens (Martin, 1993; Stokes & Baer, 1977; Stokes & Osnes, 1988, 1989). Furthermore, extended research indicated that stimuli that have no obvious punishing properties, such as the words "tree" or "right," nonetheless functioned as punishers when made contingent on stuttering (Cooper, Cady, & Robbins, 1970). "Timeout," the most successful of the response-contingent procedures (J. C. Ingham, 1993; Prins & Hubbard, 1988), reduced stuttering even when contingent presentation of the stimulus was achieved only a fraction of the time, and regardless of the duration of the time-out interval (James, 1976). These findings are difficult to reconcile with a punishment explanation and led skeptics to dismiss the effects as simply another instance of the power of "distraction" in reducing stuttering (Biggs & Sheehan, 1969; Bloodstein, 1995). Another reason for increasing dissatisfaction with the operant approach may be that it produced no serious attempt to explain the origins of stuttering except for a very preliminary analysis by Shames and Sherrick (1963). Another argument against the approach was that, with its concentration on observable behaviors, it was insensitive to the stutterer's emotions and cognitions (Murphy, 1970; Sheehan, 1970). Kuhr (1994) has suggested the more mundane explanation that clinicians found the method boring. Finally, Bloodstein has commented that the reason for the success of operant methods in reducing stuttering is far from clear:

> Almost all research findings point to the conclusion that response-contingent stimuli have a broad potential for reducing the frequency of stuttering. The reason for this reduction, however, is far from clear. What was at first widely thought to be a punishment effect that contradicted long-standing clinical assumptions about the effect of aversive reactions to stuttering now seems more and more to represent another kind of process, as yet poorly understood, in which the aversiveness of the contingent stimulus is irrelevant and which has little in common with the social penalty that often appears to increase the severity of stuttering. (Bloodstein, 1995, pp. 344–345)

Whatever the reasons for the eventual demise of the operant approach, it is noteworthy that it was not displaced by a major contending theory of comparable scope and influence. Instead, there now exist numerous theories, each productive in its own right, but also more restricted. For example, a recent textbook (Curlee & Siegel, 1997) that purports to be a representation of current thinking in the field includes numerous chapters that are theoretical in intent, encompassing genetics, brain imaging, multifactorial models, the anticipatory-struggle hypothesis, the covert repair hypothesis, and so on. In so far as theories are designed to generate testable hypotheses, these various approaches are very successful. All include sections pointing to the need for future research. But if the further purpose of a theory is to provide an overarching paradigm of the sort that Kuhn (1970) described, in which the participants share a common vocabulary, world view, and research agenda, the current theories fall far from the mark. Instead, each delineates a relatively specific and narrow domain.

By the same token, the clinical chapters are not bound by the theories. Instead, the therapy approaches that are described seem more driven by pragmatic considerations, clinical intuition, and experience. For example, the covert repair hypothesis of Kolk and Postma (1997) has attracted a great deal of interest as a psycholinguistic theory of stuttering, but of the 10 chapters in the section on "Clinical Management," only one (Chapter 12, by Conture) cites it. Apparently, clinicians have not yet found the theory useful; or perhaps it is too abstract to capture the attention of practitioners. In general, the chapters on management of stuttering seldom appeal to theory in justifying a particular clinical intervention. A comparison of the theoretical and the clinical chapters in this book reveals the extent to which the field has become fractionated, an observation made also by Perkins (e.g., 1997). There seems to be neither a need nor an inducement to use theories to justify or rationalize clinical approaches. As a consequence, it is not possible to exploit the potential value of a major theory as a filter, helping to determine where research efforts might best be directed, where the most useful therapy methods are likely to be found, and, just as importantly, which claims can confidently be ignored.

Theory provides a context for clinical procedures and that context is sometimes the difference between innovative and exploitative therapy. Many of the fluency management methods in current use have a checkered history as techniques embraced by the so-called "stuttering schools" (see Bloodstein, 1995; Van Riper, 1973). Rhythm, rate control, and prolongation were standard procedures in these schools, and were rejected by responsible clinicians because of that association. They have recently been reintroduced and now can be encompassed within the framework developed by Goldiamond.

Perkins (1997) has stated that for want of a theory, the science of stuttering has been lost, and Ingham and colleagues (Fox et al., 1996) recently commented on "the need for a unifying theory of sufficient scope to accommodate the full complexity of the observed actions and interactions of the neural systems" (p. 161). The same could be said concerning the need for a unifying theory to accommodate environmental and linguistic actions and interactions, but it seems evident that no such theory now exists.

WHAT TO DO WHILE WAITING FOR A PARADIGM

Although there is no dominant theory to set the research agenda, there are other sources that provide some guidance; three will be discussed in this concluding section. The first is the clinic. Speech pathology has a long history of providing service to stutterers. Some of the methods in current use are left over from older theories. To the extent that these methods continue to produce desirable effects, they deserve analysis and research. In fact, the experience of the clinic may help to shape the theories that are developed. Any serious theory of stuttering must ultimately account for the fact that singing, delayed auditory feedback (DAF), slowed speech, time-out, prolongation, rhythm, and shadowing all have the capability of causing significant reductions in stuttering. Research that helps identify the conditions under which various therapy approaches lead to successful outcomes provides one road to a comprehensive theory of stuttering.

Another road, quite obviously, is technology. The imaging techniques already available are dazzling in their promise of "unlocking the secrets of the brain," and there will be even more dramatic developments in the future (Ingham, see Chapter 4 of this volume). In addition to brain imaging, there is a whole new array of instruments designed to analyze speech that have greatly expanded the options for measuring and modifying speech and for evaluating the effects of such manipulations (Bakker, 1997). New technology energizes research and stimulates theory development as the data reveal puzzles that need explanation. Perkins (1997) is dismissive of research that is a "fishing expedition," and that proceeds without a theory to guide it, but that may be too narrow a view. The ways of science are not always predictable, and any activity that maintains a posture of inquiry, exploration, and curiosity has the potential to lead to an important theory.

A third stimulus to research are puzzles that arise from numerous sources, including the research itself (Kuhn, 1970). A puzzle can emerge when two experiments yield discrepant results. The stuttering literature is full of conflicting results, as even a casual reading of Bloodstein (1995) will attest, and to the constant annoyance of our students who rebel at all of the "equivocal findings" that clutter our textbooks. Often the discrepancy is dismissed as due to "methodological differences," but the attempt to resolve the discrepancy may reveal something more fundamental, as was the case with much of the early research on the effects of "penalty" on stuttering (Siegel, 1970). Sometimes puzzles emerge when a research finding is simply counterintuitive, as in the earlier example of the Cooper et al. (1970) finding that stuttering is reduced by contingent presentation of such unlikely punishers as "right" or "tree." The explanation of such findings may resolve the ambiguous status of stuttering as an operant response as well as the even more ambiguous role of "distraction" as an explanatory construct to explain reductions in stuttering.

Puzzle-solving research propagates itself. Sometimes the follow-up research seems trivial, but it is impossible to predict the influence of a particular piece of research on further thinking and experimenting. Puzzles are divining rods for researchers. They provide hints about where to begin digging and occasionally they reveal unanticipated treasures.

SUMMARY

Earlier in this century, research and therapy for stuttering were successively encompassed by broad approaches that seemed to have many of the characteristics that Kuhn (1970) identified with the major paradigms of physical sciences. Although no single approach to stuttering ever entirely vanquished all others, each, in its time, tended to dominate the field, up through the 1960s and 1970s, when Goldiamond's (1965) treatment of stuttering as operant behavior was so influential. Not surprisingly, the operant approach eventually lost much of its influence, as it has in other areas of behavioral science. What is surprising, in view of Kuhn's analysis and our own history, is that it has not been replaced by another theory of comparable scope.

There may be another difference between the current and earlier eras that relates to the personages who promulgated the early theories, and to the status of the profession early in its history. Perhaps it always seems so, but looking back it seems "there were giants in those days." In our own field, with the death of Charles Van Riper, we have seen the close of an era in which the profession was dominated by persons of great intellect, charisma, and authority. By contrast, in our own day, as Cassius remarked to Brutus about Julius Caesar, "We petty men walk under his huge legs and peep about to find ourselves dishonorable graves." In the current era, perhaps science has overtaken authority; or perhaps such authorities as we have cannot command the allegiance and loyalty of their predecessors.

In the absence of a broad theory or paradigm, clinicians and researchers turn to other sources of stimulation, such as can be found in the clinic, in technology, and in the puzzles that invite us at every turn. It may be that the next significant paradigm will come from these sources. Or it may be imported from another field, as it has in the past. In any event, if we use these sources well, there will be enough raw material to offer the next paradigm a warm welcome—and to set into motion the forces that will subsequently lead to its demise.

ACKNOWLEDGMENTS: Portions of this paper were presented to the Southwest Conference on Communication Disorders, February 23, 1996, in Albuquerque, New Mexico. Many thanks to the students of the University of New Mexico for providing the occasion to develop these observations.

REFERENCES

Bakker, K. (1997). Instrumentation for the assessment and treatment of stuttering. In R. Curlee & G. M. Siegel (Eds.), *Nature and treatment of stuttering: New directions* (2nd ed., pp. 377–397). Needham Heights, MA: Allyn & Bacon.

Biggs, B., & Sheehan, J. (1969). Punishment or distraction? Operant stuttering revisited. *Journal of Abnormal Psychology, 74*, 256–262.

Bloodstein, O. (1959). *A handbook on stuttering for professional workers.* Chicago: National Society for Crippled Children and Adults.

Bloodstein, O. (1995). *A handbook on stuttering.* San Diego: Singular Publishing Group.

Cooper, E. B., Cady, B. B., & Robbins, C. J. (1970). The effect of the verbal stimulus words *wrong, right,* and *tree* on the disfluency rates of stutterers and nonstutterers. *Journal of Speech and Hearing Research, 13,* 239–244.

Curlee, R. F. (1993). The early history of behavior modification of stuttering: From laboratory to clinic. *Journal of Fluency Disorders, 18,* 13–25.

Curlee, R. F., & Siegel, G. M. (Eds.). (1997). *Nature and treatment of stuttering: New directions* (2nd ed.). Needham Heights, MA: Allyn & Bacon.

Fox, P. T., Ingham, R. J., Ingham, J. C., Hirsch, T. B., Downs, J. H., Martin, C., Jerabek, J., Glass, T., & Lancaster, J. L. (1996). A PET study of the neural systems of stuttering. *Nature, 382,* 158–161.

Goldiamond, I. (1965). Stuttering and nonfluency as manipulatable operant response classes. In L. Krasner & L. P. Ullman (Eds.), *Research in behavior modification* (pp. 106–156). New York: Holt, Rinehart, & Winston.

Ingham, J. C. (1993). Current status of stuttering and behavior modification—I. Recent trends in the application of behavior modification in children and adults. *Journal of Fluency Disorders, 18,* 27–55.

James, J. (1976). The influence of duration on the effects of time-out from speaking. *Journal of Speech and Hearing Research, 19,* 206–215.

Johnson, W. (1956a). Stuttering. In W. Johnson, S. J. Brown, J. J. Curtis, C. W. Edney, & J. Keaster (Eds.), *Speech handicapped school children* (rev. ed., pp. 202–300). New York: Harper & Bros.

Johnson, W. (1956b). An open letter to the mother of a stuttering child. Stuttering. In W. Johnson, S. J. Brown, J. J. Curtis, C.W. Edney, & J. Keaster (Eds.), *Speech handicapped school children* (rev. ed., pp. 558–567). New York: Harper & Bros.

Johnson, W., and Associates (1959). *The onset of stuttering.* Minneapolis: University of Minnesota Press.

Johnson, W., & Leutenegger, R. R. (1955). (Eds.). *Stuttering in children and adults.* Minneapolis: University of Minnesota Press.

Johnston, J. R. (1983). What is language intervention? The role of theory. In J. Miller, D. Yoder, & R. Schiefelbusch (Eds.), Contemporary issues in language intervention. *ASHA Reports, 12,* 52–57.

Kent, R. D., & Fair, J. (1985). Clinical research: Who, where, and how. *Seminars in Speech and Language, 6,* 23–34.

Kolk, H., & Postma, A. (1997). Stuttering as a covert repair phenomenon. In R. F. Curlee & G. M. Siegel (Eds.), *Nature and treatment of stuttering: New directions* (2nd ed., pp. 182–203). Needham Heights, MA: Allyn & Bacon.

Kuhn, T. S. (1970). *The structure of scientific revolutions* (2nd ed.). Chicago: University of Chicago Press.

Kuhr, A. (1994). Rise and fall of operant programs for the treatment of stammering. *Pholia Phoniatrica et Logopaedica, 46,* 232–240.

Lincoln, M., Onslow, M., Lewis, C., & Wilson, L. (1996). A clinical trial of an operant treatment for school-age children who stutterer. *American Journal of Speech-Language Pathology, 5,* 73–85.

Martin, R. R. (1993). The future of behavior modification of stuttering: What goes around comes around. *Journal of Fluency Disorders, 18*, 81–108.

Murphy, A. T. (1970). Stuttering, behavior modification, and the person. *Conditioning in stuttering therapy: Applications and limitations* (pp. 99–109). Memphis, TN: Speech Foundation of America.

Onslow, M., Andrews, C., & Lincoln, M. (1994). A control/experimental trial of an operant treatment for early stuttering. *Journal of Speech and Hearing Research, 37*, 1244–1259.

Onslow, M., Costa, L., & Rue, S. (1990). Direct early intervention with stuttering: Some preliminary data. *Journal of Speech and Hearing Research, 55*, 405–416.

Onslow, M., Packman, A., Stocker, S., van Doorn, J., & Siegel, G. M. (1997). Control of children's stuttering with response-contingent time-out: Behavioral, perceptual, and acoustic data. *Journal of Speech, Language, and Hearing Research, 40*, 121–133.

Perkins, W. (1986). Functions and malfunctions of theories in therapies. *Asha, 28*, 31–33.

Perkins, W. (1997). Historical analysis of why science has not solved stuttering. In R. F. Curlee & G. M. Siegel (Eds.), *Nature and treatment of stuttering: New directions* (2nd ed., pp. 218–235). Needham Heights, MA: Allyn & Bacon.

Prins, D., & Hubbard, C. P. (1988). Response contingent stimulation and stuttering: Issues and implications. *Journal of Speech and Hearing Research, 31*, 696–709.

Ringel, R. L., Trachtman, L. E., & Prutting, C. (1984). The science in human communication sciences. *Asha, 26*, 33–37.

Shames, G. H., & Sherrick, C. E., Jr. (1963). A discussion of nonfluency and stuttering as operant behavior. *Journal of Speech and Hearing Disorders, 28*, 3–18.

Sheehan, J. (1970). Reflections on the behavioral modification of stuttering. *Conditioning in stuttering therapy: Applications and limitations* (pp. 123–136). Memphis, TN: Speech Foundation of America.

Siegel, G. M. (1970). Punishment, stuttering, and disfluency. *Journal of Speech and Hearing Research, 13*, 677–714.

Siegel, G. M. (1987). The limits of science in communication disorders. *Journal of Speech and Hearing Disorders, 52*, 306–312.

Siegel, G. M. (1992). Liberation thereology. In H. L. Pick, Jr., P. van den Broek, & D. C. Knill (Eds.), *Cognition: Conceptual and methodological issues* (pp. 295–303). Washington, DC: American Psychological Association.

Stokes, T. F., & Baer, D. M. (1977). An implicit technology of generalization. *Journal of Applied Behavior Analysis, 10*, 349–367.

Stokes, T. F., & Osnes, P. G. (1988). The developing applied technology of generalization and maintenance. In R. H. Horner, G. Dunlap, & R. L. Koegel (Eds.), *Generalization and maintenance: Life-style changes in applied settings.* Baltimore: Paul H. Brookes.

Stokes, T. F., & Osnes, P. G. (1989). An operant pursuit of generalization. *Behavior Therapy, 20*, 337–355.

Travis, L. E. (1931). *Speech pathology.* New York: D. Appleton-Century.

Van Riper, C. (1958). Experiments in stuttering therapy. In J. Eisenson (Ed.), *Stuttering: A symposium* (pp. 273–390). New York: Harper & Row.

Van Riper, C. (1973). *The treatment of stuttering.* Englewood Cliffs, NJ: Prentice-Hall.

Watson, B. C., & Freeman, F. J. (1997). Brain imaging contributions. In R. F. Curlee & G. M. Siegel (Eds.), *Nature and treatment of stuttering: New directions* (2nd ed., pp. 143–166). Needham Heights, MA: Allyn & Bacon.

PART II

Treatment Procedures and Outcomes

The chapters in this section address stuttering assessment and treatment more directly than the chapters in the first section. The section begins with Anne Cordes's review of reported procedures and outcomes in the stuttering treatment literature. Jill Rosenthal, Richard Curlee, and Yingyong Qi then assess whether acoustic measures might differentiate between children who stutter and those who do not. Bruce Ryan's chapter summarizes several studies from several years' worth of his treatment research with children who stutter. Elisabeth Harrison, Mark Onslow, Cheryl Andrews, Ann Packman, and Margaret Webber present and evaluate a timely new approach to prolonged speech treatment programs. Scott Yaruss discusses treatment outcome evaluation, then presents some new outcome data about one well-established adult treatment program. James Hillis and Jeanne McHugh discuss and assess some of the many cognitive and other variables that may affect the generalization and maintenance of treatment gains. Finally, Patricia Zebrowski and Edward Conture discuss variables that may alter the effectiveness of stuttering treatments; their chapter focuses on school-age children, but it has important implications for younger and older clients as well.

These chapters include a few answers about stuttering treatment, in among many questions, suggestions, and unresolved issues for future argument and future research. Despite the many remaining questions about the issues addressed in these chapters and about many other issues, the combined effect of these chapters is to create the distinctly positive impression that clinical research may yet identify some consistently and demonstrably effective treatments for stuttering.

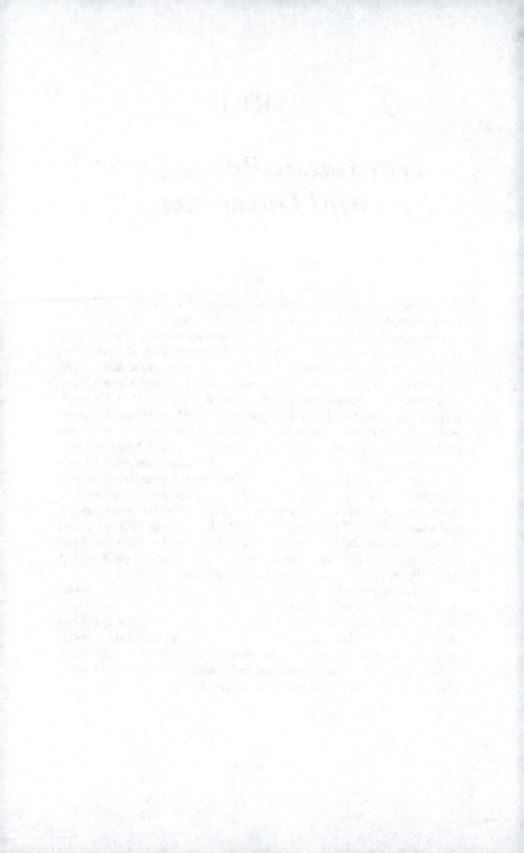

CHAPTER

6

Current Status of the Stuttering Treatment Literature

ANNE K. CORDES, Ph.D.

This review was undertaken because of a conference presentation about stuttering treatment research (Ingham, 1996) that subsequently became a book chapter (Ingham & Cordes, in press). Both the presentation and the resulting chapter argued, in uncomfortably direct terminology, that the state of stuttering treatment research as of early 1996 was abysmal; that some of the people who at that time considered themselves to be the leaders in the field had abandoned the basic scientific principles that should have formed the heart of any attempt to establish treatment efficacy; and that some of the opinions being expressed and recommendations being made about stuttering treatment at the time could be traced, relatively directly, to scientific and intellectual sloppiness. The presentation and the chapter provided specific examples, named names, and used intentionally confrontational language in several places, in part to make the point that several decades' worth of gently worded suggestions about the scientific method were already available and seemed to have had little influence on much stuttering treatment research. The message, in other words, was as simple as that children and adults who stutter deserve nothing less than rigorously tested and empirically supported treatments. The style, however, was intentionally abrasive, and the presentation was met with a mix of reactions that included everything from astonished praise to relatively predictable hostility.

The Ingham and Cordes (in press) chapter does not need to be changed, retracted, or softened, and the point of this review was certainly not to undermine the earlier one. Nevertheless, the process of creating the Ingham and Cordes chapter left its second author with the distinct and disquieting sense that perhaps there was an alternative interpretation to be aired or a larger story to be told about the stuttering treatment research literature. The main impetus for the present review, in other words, was this author's unwillingness to accept that the stuttering treatment research literature could truly be as uninterpretable or as uninformative as the Ingham and Cordes (in press) chapter had implied. The original intent of this review, therefore, was to set aside the methodological complaints that had formed the basis for the Ingham and Cordes chapter (and that form the basis for most of our work) and to examine the stuttering treatment research literature with an eye toward the extremely basic question of which stuttering treatments were reported to result in good outcomes. This approach was selected for this review not because the methodological and design issues are unimportant, but because the sheer number of current controversies about stuttering treatment and stuttering treatment research seemed to suggest that there might be some value in simply going back to the literature and starting over.

The purposes of this review, therefore, were straightforward: to examine a sample of the available professional literature on stuttering treatment and stuttering treatment research, to identify the treatment procedures that are reported to be associated with positive outcomes, and to identify the issues that appear to deserve further research or discussion. It was also an explicit purpose of this review to examine the effectiveness of treatment procedures in a way that was as independent as possible of the labels ascribed to those procedures; that is, this review incorporated an analysis of the treatment components that could be identified within larger treatment procedures or packages and regardless of the terminology used by the original researchers. The methodological adequacy of the examined studies was not intended to be of primary concern for this review, as discussed above. Despite this original intention, however, it also became obvious as this work proceeded that methodological problems are actually so pervasive in the stuttering treatment research literature that it was, to a great extent, not possible to complete a straightforward summary of reported treatment outcomes, a point that will be developed in greater detail throughout the remainder of this chapter.

IDENTIFICATION OF CHAPTERS AND ARTICLES FOR REVIEW

The first stage of this project identified peer-reviewed journal articles, including both stuttering treatment research reports and reports from laboratory investigations of stuttering treatment methods or procedures. These publications were identified from several sources: a computer-assisted library search; Bloodstein's (1995) appendix of treatment publications; treatment-related sections of Culatta and Goldberg's (1995) Research Bibliography; and a physical search of all issues of the *Journal of Speech and Hearing Research*, the *American Journal of Speech-Language Pathology*, and the *Journal of Fluency Disorders* from 1990 through 1996. Articles were selected if they were research reports (as opposed to review or theoretical articles) that met two simple selection criteria:

1. dated 1965–1996; and
2. clearly represented an assessment of a stuttering treatment technique with the implicit or explicit goal of change beyond experimental conditions (usually including the title word "treatment" or "therapy").

Articles from before 1965 were excluded so that this review might concentrate on treatments developed and used since the advent of delayed auditory feedback and prolonged speech procedures, and since the widespread incorporation of methods from behavioral psychology. Assessments of pharmacological interventions for stuttering were also excluded from this review (see Brady, 1991), as were articles that were not available in English.

This first search identified approximately 100 papers for potential review. Of those, several were not readily available, several were determined to be preliminary or narrative reports rather than data-based research reports, and many were determined to be reports of research about fluency-inducing conditions but not research about treatment procedures as such (e.g., investigations by Adams, Lewis, & Besozzi, 1973; Cross & Cooper, 1976). In addition, several papers were identified that were based to some extent on treatment data but that focused on other analyses, such as Onslow, Hayes, Hutchins, and Newman's (1992) investigation of speech naturalness. There were 64 papers that were readily available and that presented relatively complete reports of treatment research; these 64 papers, identified in the References section, were selected to serve as the sample of the stuttering treatment literature that would be analyzed for this review.

Even before any formal review had been completed, however, the general content of these papers suggested an important conclusion. This set of 64 papers did not appear to meet a face validity criterion of representing the treatments that are currently in widespread use or the treatments that are currently discussed and recommended in forums outside the primary research literature. To test this hypothesis, and to assure that the papers surveyed would represent a wide range of treatments, at this point the literature search was extended to create a second set of papers. The second set, referred to as the Recommendations Subgroup, consisted entirely of all treatment articles or chapters in three recent collections of treatment recommendations for stuttering: two "Current Therapy of Communication Disorders" collections devoted to fluency disorders (Curlee, 1993b; Perkins, 1984a), and the April 1995 issue of *Language, Speech, and Hearing Services in Schools*. The Recommendations Subgroup contained 24 chapters or articles (see References) that recommended 27 treatments.[1]

SURVEY OF IDENTIFIED CHAPTERS AND ARTICLES

Review of the 88 selected publications was completed by three experimenters using a written survey. Two to four independent surveys were completed, by one to three experimenters, for each publication. The surveys of each publication were then compared, and disagreements among them were resolved by the most experienced of the three reviewers (the author). Most disagreements among the surveys represented errors of underidentification by an experimenter and were easily resolved; others stemmed from differences in how the experimenters had interpreted vague or incomplete information from a publication. Some of the final decisions incorporated into this review unquestionably represent this author's interpretations, and interested readers are encouraged to complete their own review of these articles.

The survey required reviewers to identify and describe the treatment techniques in each article and then to summarize the reported results. Each treatment was described both by copying verbatim the terminology used by the author of the report and by judging whether that treatment incorporated any or all of seven individual treatment elements: reduced utterance length at the beginning of treatment; reduced speech rate at the beginning of treatment; controlled breathing patterns; easy onsets to sounds, words, or phrases; altered vocalization; gentle or modified articulatory gestures; or any verbal or other consequence that

---

[1] Many of the articles and chapters in the Recommendations Subgroup reported summarized results of treatment research, were based on a treatment research program, or were otherwise connected to stuttering treatment research. Their designation here as "Recommendations" papers rather than as "Research" papers does not necessarily imply the absence of a research base; it suggests only that these particular chapters and articles, by their intent and design, were meant to summarize or recommend a treatment approach rather than to present original research results.

immediately followed a stutter. These seven elements were selected for this review based on previous reviews of the techniques used most commonly for the direct treatment of stuttering (e.g., Culatta & Goldberg, 1995). Results of each treatment were summarized where possible by copying the authors' reports of their treatment outcome data along with a description of the speech samples or other source from which those data were collected. For reports that did not include such information, judges were to make estimates from figures or copy verbatim the description of any measured or described outcomes that appeared to be intended to convey the results of the treatment.

Types of Researched and Recommended Stuttering Treatment

The 64 papers identified from the primary literature—now labeled the Research Subgroup—reported investigations of 81 different treatments (see Table 6–1 and References). The frequency with which certain treatments were investigated varied widely. There was one report each of play therapy (Wakaba, 1983), acupuncture (Craig & Kearns, 1995), reinforcing fluency (with no other procedures; Shaw & Shrum, 1972), self-recording of stuttering (with no other procedures; La Croix, 1973), delayed auditory feedback (with no instruction as to speech modifications or discussion of altered speech pattern; Martin & Haroldson, 1979) (see also Watts, 1971), electromyographic feedback (as the primary treatment technique in one condition; Craig et al., 1996), recorded "self-modelling" of nonstuttered speech (Bray & Kiehle, 1996), and "programmed traditional" (Ryan & Ryan, 1983) treatment. There were, in contrast, 13 investigations of prolonged (or smooth) speech, and there was also a relatively large number of investigations of desensitization or cognitive procedures, airflow or regulated breathing therapies, and response-contingent time-out.

The pattern of treatments represented among the Recommendations publications differed in some interesting ways from the pattern observed in the Research Subgroup (Table 6–2). Comparison of Tables 6–1 and 6–2 shows that one difference is in the prevalence of operant approaches: Only 2 of the 27 Recommendations were for response-contingent time-out, and both of those were from the same author (Costello, 1984; Ingham, 1993). In contrast, 20 of the 81 treatments analyzed in the Research publications could be classified as operant: time-out or other punishers, or reinforcing fluency, or combinations of reinforcement and punishment.

Another important difference between the Research Subgroup and the Recommendations Subgroup appeared in the emphasis on cognitive or cognitive-emotional treatment procedures. Fourteen of the 27 Recommendations, more than half, were exclusively cognitive or relied heavily on cognitive procedures, but only 10 of the 81 Research reports

Table 6–1. Treatment Procedures Investigated in the Research Subgroup.

1 Study Each

play therapy
acupuncture
reinforce fluency
self-recording
recorded self-models
delayed auditory feedback
electromyographic feedback
"programmed traditional"

3–5 Studies Each

Precision Fluency Shaping (3)
prolonged speech plus cognitive (3)
parent-administered operant (3)
parental change (3)
other packages (3)
masking (3)
punishment (4)
GILCU/ELU (4)
rhythmic speech (5)

7–13 Studies Each

desensitization/cognitive (7)
airflow and regulated breathing (10)
response contingent time-out (12)
prolonged/smooth speech (13)

Note: The Research Subgroup included 64 publications from the primary research literature; some publications investigated more than one treatment procedure. Publications included in this table are marked "[RES]" in the References section.

involved cognitive/emotional procedures. A third interesting difference between the two Subgroups was the complete absence of airflow or regulated breathing therapies from the Current Therapy and *Language, Speech, and Hearing Services in the Schools* recommendations, even though airflow was one of the most common procedures in the Research Subgroup. Breathing or breath management skills were certainly included within some of the recommended prolonged speech or fluency-shaping treatments, as discussed in further detail below, but the Recommendations Subgroup included no recommendations of regulated breathing therapies per se or of airflow therapies that were described as such by the authors.

Table 6–2. Treatment Procedures Discussed in the Recommendations Subgroup.

1–3 Chapters Each

parental change plus speech rate and utterance length (1)
GILCU/ELU (2)
response contingent time-out (2)
parental change (3)

5–9 Chapters Each

desensitization/cognitive (5)
prolonged speech/related fluency skills (5)
prolonged speech plus cognitive (9)

Note: The Recommendations Subgroup included 24 publications from two "Current Therapy of Communication Disorders" collections devoted to fluency disorders (Curlee, 1993b; Perkins, 1984a) and from the April 1995 issue of *Language, Speech and Hearing Services in Schools.* Some publications mentioned more than one treatment procedure. Publications included in this table are marked "[REC]" in the References section.

There could certainly be many reasons for differences between the number of research reports about a particular treatment technique and the number of times that that treatment technique is recommended; in fact, it would not be meaningful or reasonable to expect a particular relationship between the two. This finding might suggest, for example, that treatment researchers are establishing that certain treatments do not work and that those treatments are then, quite appropriately, not being recommended. It might suggest that the existence of a research base, as reflected in a history of publications, is simply not an important factor for authors making treatment recommendations. It might provide some comment on the division between research and politics in stuttering treatment, because the Recommendations Subgroup must be assumed to reflect the positions or preferences of the authors who were invited to contribute to these collections (who might, in turn, be assumed to reflect the judgments of the editors of those collections as to which authors or which positions needed to be represented in a collection of treatment recommendations). The differences between the two Subgroups might also reflect nothing more than the fact that a set of recommendations is often purposely designed to include one chapter about each possibility, whereas any given set of research papers will include multiple investigations about some topics and few or none about other topics.

One important conclusion that must be drawn from this review, however, is simply that the treatments that were the most often recommended in these papers were not the treatments that had been the most comprehensively researched. This conclusion represents a major weakness in the overall stuttering treatment literature if the treatments that are being recommended have been shown to be ineffective. It represents a potential weakness in the literature if treatments that have been shown to be effective are not being recommended, and it represents a potential weakness if the treatments being recommended have not been studied in the research literature and therefore have not been shown to be either effective or ineffective. The next question to be answered, then, involves the reported effectiveness of the treatments identified in the Research Subgroup and in the Recommendations Subgroup: Are researchers investigating, and are authors recommending, effective treatments for children and adults who stutter?

Effectiveness of Researched and Recommended Stuttering Treatments

Establishing Treatment Effectiveness

One standard measure of the effectiveness of stuttering treatment involves whether the frequency of overt, observer-judged stutterings in speech has been reduced. To some authors, such a reduction in overt stutterings represents the bare minimum that must be expected of any treatment (Ingham & Cordes, in press); to others, it represents one of many important goals of treatment (Starkweather, 1993); to still others, it represents a misplaced emphasis that ignores more important aspects of the disorder and of the treatment process (Cooper, 1986). In the papers in the Research Subgroup, frequency of stuttering was the most frequently reported dependent variable: 59 of the 64 articles were based on data about frequency of stuttering, including data gathered through observers' counts, stuttering severity scales, and subjects' reports of their own stuttering frequency or severity. Four articles reported data solely in terms of fluent or disfluent speech, rather than in terms of stuttered or nonstuttered speech, but only one article in the Research Subgroup provided essentially no discussion of speech performance (Wakaba, 1983). All of the desensitization or other cognitive studies in the primary literature included data about stuttering frequency, a point that seemed especially noteworthy.

The Recommendations Subgroup, in contrast, included 22 discussions that mentioned stuttering frequency or discussed their treatment goals in terms of stuttering frequency and 5 discussions that addressed almost exclusively cognitive goals for stuttering treatment. Gregory and Hill's (1993) presentation is representative of the latter group: They reported that children are successful with their program if they "gain confidence sufficient to be comfortable about communication and are able to speak easily in most situations" (Gregory & Hill, 1993, p. 42). The presence of such perspectives as Gregory and Hill's is acknowledged, but the following analyses of treatment results used stuttering frequency as a primary dependent variable for two reasons: because the majority of reports in the Research Subgroup used stuttering frequency as a primary dependent variable, making this a common variable for comparisons, and because it is this author's bias that a low (or zero) frequency of stuttering is a necessary outcome of any stuttering treatment, whether it is a sufficient outcome or not. In these terms, then, the question of treatment effectiveness became, for this review, the question of whether these treatments were reported to reduce observer-judged stutters in speech.

In keeping with the general purposes of this review, the data from each study (or from each treatment within a treatment-comparison study) were summarized in terms of relatively broad categories, using decision rules that were intended to allow false positive errors (over-identification of positive treatment outcomes) rather than false negative errors (underidentification of positive treatment outcomes). Thus, treatments were divided into those for which mean or overall frequency of stuttering immediately posttreatment fell below 1% syllables or words stuttered, fell between 1% and 3% syllables or words stuttered, fell above 3% syllables or words stuttered, or could not be summarized in this form ("other" in Tables 6–3 through 6–6). In any case where it was difficult to determine how to categorize a given set of treatment results, the most lenient decision was made; that is, studies were placed into the best or most effective category into which they could possibly be placed.

The fact that some studies were difficult to categorize was an important finding of this review in itself, and it deserves some further comment. In some cases, for example, the data that were summarized or provided by the authors of these papers simply did not show whether posttreatment frequency of stuttering fell above or below the cut-off frequencies selected for this review (e.g., data presented as number of stutters per session). In other cases, the present experimenters were forced to estimate stuttering frequency from graphs that did not have the resolution necessary to support such estimates. The lack of standardized measurement systems for stuttering also meant that this review includes some inaccurate comparisons between percent of syllables stuttered and percent of words stuttered, which are not the same metric at all. Similar measurement difficulties were raised by studies that presented data in terms of other metrics such as stuttered words per minute; where possible, such data were converted to rough estimates of percent of words stuttered using available speech rate data. Many studies are represented in the following discussions by a group mean score that ignores the substantial variability that was obtained across subjects;

worse yet, variability information is unknown for some of these reports, because some authors provided mean data without providing any data about within- or across-subject variability. Many papers provided data without providing an adequate description of the speech tasks from which those data were recorded; some papers provided data from unacceptably short speech samples; most provided data from unacceptably few speech samples from unacceptably few speaking situations.

These and several other methodological issues were precisely the sorts of questions that this review was originally designed to avoid, in favor of a straightforward summary of reported treatment outcomes. Even with no methodological criteria or expectations, however, there were some studies for which it was literally not possible, without relying on the authors' interpretations, to determine whether the reported results meant that stuttering frequency had been reduced by the treatment or not. The more common problem, encountered in the Research Subgroup as well as in the Recommendations Subgroup, was that many of these papers clearly did not meet even the most minimal measurement or design standards of providing well-defined measures of central tendency and variability from well-described and adequately representative experimental conditions. One of the greatest weaknesses of the analyses presented in the remainder of this chapter, in fact, reflects one of the greatest difficulties with the stuttering treatment literature itself: A report that provided little more than averaged and summarized results from one short within-clinic posttreatment speech sample must somehow be compared to reports such as that of Onslow, Andrews, and Lincoln (1994), who provided data from over 75,000 syllables of carefully described and analyzed speech from multiple recordings from multiple subjects.

Reduction of Stuttering Reported in the Research Subgroup

All such methodological complexities aside, Tables 6–3 and 6–4 summarize the types of treatments and the reported results of those treatments from the Research Subgroup. It appears from these tables, and especially from Table 6-4, that some of the treatments being researched can be described as effective, if one chooses to define a successful result as a mean below 1% stuttering or a mean below 3% stuttering.

One of the more interesting findings, and the driving force behind the organization of these tables, lies in the sorts of treatments that were identified. There were nine types of treatments for which the Research Subgroup included at least one report of mean levels of stuttering of 1% or less immediately posttreatment, referred to below as the highly effective treatments (Table 6–4): self-recording of stutterings, response contingent time-out, punishment other than time-out, a parent-

Table 6–3. Posttreatment Stuttering Frequency in Selected Studies from the Research Subgroup.

Treatment Type	Stuttering Frequency			
	0–1%	1–3%	>3%	Other
EMG feedback		1		
Recorded self-models			1	
Reinforce fluency[a]			1	
Delayed auditory feedback			1	
Acupuncture				1
Play therapy				1
Rhythmic speech		1	3	1
Precision fluency shaping			2	1
Other packages		1	1	1
Parental change			2	1
Desensitization/cognitive			2	5

Note: Entries represent the number of reports in the Research Subgroup for which mean percent of syllables or words stuttered immediately posttreatment fell between 1% and 3%, fell above 3%, or was reported in other terms. This table includes only those treatments for which the Research Subgroup included no report of mean %SS or %WS below 1% immediately posttreatment (cf. Table 6–4). Publications included in Table 6–3 are marked "[RES 6–3]" in the References section.

[a]Manning, Trutna, and Shrum (1976), not represented in this table, also reported positive results from their study of reinforcing fluent and stuttered speech intervals in three children.

administered operant package (the work of Onslow and colleagues), Gradual Increase in Length and Complexity of Utterance (GILCU; Ryan, 1974), programmed traditional treatment (Ryan & Ryan, 1983), masking (and masking plus shadowing; Peins, Lee, & McGough, 1970), airflow or regulated breathing, and prolonged or smooth speech. These are not nine different treatments at all, a point that becomes even more obvious from an analysis of the individual treatment components that could be identified in these reports.

Treatment Components Identified Within Highly Effective Treatments in the Research Subgroup

As described above, the survey that was completed for each article required the present experimenters to identify the individual treatment elements that they judged to exist in these treatments (reduced utterance

Table 6–4. Posttreatment Stuttering Frequency in Selected Studies from the Research Subgroup.

Treatment Type	Stuttering Frequency			
	0–1%	**1–3%**	**>3%**	**Other**
Self-recording of stutters	1			
Response contingent time-out	5	4	3	
Other punishment	2		2	
Parent-administered operant	3			
GILCU/ELU	3			1
Programmed traditional	1			
Masking	1	1	1	
Airflow/regulated breathing	2	4	3	1
Prolonged/smooth speech	8	3	1	1
Prolonged speech plus cognitive	1	1		1

Note: Entries represent the number of reports in the Research Subgroup for which mean percent of syllables or words stuttered immediately posttreatment fell below 1%, fell between 1% and 3%, fell above 3%, or was reported in other terms. This table includes only those treatments for which the Research Subgroup included at least one report of mean %SS or %WS below 1% immediately posttreatment (cf. Table 6–3). Publications included in Table 6–4 are marked "[RES 6–4]" in the References section.

length at the beginning of treatment; reduced speech rate at the beginning of treatment; controlled breathing patterns; easy onsets to sounds, words, or phrases; altered vocalization; gentle or modified articulatory gestures; or any verbal or other consequence that immediately followed a stutter). Two of the treatments identified above as having at least one report of mean stuttering below 1% immediately posttreatment were removed from the analyses reported here; this level of success was reported for self-recording and for masking in only one narrative and preliminary description each, with very little methodological detail available (LaCroix, 1973; Peins et al., 1970). The seven remaining treatments could be clearly divided into one investigation of "programmed traditional" treatment (Ryan & Ryan, 1983) and three further subgroups.

The first subdivision of the highly effective Research articles included 19 reports of response contingent time-out and other operant controls (see Table 6–4). For 15 of these 19 reports, the only identifiable treatment element was the response contingent consequence for stuttering. For one condition reported by Ingham and Packman (1977), response contingencies were combined with reduced speech rate, and the final three reports combined response contingent punishers with other procedures, including reinforcers for fluent speech and overcorrection, to create a parent-administered program for children (Lincoln, Onslow, Lewis, & Wilson, 1996; Onslow et al., 1994; Onslow, Costa, & Rue, 1990).

A second subdivision included four reports that were primarily reports of treatments that controlled the length and/or complexity of clients' utterances. For two of these, control of utterance length or complexity was the only identifiable treatment element (Ratner & Sih, 1997; Rustin, Ryan, & Ryan, 1987); the other two combined control of utterance length plus immediate consequences for stutterings (Ryan & Ryan, 1983, 1995).

The third and final subdivision of these highly effective treatments within the Research Subgroup included 26 reports of treatments referred to by their authors as breathstream management, airflow techniques, prolonged speech, or smooth speech. These treatments were distinguished from those in the first two subdivisions by a larger number of individually identifiable elements, with between two and six of the seven components identified in each treatment. In addition, these treatments tended to depend on the same sorts of procedures, usually including the combination of an initial reduction in speech rate, some change to phonatory patterns, and some change to respiratory patterns. It was especially interesting to note that most of these treatments also incorporated one or both of the procedures that constituted the first two subdivisions of effective treatments: either reduced utterance length in initial stages of treatment, or contingencies for stuttering, or both. There were, in summary, a few individual procedures or components that were associated in the Research Subgroup with the reduction of stuttering to below 1%: contingencies for overt stutterings, beginning treatment with a reduced utterance length, beginning treatment with a reduced rate, and making some change to the use of respiratory and phonatory systems.

Reduction of Stuttering and Treatment Components in the Recommendations Subgroup

Seventeen of the 27 Recommendations provided evidence of the effectiveness of the recommended treatment or discussed treatment outcomes. Of those, stuttering was claimed to fall to approximately 1% or lower according to the authors of two reports about GILCU (Ryan, 1984) or extended length of utterance (ELU; Costello, 1984) procedures, two reports that combined elements of prolonged speech with cognitive procedures and goals (Boberg, 1984; Shine, 1984), and one discussion of changing parental demands (Gottwald & Starkweather, 1995). Because these chapters were intended to provide discussion and recommendations rather than research results, the evidence provided or cited to support these assertions of treatment success ranged from relatively strong to essentially nonexistent. Both Shine (1984) and Boberg (1984), interestingly, also mentioned some work with reduced utterance length and immediate consequences for stuttering, factors that were associated in the Research Subgroup with the reduction of stuttering.

Maintenance of Treatment Effects

It was not an original intention of this review to address the question of treatment maintenance; indeed, some articles were originally excluded from the Research Subgroup because they addressed maintenance questions rather than establishment questions. Maintenance of treatment gains is such a critical issue for stuttering treatment, however, that it seemed to be of some interest to examine the limited maintenance data that were available in the treatment literature. Of the 81 reports of treatment effects in the 64 Research articles, only 40 included any follow-up or maintenance data. Of those 40, only 8 reported or included data to show that treatment effects of stuttering below approximately 1% were maintained for *any* measured period of time after the end of treatment (Tables 6–5 and 6–6). This number of reports is extremely small and does not serve as a strong basis for any conclusion other than a repeated call for long-term treatment outcome data.[2]

SUMMARIES, ADDITIONAL CONSIDERATIONS, AND FUTURE RESEARCH

Most of the findings of this review were straightforward and do not represent new or surprising insights. One of the primary findings, for example, was simply that the stuttering treatment literature includes investigations and recommendations of many procedures, with some more frequently investigated and some more frequently recommended than others. It also appeared that the stuttering treatment literature in general, and the Recommendations papers in particular, placed some noticeable emphasis on cognitive and emotional variables, but the primary dependent variable in the treatment research literature still seems

---

[2]Investigations of treatment maintenance excluded from this review also support the general impression created by Tables 6–5 and 6–6 that specific maintenance-oriented planning and programming, including especially the use of performance contingent procedures or schedules, are important to the maintenance of treatment gains (Blood, 1995a, 1995b; Ingham, 1980, 1982; Prins, 1970).

Table 6–5. Maintenance Phase Stuttering Frequency in Selected Studies from the Research Subgroup.

| Treatment Type | Stuttering Frequency | | | |
	0–1%	1–3%	>3%	Other
EMG feedback		1		
Recorded self-models			1	
Reinforce fluency				
Delayed auditory feedback				
Acupuncture				
Play therapy				
Rhythmic speech				2
Precision fluency shaping				2
Other packages				1
Parental change				
Desensitization/cognitive			1	2

Note: Entries represent the number of articles for which mean percent of syllables or words stuttered fell between 1% and 3%, fell above 3%, or was reported in other terms after any maintenance phase. Treatments with no entry did not report maintenance data. This table includes only those treatments for which the Research Subgroup included no report of mean %SS or %WS below 1% immediately posttreatment (from Table 6–3; compare Tables 6–4 and 6–6).

to be frequency of stuttering. The individual treatment components that are associated with reduced stuttering frequency appeared to be relatively few, although not so few as to lead to any truly innovative conclusions. The primary conclusion about maintenance of treatment gains that must be drawn from this review, finally, is simply that our treatment research does not tend to report maintenance data.

Of these results, the most intriguing may be that the primary stuttering treatment literature investigated different procedures than those recommended in the secondary collections. The suggestion was made earlier in this chapter that such a relationship between research and recommendations is necessarily problematic only if the widely recommended treatments have been shown to be ineffective. In other words, neither the finding that some effective treatments are not being widely recommended, nor the finding that unstudied treatments are being widely recommended, is necessarily cause for concern. The first might be unfortunate, if effective treatments are being ignored; if equally effective treatments are being recommended, however, then the goal of

Table 6–6. Maintenance Phase Stuttering Frequency in Selected Studies from the Research Subgroup.

Treatment Type	Stuttering Frequency			
	0–1%	1–3%	>3%	Other
Self-recording of stutters				
Response contingent time-out	3			
Other punishment				
Parent-administered operant	2	1		
GILCU/ELU	2			
Programmed traditional				
Masking[a]				
Airflow/regulated breathing		4	5	1
Prolonged/smooth speech	1	8	2	

Note: Entries represent the number of articles for which mean percent of syllables or words stuttered fell below 1%, fell between 1% and 3%, fell above 3%, or was reported in other terms after any maintenance phase. Treatments with no entry did not report maintenance data. This table includes only those treatments for which the Research Subgroup included at least one report of mean %SS or %WS below 1% immediately posttreatment (from Table 6–4; compare Tables 6–3 and 6–5).

[a]Peins et al. (1970), not represented in this table, reported maintenance of less than 1% words stuttered after a program that combined masking and shadowing, for one subject who had also received other treatments.

providing effective treatments to clients who need them can obviously be met. The second might be unremarkable, if the recommended and as-yet-unstudied treatments are eventually shown to be effective in controlled research. The second might present an important problem, however, if recommended but unstudied treatments are later found to be ineffective—especially if effective alternatives were ignored in the meantime.

This review found evidence of multiple such problems and potential problems in the stuttering treatment literature. Response contingent treatments and GILCU- and ELU-type treatments, for example, have been shown to be highly effective (defined for this chapter as stuttering reduced to below 1%) and to be associated with posttreatment maintenance of treatment gains, but these treatments were mentioned only infrequently in the Recommendations literature. This situation is unfortunate, because effective treatments are being ignored or underutilized, but it is not necessarily a major problem in itself, as discussed in the preceding paragraph. Papers in the Research Subgroup also supported the effectiveness of such alterations to the manner of speech as reduced rate plus certain changes in phonatory and respiratory behavior, or the combination of factors that is usually referred to as prolonged speech or fluency skills training; prolonged-speech-type treatments were also relatively frequently recommended. This combination of recommending an effective treatment is clearly not cause for concern.

One important problem identified by this review involves those treatments that were collectively referred to as desensitization and other cognitive, counselling, or emotional treatments. The most frequently Recommended treatments, by far, combined elements of prolonged speech or related fluency skills with cognitive or emotional emphases (Table 6–2). The Research literature provides relatively little evidence that cognitive or emotional procedures are necessary to the success of prolonged speech treatments (Tables 6–3 and 6–4), although one direct comparison did report better maintenance for clients who completed a combination of prolonged speech and personal construct therapy than for clients who completed the same prolonged speech program and then received extra speech practice (Evesham & Fransella, 1985). Thus, the frequent recommendation of combined treatments (prolonged speech plus cognitive emphases) represents a potential problem that may or may not be realized, depending on whether such combined treatments are eventually shown to be more or less effective or efficient than prolonged speech on its own.

An even more critical finding from this review is that desensitization and related cognitive procedures, on their own, were recommended as frequently as prolonged speech in the Recommendations Subgroup, but were shown within the Research Subgroup not to be associated with reduced stuttering (Table 6–3). The importance of this conclusion may be mitigated by the fact that the goal of desensitization and related cognitive procedures might not be to reduce stuttering, but this situation obviously represents a case where treatments that have been shown to be ineffective, by at least one definition, are nevertheless being widely recommended.

Three final issues are relevant to this discussion, all of which suggest important future directions for stuttering treatment research. The first is straightforward: In addition to the differences between the Research papers and the Recommendations papers, there are clear differences between most treatment procedures and the current emphases on studying the nature of stuttering as a physiological, neurophysiological, or neurolinguistic disorder (see Curlee & Siegel, 1997; Hulstijn, Peters, & van Lieshout, 1997). One obvious avenue for treatment research, then, would be to determine whether better treatment outcomes for stuttering might be obtained not only from more direct relationships between treatment research and treatment recommendations, but also from more direct relationships between basic research and treatment techniques.

The second issue is equally straightforward. Both the immediate consequences for stuttering that constitute response contingent treatments, and the standard clinical progression from shorter response units to longer ones that constitutes GILCU- and ELU-type programs, were identified as effective in isolation and were also identified as components of many other treatments. Such a finding suggests that stuttering treatment researchers might profitably consider investigating the contribution that these two procedures make to those fluency-skills or prolonged-speech treatment packages that combine specific speech-motor alterations or fluency skills, plus feedback about stutterings, plus a progression from syllable- or word-level responses to phrase- or sentence-level responses. It would appear to be possible that the functional component of some mixed treatments, for some clients, might be simply the straightforward identification and punishment of stutterings within a progression from shorter response units to longer ones.

The third and final issue that must be addressed is more complex and involves the methodological adequacy of the reports reviewed here and, therefore, the validity of the conclusions drawn here. Reports were incorporated into this Research Subgroup with essentially no methodological exclusion criteria; if an article claimed to present the results of treatment research, it was reviewed as interpretable treatment research. Such an approach prevents the problem of selecting reports in a way that might bias the findings of the review,[3] but it may also allow methodologically unsound reports to remain in the review pool. Because the methodological quality of these reports did vary, the possibility exists that very different conclusions might have been drawn from this review if included reports had been required to meet some criteria for methodological adequacy. The methodological questions that surround treatment evaluation have been addressed well and repeatedly elsewhere; in one sense, the answer to these questions is as simple as expecting that, at the very least, a claim of treatment success should be supported by the same evidence of internal validity that would be expected of any other research report. The report that a given treatment procedure has produced a given result, therefore, should be accepted only if the study's design can methodologically support the conclusion that it was the treat-

---

[3] Requiring data from groups of a certain size, for example, can have the effect of eliminating studies of operant procedures, which have often been tested in single-subject experimental designs (Ingham, 1990). This factor also provides one explanation for the differences between the conclusions reached by this review and the conclusions reached by Andrews, Guitar, and Howie (1980).

ment, and not some other factor, that caused the obtained result or the obtained difference between treatment and no-treatment conditions. In addition, evidence should be available that the obtained results accurately reflect that which they are meant to reflect; this requirement refers simply to reliability and validity of measurements and interpretations. Such requirements of design and measurements are not specific to stuttering treatment research; they merely represent the basic expectation of internal validity for any research result.

Ingham and Cordes (in press) described one set of measurement and design standards for stuttering treatment research: repeated measurements of speech-related performance before, during, and after treatment; measurements of speech-related performance in both within-clinic and beyond-clinic conditions; and assessments of stuttering frequency, speech rate, and speech quality, with some evidence that measurement reliability is sufficient to support whatever conclusions are drawn. These requirements are minimal and cannot, on their own, ensure a trustworthy result; studies that do not meet them, however, are clearly threatened by the possibility that they are describing little more than clinic-bound fluency or the natural variability of stuttering frequency. To assess the reports that served as the basis for this review's conclusions, the standards suggested by Ingham and Cordes (in press) were relaxed even further, to require only data about stuttering frequency and speech rate, with at least central tendency and variability reported in each case, and with the reliability of those data assessed in any way (Data, in Table 6–7); at least two measurements of speech-related performance before treatment and at least two after treatment (Repeated Measures, in Table 6–7); and measurements of speech-related performance in within-clinic and beyond-clinic conditions both before and after treatment (Beyond Clinic, in Table 6–7). Only the first of these (Data) specifically required the presence of stuttering frequency data; the other two could have been satisfied, for example, by repeated assessments of clients' satisfaction with their communicative skills in beyond-clinic conditions.

As shown in Table 6–7, assessments of measurement and methodological adequacy were completed for the Research papers that reported maintained stuttering below 1% (see Table 6–6) and also for the Research papers that were related to (and assumed to provide the empirical support for) the most frequently Recommended treatments (see Table 6–2). The extent to which these articles satisfied the methodological and measurement criteria varied, with only the selected highly effective articles from the Research Subgroup and the prolonged speech articles from the Research Subgroup tending to meet these criteria (one highly effective article was a prolonged speech study: Ryan & Van Kirk, 1974). The articles from the Research Subgroup that addressed cognitive

Table 6–7. Number and Percent of Reports That Met Three Measurement and Design Requirements.

Reports	Data[a]	Repeated Measures[b]	Beyond Clinic[c]
Articles in Research Subgroup with <1% stuttering maintained over any maintenance phase	6/8 (75.0%)	8/8 (100.0%)	7/8 (87.5%)
Articles in Research Subgroup related to most frequently Recommended treatments			
Prolonged speech	7/14 (50.0%)	9/14 (64.3%)	6/14 (42.9%)
Cognitive/emotional	0/6 (0.0%)	1/6 (16.7%)	0/6 (0.0%)
Prolonged speech with cognitive/emotional elements	0/3 (0.0%)	2/3 (66.7%)	0/3 (0.0%)

Note: These data are for selected articles and reports only; see text.

[a]The Data criterion required data for at least stuttering frequency and speech rate, with at least central tendency and variability reported for each, and required evidence of any attempt to establish judgment reliability.

[b]The Repeated Measures criterion required that stuttering-related measurements be provided for at least two occasions before treatment and at least two occasions after treatment.

[c]The Beyond Clinic criterion required that stuttering-related measurements be provided from beyond-clinic conditions before treatment and after treatment.

or emotional procedures, or the combination of prolonged speech with cognitive or emotional procedures, tended not to meet these criteria.

The information presented in Table 6–7 suggests that the methodological adequacy of some of the reports included in this review may have been questionable, but it does not suggest the need to change the primary conclusions drawn from this review. It also seems reasonable to speculate that the methodological weaknesses revealed in Table 6–7, and the differences between Research and Recommendations that were identified by this review, might both be related to the general dissatisfaction that is often expressed about the effectiveness of stuttering treatments. The integrity of a clinical discipline depends, in part, on whether its popular or frequently recommended treatments are those that have been carefully, reliably, and validly demonstrated to result in satisfactory and well-maintained treatment effects. If, as appears may be the case for stuttering treatment, the most frequently recommended treatments are supported by methodologically questionable research, or not supported by a research base at all, then it should come as no surprise that, as also appears to be the case for stuttering treatment, an almost irreparable split might occur within the field. On the one side might gather proponents of the Recommended treatments who are not influenced by the Research findings. These people might insist that the goals and the methods addressed in the Research literature are unimportant or irrelevant: Cognitive or emotional treatments may not reduce the frequency of observer-judged stutters in controlled research, and they may not add to the ability of prolonged-speech procedures to reduce the frequency of observer-judged stutters, but they are believed to be effective in other ways or for other reasons. On the other side might gather those researchers and clinicians who favor the Researched treatments and are not influenced by the weight or the number of the Recommendations papers. This group might insist that, whatever else a stuttering treatment is designed to do or believed to do, it must first be able to show an experimentally trustworthy change in stuttered speech.

Reunifying two such disparate views will be difficult. One solution might be for the primary research literature to investigate the treatments that are being recommended; alternatively, the secondary literature could recommend the treatments that have been thoroughly researched and found to be satisfactory. Whether stuttering treatment researchers, clinicians, and persons who stutter select one of these options or select a third, there obviously remains much work to be done in developing and validating effective management procedures for all the complexities that are associated with stuttering.

REFERENCES[4]

Adams, M. R., & Hotchkiss, J. (1973). Some reactions and responses of stutterers to a miniaturized metronome and metronome-conditioning therapy: Three case reports. *Behavior Therapy, 4,* 565–569. [RES 6–3]

---

[4]All publications that were included in the literature review are listed here, whether they were cited individually in the text or not. Publications in the Research Subgroup that are included in Table 6–3 are identified as [RES 6–3]; publications in the Research Subgroup that are included in Table 6–4 are identified as [RES 6–4]; publications in the Recommendations Subgroup are identified as [REC]. In addition, the three subdivisions of investigations described in the discussion of treatment components are identified here: 16 reports of response contingent procedures ([RES 6–4 RC]), 4 reports of controlling length or complexity of utterance ([RES 6–4 LC]), and 26 reports of prolonged speech or airflow techniques ([RES 6–4 PA]). Some publications included investigations of multiple treatment procedures.

Adams, M. R., Lewis, J. I., & Besozzi, T. E. (1973). The effect of reduced reading rate on stuttering frequency. *Journal of Speech and Hearing Research, 16,* 671–675.

Adams, M. R., & Popelka, G. (1971). The influence of "time-out" on stutterers and their dysfluency. *Behavior Therapy, 2,* 334–339. [RES 6–4 RC]

Andrews, G., & Feyer, A. (1985). Does behavior therapy still work when the experimenters depart? An analysis of a behavioral treatment program for stuttering. *Behavior Modification, 9,* 443–457. [RES 6–4 PA]

Andrews, G., Guitar, B., & Howie, P. (1980). Meta-analysis of the effects of stuttering treatment. *Journal of Speech and Hearing Disorders, 45,* 287–307.

Andrews, G., & Tanner, S. (1982). Stuttering: The results of 5 days treatment with an airflow technique. *Journal of Speech and Hearing Disorders, 47,* 427–429. [RES 6–4 PA]

Azrin, N. H., Nunn, R. G., & Frantz, S. E. (1979). Comparison of regulated-breathing versus abbreviated desensitization on reported stuttering episodes. *Journal of Speech and Hearing Disorders, 44,* 331–339. [RES 6–3; RES 6–4 PA]

Berecz, J. M. (1973). The treatment of stuttering through precision punishment and cognitive arousal. *Journal of Speech and Hearing Disorders, 38,* 256–267. [RES 6–3]

Berkowitz, M., Cook, H., & Haughey, M. J. (1994). A non-traditional fluency program developed for the public school setting. *Language, Speech, and Hearing Services in Schools, 25,* 94–99. [RES 6–3]

Blood, G. W. (1995a). A behavioral-cognitive therapy program for adults who stutter: Computers and counseling. *Journal of Communication Disorders, 28,* 165–180. [RES 6–3]

Blood, G. W. (1995b). Power2: Relapse management with adolescents who stutter. *Language, Speech, and Hearing Services in Schools, 26,* 169–179. [REC]

Bloodstein, O. (1995). *A handbook on stuttering.* San Diego: Singular Publishing Group, Inc.

Boberg, E. (1984). Intensive adult/teen therapy program. In W. H. Perkins (Ed.), *Stuttering disorders* (pp. 161–171). New York: Thieme-Stratton. [REC]

Boberg, E., & Kully, D. (1994). Long-term results of an intensive treatment program for adults and adolescents who stutter. *Journal of Speech and Hearing Research, 37,* 1050–1055. [RES 6–4 PA]

Brady, J. P. (1991). The pharmacology of stuttering: A critical review. *American Journal of Psychiatry, 148,* 1309–1316.

Bray, M. A., & Kiehle, T. J. (1996). Self-modeling as an intervention for stuttering. *School Psychology Review, 25,* 358–369. [RES 6–3]

Conture, E. G., Louko, L. J., & Edwards, M. L. (1993). Simultaneously treating stuttering and disordered phonology in children: Experimental treatment, preliminary findings. *American Journal of Speech-Language Pathology, 2,* 72–81. [RES 6–3]

Cooper, E. B. (1986). Treatment of disfluency: Future trends. *Journal of Fluency Disorders, 11,* 317–328.

Coppola, V. A., & Yairi, E. (1982). Rhythmic speech training with preschool stuttering children: An experimental study. *Journal of Fluency Disorders, 7,* 447–457. [RES 6–3]

Costello, J. (1975). The establishment of fluency with time-out procedures: Three case studies. *Journal of Speech and Hearing Disorders, 40*, 216–231. [RES 6–4 RC]

Costello, J. M. (1984). Operant conditioning and the treatment of stuttering. In W. H. Perkins (Ed.), *Stuttering disorders* (pp. 107–127). New York: Thieme-Stratton. [REC]

Craig, A., Hancock, K., Chang, E., McCready, C., Shepley, A., McCaul, A., Costello, D., Harding, S., Kehren, R., Masel, C., & Reilly, K. (1996). A controlled clinical trial for stuttering in persons aged 9 to 14 years. *Journal of Speech and Hearing Research, 39*, 808–826. [RES 6–3; RES 6–4 PA]

Craig, A. R., & Kearns, M. (1995). Results of a traditional acupuncture intervention for stuttering. *Journal of Speech and Hearing Research, 38*, 572–578. [RES 6–3]

Cross, D. E., & Cooper, E. B. (1976). Self-versus investigator-administered presumed fluency reinforcing stimuli. *Journal of Speech and Hearing Research, 19*, 241–246.

Culatta, R., & Goldberg, S. A. (1995). *Stuttering therapy: An integrated approach to theory and practice.* Boston: Allyn and Bacon.

Curlee, R. F. (1984). Counseling with adults who stutter. In W. H. Perkins (Ed.), *Stuttering disorders* (pp. 153–159). New York: Thieme-Stratton. [REC]

Curlee, R. F. (1993a). Identification and management of beginning stuttering. In R. F. Curlee (Ed.), *Stuttering and related disorders of fluency* (pp. 1–22). New York: Thieme Medical. [REC]

Curlee, R. F. (Ed.) (1993b). *Stuttering and related disorders of fluency.* New York: Thieme Medical.

Curlee, R. F., & Perkins, W. H. (1969). Conversational rate control therapy for stuttering. *Journal of Speech and Hearing Disorders, 34*, 245–250. [RES 6-4 PA]

Curlee, R. F., & Siegel, G. M. (Eds.) (1997). *Nature and treatment of stuttering: New directions* (2nd ed.). Boston: Allyn & Bacon.

Daly, D. A., Simon, C. A., & Burnett-Stolnack, M. (1995). Helping adolescents who stutter focus on fluency. *Language, Speech, and Hearing Services in Schools, 26*, 162–168. [REC]

Dell, C. W. (1993). Treating school-age stutterers. In R. F. Curlee (Ed.), *Stuttering and related disorders of fluency* (pp. 45–67). New York: Thieme Medical. [REC]

De Nil, L. F., & Kroll, R. M. (1995). The relationship between locus of control and long-term stuttering treatment outcome in adult stutterers. *Journal of Fluency Disorders, 20*, 345–364. [RES 6–3]

Dewar, A., Dewar, A. D., Austin, W. T. S., & Brash, H. M. (1979). The long term use of an automatically triggered auditory feedback masking device in the treatment of stammering. *British Journal of Disorders of Communication, 14*, 219–229. [RES]

Evesham, M., & Fransella, F. (1985). Stuttering relapse: The effect of a combined speech and psychological reconstruction program. *British Journal of Disorders of Communication, 20*, 237–248. [RES 6–4 PA]

Evesham, M., & Huddleston, A. (1983). Teaching stutterers the skill of fluent speech as a preliminary to the study of relapse. *British Journal of Disorders of Communication, 18*, 31–38. [RES 6–4 PA]

Falkowski, G. L., Guilford, A. M., & Sandler, J. (1982). Effectiveness of a modified version of airflow therapy: Case studies. *Journal of Speech and Hearing Disorders, 47*, 160–164. [RES 6–4 PA]

Gagnon, M., & Ladouceur, R. (1992). Behavioral treatment of child stutterers: Replication and extension. *Behavior Therapy, 23*, 113–129. [RES 6–4 PA]

Gottwald, S. R., & Starkweather, C. W. (1995). Fluency intervention for preschoolers and their families in the public schools. *Language, Speech, and Hearing Services in Schools, 26*, 117–126. [REC]

Gray, B. B., & England, G. (1972). Some effects of anxiety deconditioning upon stuttering frequency. *Journal of Speech and Hearing Research, 15*, 114–122. [RES 6–3]

Gregory, H. H. (1972). An assessment of the results of stuttering therapy. *Journal of Communication Disorders, 5*, 320–334. [RES 6–3]

Gregory, H. H., & Hill, D. (1984). Stuttering therapy for children. In W. H. Perkins (Ed.), *Stuttering disorders* (pp. 77–93). New York: Thieme-Stratton. [REC]

Gregory, H. H., & Hill, D. (1993). Differential evaluation-differential therapy for stuttering children. In R. F. Curlee (Ed.), *Stuttering and related disorders of fluency* (pp. 23–44). New York: Thieme Medical. [REC]

Guitar, B., & Bass, C. (1978). Stuttering therapy: The relation between attitude change and long-term outcome. *Journal of Speech and Hearing Disorders, 43*, 392–400. [RES 6–4 PA]

Guitar, B., Schaefer, H. K., Donahue-Kilburg, G., & Bond, L. (1992). Parent verbal interactions and speed rate: A case study in stuttering. *Journal of Speech and Hearing Research, 35*, 742–754. [RES 6–3]

Hanson, B. R. (1978). The effects of a contingent light-flash on stuttering and attention to stuttering. *Journal of Communication Disorders, 11*, 451–458. [RES 6–4 RC]

Haroldson, S. K., Martin, R. R., & Starr, C. D. (1968). Time-out as a punishment for stuttering. *Journal of Speech and Hearing Research, 11*, 560–566. [RES 6–4 RC]

Hasbrouck, J. M., Doherty, J., Mehlmann, M. A., Nelson, R., Randle, B., & Whitaker, R. (1987). Intensive stuttering therapy in a public school setting. *Language, Speech, and Hearing Services in Schools, 18*, 330–343. [RES 6–4 PA]

Hasbrouck, J. M., & Lowry, F. (1989). Elimination of stuttering and maintenance of fluency by means of airflow, tension reduction, and discriminative stimulus control procedures. *Journal of Fluency Disorders, 14*, 165–183. [RES 6–4 PA]

Healey, E. C., & Scott, L. A. (1995). Strategies for treating elementary school-age children who stutter: An integrative approach. *Language, Speech, and Hearing Services in Schools, 26*, 151–161. [REC]

Helps, R., & Dalton, P. (1979). The effectiveness of an intensive group speech therapy programme for adult stammerers. *British Journal of Disorders of Communication, 14*, 17–30. [RES 6–3; RES 6–4 PA]

Howie, P. M., Tanner, S., & Andrews, G. (1981). Short- and long-term outcome in an intensive treatment program for adult stutterers. *Journal of Speech and Hearing Disorders, 46*, 104–109. [RES 6–4 PA]

Hulstijn, W., Peters, H. F. M., & van Lieshout, P. H. H. M. (1997). *Speech production: Motor control, brain research and fluency disorders.* Amsterdam: Elsevier.

Ingham, J. C. (1993). Behavioral treatment of stuttering children. In R. F. Curlee (Ed.), *Stuttering and related disorders of fluency* (pp. 68–89). New York: Thieme Medical. [REC]

Ingham, R. J. (1980). Modification of maintenance and generalization in stuttering treatment. *Journal of Speech and Hearing Research, 23,* 732–745.

Ingham, R. J. (1982). The effects of self-evaluation training on maintenance and generalization during stuttering treatment. *Journal of Speech and Hearing Disorders, 47,* 271–280.

Ingham, R. J. (1990). Research on stuttering treatment for adults and adolescents: A perspective on how to overcome a malaise. In J. A. Cooper (Ed.), *Research needs in stuttering: Roadblocks and future directions, ASHA Reports, 18,* 91–95.

Ingham, R. J. (1996, May). *On watching a discipline shoot itself in the foot: Some observations on current trends in stuttering treatment research.* Paper presented at the meeting of the American Speech-Language-Hearing Association Special Interest Division 4, Monterey, CA.

Ingham, R. J., & Cordes, A. K. (in press). On watching a discipline shoot itself in the foot: Some observations on current trends in stuttering treatment research. In C. Healey & N. Ratner (Eds.), *Stuttering treatment efficacy.* New York: Lawrence Erlbaum.

Ingham, R. J., & Packman, A. (1977). Treatment and generalization effects in an experimental treatment for a stutterer using contingency management and speech rate control. *Journal of Speech and Hearing Disorders, 42,* 394–407. [RES 6–4 RC]

James, J. E. (1983). Parameters of the influence of self-initiated time-out from speaking on stuttering. *Journal of Communication Disorders, 16,* 123–132. [RES 6–4 RC]

James, J. E., & Ingham, R. J. (1974). The influence of stutterers' expectancies of improvement upon response to time-out. *Journal of Speech and Hearing Research, 17,* 86–93. [RES 6–4 RC]

James, J. E., Ricciardelli, L. A., Rogers, P., & Hunter, C. E. (1989). A preliminary analysis of the ameliorative effects of time-out from speaking on stuttering. *Journal of Speech and Hearing Research, 32,* 604–610. [RES 6–4 PA]

Johnson, L. (1984). Facilitating parental involvement in therapy of the preschool disfluent child. In W. H. Perkins (Ed.), *Stuttering disorders* (pp. 29–39). New York: Thieme- Stratton. [REC]

Kuhr, A., & Rustin, L. (1985). The maintenance of fluency after intensive inpatient therapy: Long-term follow-up. *Journal of Fluency Disorders, 10,* 229–236. [RES 6–4 PA]

LaCroix, Z. E. (1973). Management of disfluent speech through self-recording procedures. *Journal of Speech and Hearing Disorders, 38,* 272–274. [RES]

Ladouceur, R., Cote, C., Leblond, G., & Bouchard, L. (1982). Evaluation of regulated-breathing method and awareness training in the treatment of stuttering. *Journal of Speech and Hearing Disorders, 47,* 422–426. [RES 6–4 PA]

Ladouceur, R., & Saint-Laurent, L. (1986). Stuttering: A multidimensional treatment and evaluation package. *Journal of Fluency Disorders, 11*, 93–103. [RES 6–4 PA]

Lincoln, M., Onslow, M., Lewis, C., & Wilson, L. (1996). A clinical trial of an operant treatment for school-age children who stutter. *American Journal of Speech-Language Pathology, 5*, 73–85. [RES]

Mallard, A. R. (1977). The effects of syllable-timed speech on stuttering behavior: An audiovisual analysis. *Behavior Therapy, 8*, 947–952. [RES 6–3]

Mallard, A. R., & Kelley, J. S. (1982). The precision fluency shaping program: Replication and evaluation. *Journal of Fluency Disorders, 7*, 287–294. [RES 6–3]

Manning, W. H., Trutna, P. A., & Shaw, C. K. (1976). Verbal versus tangible reward for children who stutter. *Journal of Speech and Hearing Disorders, 41*, 52–62.

Martin, R. R., & Haroldson, S. K. (1969). The effects of two treatment procedures on stuttering. *Journal of Communication Disorders, 2*, 115–125. [RES 6–3; RES 6–4 RC]

Martin, R. R., & Haroldson, S. K. (1979). Effects of five experimental treatments on stuttering. *Journal of Speech and Hearing Research, 22*, 132–146. [RES 6–3; RES 6–4 RC]

Martin, R. R., & Haroldson, S. K. (1982). Contingent self-stimulation for stuttering. *Journal of Speech and Hearing Disorders, 47*, 407–413. [RES 6–4 RC]

Martin, R. R., Kuhl, P., & Haroldson, S. (1972). An experimental treatment with two preschool stuttering children. *Journal of Speech and Hearing Research, 15*, 743–752. [RES 6–4 RC]

Miltenberger, R. G., Wagaman, J. R., & Arndorfer, R. E. (1996). Simplified treatment and long-term follow-up for stuttering in adults: A study of two cases. *Journal of Behavior Therapy and Experimental Psychiatry, 27*, 181–188. [RES 6–3]

Neilson, M., & Andrews, G. (1993). Intensive fluency training of chronic stutterers. In R. F. Curlee (Ed.), *Stuttering and related disorders of fluency* (pp. 139–165). New York: Thieme Medical. [REC]

Onslow, M., Andrews, C., & Lincoln, M. (1994). A control/experimental trial of an operant treatment for early stuttering. *Journal of Speech and Hearing Research, 37*, 1244–1259. [RES]

Onslow, M., Costa, L., Andrews, C., Harrison, E., & Packman, A. (1996). Speech outcomes of a prolonged-speech treatment for stuttering. *Journal of Speech and Hearing Research, 39*, 734–749. [RES 6–4 PA]

Onslow, M., Costa, L., & Rue, S. (1990). Direct early intervention with stuttering: Some preliminary data. *Journal of Speech and Hearing Disorders, 55*, 405–416. [RES]

Onslow, M., Hayes, B., Hutchins, L., & Newman, D. (1992). Speech naturalness and prolonged-speech treatments for stuttering: Further variables and data. *Journal of Speech and Hearing Research, 35*, 274–282.

Peins, M., Lee, B. S., & McGough, W. E. (1970). A tape-recorded therapy method for stutterers: A case report. *Journal of Speech and Hearing Disorders, 35*, 188–193. [RES]

Perkins, W. H. (Ed.). (1984a). *Stuttering disorders*. New York: Thieme-Stratton.

Perkins, W. H. (1984b). Techniques for establishing fluency. In W. H. Perkins (Ed.), *Stuttering disorders* (pp. 173–181). New York: Thieme-Stratton. [REC]

Perkins, W. H., Rudas, J., Johnson, L., Michael, W. B., & Curlee, R. F. (1974.) Replacement of stuttering with normal speech. III: Clinical effectiveness. *Journal of Speech and Hearing Disorders, 39*, 416–428. [RES 6–4 PA]

Prins, D. (1970). Improvement and regression in stutterers following short-term intensive therapy. *Journal of Speech and Hearing Disorders, 35*, 123–135.

Prins, D. (1993). Management of stuttering: Treatment of adolescents and adults. In R. F. Curlee (Ed.), *Stuttering and related disorders of fluency* (pp. 115–138). New York: Thieme Medical. [REC]

Ramig, P. R., & Bennett, E. M. (1995). Working with 7- to 12-year-old children who stutter: Ideas for intervention in the public schools. *Language, Speech, and Hearing Services in Schools, 26*, 138–150. [REC]

Ratner, N. B. (1995). Treating the child who stutters with concomitant language or phonological impairment. *Language, Speech, and Hearing Services in Schools, 26*, 180–186. [REC]

Ratner, N. B., & Sih, C. C. (1987). Effects of gradual increases in sentence length and complexity on children's dysfluency. *Journal of Speech and Hearing Disorders, 52*, 278–287. [RES 6–4 LC]

Reed, C. G., & Godden, A. L. (1977). An experimental treatment using verbal punishment with two preschool stutterers. *Journal of Fluency Disorders, 2*, 225–233. [RES 6–4 RC]

Runyan, C. M., & Runyan, S. E. (1993). Therapy for school age stutterers: An update on the fluency rules program. In R. E. Curlee (Ed.), *Stuttering and related disorders of fluency* (pp. 101–114). New York: Thieme Medical. [REC]

Rustin, L., & Cook, F. (1995). Parental involvement in the treatment of stuttering. *Language, Speech, and Hearing Services in Schools, 26*, 127–137. [REC]

Rustin, L., Ryan, B. P., & Ryan, B. V. (1987). Use of the Monterey programmed stuttering therapy in Great Britain. *British Journal of Disorders of Communication, 22*, 151–162. [RES 6–4 LC, PA]

Ryan, B. P. (1974). *Programmed therapy for stuttering in children and adults.* Springfield, IL: Charles C. Thomas.

Ryan, B. P. (1984). Treatment of stuttering in school children. In W. H. Perkins (Ed.), *Current therapy of communication disorders: Stuttering Disorders* (pp. 95–105.) New York: Thieme-Stratton. [REC]

Ryan, B. P., & Ryan, B. V. (1983). Programmed stuttering therapy for children: Comparison of four establishment programs. *Journal of Fluency Disorders, 8*, 291–321. [RES 6–4 RC, LC, PA]

Ryan, B. P., & Ryan, B. V. (1995). Programmed stuttering treatment for children: Comparison of two establishment programs through transfer, maintenance, and follow-up. *Journal of Speech and Hearing Research, 38*, 61–75. [RES 6–4 LC]

Ryan, B. P., & Van Kirk, B. (1974). The establishment, transfer, and maintenance of fluent speech in 50 stutterers using delayed auditory feedback and operant procedures. *Journal of Speech and Hearing Disorders, 39*, 3–10. [RES 6–4 PA]

Schwartz, D., & Webster, L. M. (1977). More on the efficacy of a protracted precision fluency shaping program. *Journal of Fluency Disorders, 2*, 205–215. [RES 6–3]

Shaw, C. K., & Shrum, W. F. (1972). The effects of response-contingent reward on the connected speech of children who stutter. *Journal of Speech and Hearing Disorders, 37,* 75–88. [RES 6–3]

Sheehan, J. G., & Sheehan, V. M. (1984). Avoidance-reduction therapy: A response suppression hypothesis. In W. H. Perkins (Ed.), *Stuttering disorders* (pp. 147–151). New York: Thieme-Stratton. [REC]

Shine, R. E. (1984). Direct management of the beginning stutterer. In W. H. Perkins (Ed.), *Stuttering disorders* (pp. 57–75). New York: Thieme-Stratton. [REC]

Starkweather, C. W. (1984). A multiprocess behavioral approach to stuttering therapy. In W. H. Perkins (Ed.), *Stuttering disorders* (pp. 129–145). New York: Thieme-Stratton. [REC]

Starkweather, C. W. (1993). Issues in the efficacy of treatment for fluency disorders. *Journal of Fluency Disorders, 18,* 151–168.

Starkweather, C. W., & Gottwald, S. R. (1993). A pilot study of relations among specific measures obtained at intake and discharge in a program of prevention and early intervention for stuttering. *American Journal of Speech-Language Pathology, 2,* 51–58. [RES 6–3]

Tyre, T. E., Maisto, S. A., & Companik, P. J. (1973). The use of systematic desensitization in the treatment of chronic stuttering behavior. *Journal of Speech and Hearing Disorders, 38,* 514–519. [RES 6–3]

Wakaba, Y. Y. (1983). Group play therapy for Japanese children who stutter. *Journal of Fluency Disorders, 8,* 93–118. [RES 6–3]

Watts, F. (1971). The treatment of stammering by the intensive practice of fluent speech. *British Journal of Disorders of Communication, 6,* 144–147.

Zebrowski, P. M., Weiss, A. L., Savelkoul, E. M., & Hammer, C. S. (1996). The effect of maternal rate reduction on the stuttering, speech rates and linguistic productions of children who stutter: Evidence from individual dyads. *Clinical Linguistics and Phonetics, 10,* 189–206. [RES 6–3]

CHAPTER

Acoustic Analyses of the Stutter-Free Utterances of Children Who Do and Do Not Stutter

JILL I. ROSENTHAL, M.S.,
RICHARD F. CURLEE, Ph.D.,
and YINGYONG QI, Ph.D.

Many comparisons of the speech of people who do and do not stutter have limited their examinations to the disfluent events that disrupt perceptually fluent speech. This research focus on disfluencies is understandable; they are, after all, the obligatory, diagnostic signs of stuttering disorders. An exclusive focus on disfluency might imply that the speech production process of children and adults who stutter is normal except for the disruptions in speech that are perceived as stutters. Moreover, this assumption has been used to support the importance of early stuttering intervention with children. Interestingly, limited empirical support is available.

For more than three decades it has been known that the stutter-free portions of speech of some adults who stutter may differ perceptually from that of adults who do not stutter (Wendahl & Cole, 1964; Young, 1964, 1984). Both sophisticated and unsophisticated listeners have been able to distinguish stuttering from nonstuttering adults from audio recordings of their fluent speech (Runyan & Adams, 1978, 1979). Likewise, acoustic studies that have compared the perceptually fluent speech of groups of stuttering and nonstuttering adults have reported more frequent and longer inter- and intraword pauses (Love & Jeffress, 1971), longer voice onset times (Healey & Gutkin, 1984; Hillman & Gilbert, 1977), slower articulatory rates (Prosek & Runyan, 1982; Ramig, Krieger, & Adams, 1982) and centralized vowels (Howell & Vause, 1986; Klich & May, 1982). These acoustic findings appear to parallel the findings from electromyographic (Freeman, 1984) and electroglottographic studies (Conture, 1984) of vocal fold activity and of kinematic studies of articulator activity (Zimmerman, 1980). In addition, Metz, Samar, and Sacco (1983) reported significant, positive correlations between the frequency of stuttering and the absence of voicing and frication within the intervals following the release of stop consonants in CV and CVC words and between stuttering frequency and the length of the intervals between the release of stops and peak air flow (Samar, Metz, & Sacco, 1986).

The extent to which these perceptual and acoustic differences characterize the fluent speech of stuttering adults, and apply to all speech production tasks, is uncertain because follow-up studies have reported mixed findings (e.g., Few & Lingwall, 1972; Gronhovd, 1977; Watson & Alphonso, 1982). Some failures to replicate may have resulted from the use of different samples, speech tasks, methodologies, measures, and data analysis procedures. Following an extensive review of this research, however, Bloodstein (1987, p. 31) concluded that "the weight of the evidence strongly suggests that what observers consider to be the fluent speech of stutterers frequently reveals features on careful study that are not to be found, at least in the same degree, in the speech of nonstutterers when measuring disfluency." Overlaps in the data obtained from subjects who do and do not stutter will be seen, even when significant group differences are present (Young, 1993). Indeed, overlapping data sets can be considered a hallmark of most empirical comparisons of these two groups.

Substantially fewer studies have compared the fluent utterances of stuttering and nonstuttering children. Except for several recent studies (e.g., Ohashi, Kenjo, & Ozawa, 1994; Walker, Shine, & Hume, 1994), most perceptual and acoustic comparisons have reported few reliable differences in their fluent speech in contrast with similar studies performed with adult subjects (Colcord & Gregory, 1987; Krikorian & Runyan, 1983; Winkler & Ramig, 1986; Zebrowski, Conture, & Cudahy, 1985). Two perceptual studies asked listeners to differentiate children who stutter from those who do not using audio recordings of their fluent speech. Krikorian and Runyan (1983) used the "Sounds in Sentences" portion of the Goldman Fristoe Test of Articulation to elicit perceptually fluent utterances from 15 stuttering and 15 age-, grade-, and gender-matched nonstuttering children, ages 4:2 to 6:11. Ten graduate students and faculty members in speech-language pathology listened to pairs of utterances, matched for content and length, but only 1 of the 15 stuttering children was correctly identified at greater than chance levels ($p<.01$). In the other study, Colcord and Gregory (1987) trained nine pairs of age- and gender-matched, stuttering and nonstuttering children to use four agent-action-object sentences to describe four pictures. Fluent productions of these sentences were presented to 12 judges in single- and paired-stimulus listening formats. The paired-stimulus condition produced higher percentages of correct identifications of several children who stuttered, but neither listening format permitted listeners to reliably differentiate the two groups.

Four acoustic studies comparing the fluent speech of stuttering and nonstuttering children were found (Ohashi, Kenjo, & Ozawa, 1994; Walker, Shine, & Hume, 1994; Winkler & Ramig, 1986; Zebrowski et al., 1985). In the earliest study, Zebrowski and her colleagues (1985) used an interactive computer program designed to analyze video-sound spectrograms to compare nine temporal measures of the fluent speech of 11 matched pairs of stuttering and nonstuttering children (age range = 3:1—6:8). No significant between-group differences were found in vowel-consonant transition duration, vowel consonant transition rate, stop-gap duration, frication duration, aspiration duration, voice onset time, consonant-vowel transition duration, consonant-vowel transition rate, or steady-state vowel duration.

In contrast, the three remaining acoustic studies found significant between-group differences. Winkler and Ramig (1986) reported that a group of nine stuttering children had significantly longer pause times than did their nonstuttering controls on both sentence repetition and story retell tasks. In addition, the stuttering children's vowel durations were longer on a sentence repetition task. At the World Congress on Fluency Disorders, Ohashi et al. (1994) presented findings from an acoustic study of the fluent productions of three-syllable words and "nonsense words" by 14 age- and gender-matched, stuttering and non-stuttering, Japanese children (age range = 3:8–9:5). They found significant between-group differences in fundamental frequency, segment duration, and stop-gap duration. At that same conference, Walker et al. (1994) reported that the absolute differences in nine acoustic measures between two repetitions of 10 fluently spoken sentences were larger, "statistically and descriptively," for the children who stuttered than for the matched, nonstuttering control group. Published abstracts of these presentations provide few details of either study's findings, but it is doubtful that their findings are compatible with those of the perceptual studies of Krikorian and Runyan (1983) or Colcord and Gregory (1987), which were reviewed above, or some of the acoustic findings reported by Zebrowski et al. (1985). This sample of studies suggests acoustic analyses may be better able than perceptual studies to detect any differences that may distinguish the perceptually fluent speech of children who stutter from that of nonstuttering peers.

It is possible that some of the acoustic differences reported in the stutter-free speech of children who stutter may be precursors of some of the differences that have been found in the fluent speech of adults who stutter (e.g., Prosek & Runyan, 1982). It is also possible that one or more of these differences may be indicators of a child's risk for continuing to stutter. Such acoustic differences may reflect the physiology of deviant linguistic and motor system functions which make some children's spoken language more vulnerable to speech disruptions that are perceived as stutters. Current research findings do not allow conclusions to be drawn about these speculations, but further empirical study is clearly needed.

This chapter reports findings from a series of exploratory acoustic analyses which searched for differences in the fluent vowel, diphthong, and word-initial plosive productions of children who do and do not stutter. These explorations of stutter-free speech were based on the hypothesis that the physiological functions responsible for episodes of stuttering in children might distinguish stutter-free as well as stuttered speech. Acoustic analyses were used because it seemed likely that these measures would be better able to detect any such differences that might exist in stutter-free speech samples of young children. Formant frequencies of vowels and diphthongs were selected for analysis as they may represent possible precursors to the findings that stuttering adults appear to centralize vowels (Howell & Vause, 1986; Klich & May, 1982). In addition there was an absence of data regarding formant frequencies of vowels and dipthongs for children who stutter. Energy levels of word-initial plosives in utterance-initial positions were examined because of the frequency with which stuttering occurs at this site, especially among children, and the suspicion that high oral pressure phonemes, in particular, might evidence intensity differences at this site among children who stutter.

METHOD

The recorded speech samples analyzed were a subset of those used in the perceptual study reported by Colcord and Gregory (1987) summarized earlier. These samples were selected for acoustic analyses in the present study because they had been established as utterances of age- and gender-matched stuttering and nonstuttering children which were free of disfluencies and which listeners had been unable to reliably assign to either group of children. Four of the nine pairs of children used

Table 7–1. Gender, Age, and Percentage of Stutter-like Disfluency of the Four Pairs of Stuttering (Ss) and Nonstuttering (Ns) Children.

Subject	Gender	Age	% Disfluent
1Ss	M	6.0	17
1Ns	M	6.5	0
2Ss	M	9.6	17
2Ns	M	9.0	0
3Ss	M	7.9	11
3Ns	M	7.9	0
4Ss	F	6.0	20
4Ns	F	6.5	0

by Colcord and Gregory were selected for the present study. One pair was not selected, because the stuttering child did not meet the 3% or more stutterlike disfluences criterion commonly used to identify young children who stutter (e.g., Conture, 1997). An additional four subject pairs were excluded because one or more of their sentences added, substituted, or omitted phonemic segments which could affect acoustic comparison measures.

Subjects

All of the children who stuttered were enrolled in therapy at Northwestern University Speech and Language Clinic when their speech samples were recorded. All were reported to be otherwise free of any speech or hearing problem, as were all of the nonstuttering control children (Colcord & Gregory, 1987). Descriptions of the stuttering children's treatment were not available. Thus, it is not known if any were being trained to speak slightly slower with more relaxed, smoother movements, a common treatment approach of that clinic (Gregory & Hill, 1993). Table 7–1 presents the gender, age, and percentage of stutter-like disfluencies of the four pairs of subjects as reported by Colcord and Gregory (1987).

Recordings

Each child was trained to describe each of four action pictures using the same agent-action-object sentence for each picture, which were then audio recorded (Ampex, Model 440). Recordings were made using a head worn microphone with a mouth to microphone distance of 5 cm (Shure, Model SM12). To make certain that each sentence was free of disfluencies, the audiorecordings were examined by two certified speech-language pathologists who were instructed to listen for "any instances of sound, syllable, word, or phrase repetition, sound prolongation, hesitation, revision, sound or word interjection, unfinished word, or incomplete phrase" (Colcord & Gregory, 1987, pp. 186–187). Twenty-six of the 36 sentences that were recorded (i.e., 9 pairs of children × 4 sentences) were later judged to have no disfluencies and to be of acceptable quality for presentation to a panel of 12 graduate students in speech-language pathology, each of whom had some previous clinical exposure to stuttering. The panel was told that only fluent sentences would be presented in single- and paired-stimulus listening conditions. Each listener was instructed to identify which sentences were produced by a child who stutters and then to list the cues used in making that identification. Statistical analyses found that the panel "could not discriminate between the two groups" (p. 190) and that "there were no unique cues" listed for the correctly identified stutterers or incorrectly identified nonstutterer in either listening condition (Colcord & Gregory, 1987, p. 192).

Twenty-four of the 26 sentences just described were selected for the present study (4 child pairs × 3 sentences). Their selection was based on obtaining the largest number of matched pairs of subjects whose fluent utterances were phonemically identical. The sentences meeting this criterion were: "Ann is drinking milk," "Billy is buying candy," and "Karen is helping mommy." Each child's productions of these sentences were copied from the original recording onto an audiocassette and low-pass filtered (7.5 kHz cut-off) before being digitized by a Sun computer (Sparc 10/30) at a sampling frequency of 16 kHz and quantization level of 16 bits. The beginning and ending of each sentence were auditorily located from digital playbacks, then checked by visual inspection of the waveform. Fourteen linear predictive (LP) coefficients were computed for each signal frame using autocorrelation methods (Markel & Gray, 1976; Qi, 1990), and hamming window and pre-emphasis were used for each LP analysis. Frame length was established at 20 ms, and frame step-size was 10 ms. Formant frequencies were computed from roots of the polynomial of the LP coefficients. Only conjugate poles with large bandwidths (i.e., >500 Hz) and frequencies (i.e., >2500 Hz) were removed (Wong et al., 1979; Qi, 1990). Computations were performed using Matlab (Matlab-4.0, Mathworks). The speakers of dubbed samples were not identified until all measurements and reliability checks were completed.

Of the many vowels available, two were selected for analysis. The /æ/ in "Ann," "candy," and "Karen" and the /ɪ/ in "Billy" and "milk" were selected because of their frequency of occurrence in this sample. The diphthong, /aɪ/ in "buying," was also selected to gain information on this phoneme when produced by children. The word- and utterance-initial plosives, /b/ in "Billy" and /k/ in "Karen," were selected because of the frequency with which stuttering occurs at this site among children, and the /b/ in "buying" and /k/ in "candy" to see if utterance-position is associated with acoustic differences for the same two word-initial phonemes when they appear later in utterances.

Analyses

Each selected vowel was visually determined from spectrographic and waveform displays of the frequencies of the first and second formants in the 60 ms following vowel onset. The 60 ms analysis window from the apparent onset of each vowel was used for all of these measures because the endings of some vowels could not be identified reliably. The final boundary of the diphthong, /aɪ/, could not always be identified reliably either, so a 200 ms window after apparent onset was used to measure first and second formant frequencies steady states and transitions. Only first and second formants were measured because they provide most of the information required for the correct identification of vowels and diphthongs. LP analyses and root-solving procedures were used to estimate formant frequencies, and a dynamic formant tracking algorithm was employed to smooth and trace estimated formant frequencies, which were later verified by Fourier spectrum peak comparisons.

Each selected plosive was determined visually from spectrographic and waveform displays from the ending of implosion silence to the end of burst release. The resolution of all temporal measures was 62.5 μs (sampling frequency = 16 kHz). Then, the remainder of each word, from the end of the burst release to the end of voicing on the word's final phoneme, was determined. Voicing was determined through visual identification of the waveform segment having regular glottal impulses, and the beginning of voicing by the peak location of the first identifiable glottal impulse (Qi & Hunt, 1993; Rabiner & Sambur, 1977). The root mean square energy of each plosive and of the remaining portion of the word were measured.

Half of the samples were selected at random for remeasurement of all time and frequency measures at least 1 week after initial measures were completed. Each remeasure was within 10% of the initial measures, which resulted in a correlation coefficient of $r = 0.999$.

RESULTS

Group effects on the first and second formants of vowels and on the energy of word-initial plosives and the remainder of the word were evaluated with Analyses of Variance (ANOVA) using Statistical Analysis Software programs. A Multivariate Analysis of Variance (MANOVA) was

Table 7–2. First (F1) and Second (F2) Formant Frequencies (Hz) of /ɪ/ and /æ/, in Selected Fluent Words, Produced by Matched Pairs of Stuttering (Ss) and Nonstuttering Children (Ns).

Vowel	Word	Pair	Ss F1	Ss F2	Ns F1	Ns F2
/ɪ/	Bill	1	520	1704	484	1715
		2	499	1786	455	2141
		3	580	2105	526	2312
		4	525	2091	482	2286
	milk	1	451	2057	638	2209
		2	527	2075	546	2282
		3	482	2297	545	1908
		4	375	1739	450	2090
/æ/	Ann	1	552	2616	640	2612
		2	607	2268	623	2415
		3	615	2244	569	2854
		4	467	2280	697	2274
	candy	1	554	3277	587	2482
		2	582	2297	469	3114
		3	635	2114	544	3140
		4	487	2454	627	2224
	Karen	1	705	2319	528	2354
		2	537	2438	493	2570
		3	514	2861	517	2741
		4	521	2485	435	2172

used to evaluate the acoustic measures of diphthongs. In each of these analyses, subjects were considered to be a factor nested within each group to estimate error components. Post-hoc t-tests for independent means were used to clarify some significant ANOVA results.

Vowels

The first and second formants were evaluated as a function of group, vowel, and word and their interactions. Table 7–2 presents both formant frequencies for each subject for both /ɪ/ and /æ/. The only significant ANOVA result was the three-way interaction among group, vowel, and word for the first formant ($[F_{(3,39)} = 3.95, p = 0.02$). Follow-up, post-hoc t-tests indicated that the mean first formant frequency for /ɪ/ in "Billy" was significantly higher for the group of stuttering children ($p < 0.05$)

than for the nonstuttering children. Although the mean of the second formant frequency was higher for /ɪ/ in "Billy," and the mean of the first formant frequency of /ɪ/ in "milk" was lower for the group of children who stutter, neither difference was statistically significant ($p > 0.05$).

Diphthongs

The formant trajectory of each diphthong was traced using a dynamic programming procedure (Nemhauser, 1966; Qi, 1992). Formant traces were obtained by minimizing the global cost function for connecting candidate formant frequencies. The cost for each step was computed as the frequency difference between two neighboring candidate formant frequencies. Table 7–3 displays the three acoustic measures that characterized the four pairs of subjects' productions of /aɪ/ in "buying." The MANOVA evaluation of these data found a significant group effect ($F_{(1,36)} = 14.77$, $p = 0.0085$). The formant tracings depicting these means are shown in Figure 7–1.

As can be seen, the first formant transition between the /a/ and /ɪ/ portions of the diphthong is somewhat more linear for the children who stutter than for control children. The tracing of their second formant transition, however, is clearly steeper than that of the nonstuttering group. The F1 and F2 intercepts (Hz) were also higher for the children who stutter.

Plosives

The root mean square energy, in decibels (dB), of each subject's word- and utterance-initial plosives, /b/ in "Billy" and /k/ in "Karen," and of the word-initial /b/ in "buying" and /k/ in "candy," which occurred later in utterances, are presented in Table 7–4. The root mean square energy in the remaining portions of each word for each pair of subjects is shown in Table 7–5. The energy in both plosives and in the remaining portions of the four words they initiated were evaluated using two-way, group by word ANOVAS, neither of which detected statistically significant differences.

To control for age differences across subjects, the energy measures of each nonstuttering child's plosive were subtracted from those of the paired child who stutters. Likewise, each nonstuttering child's measure of the energy remaining in each of the four words following word-initial plosives were subtracted from those of the paired stuttering child. These data are presented in Table 7–6. Two t-tests for independent means were used to determine if the differences in energy in the two plosives or in the remaining portions of words differed between the four pairs of subjects. Even though more difference scores were negative, suggesting

Table 7–3. The Curve (C), Slope (S), and Intercept (I) of the First (F1) and Second (F2) Formant Frequencies (Hz) of /aɪ/ in Fluent Productions of "Buying" of Four Matched Pairs of Stuttering (Ss) and Nonstuttering (Ns) Children.

Formant	Pair	Ss			Ns		
		C	S	I	C	S	I
F1	1	−1.30	0.13	780	−1.32	0.11	550
	2	−0.07	0.03	880	−2.13	0.17	430
	3	−0.80	0.05	680	−0.72	0.04	690
	4	−0.72	0.04	690	−2.69	0.23	550
F2	1	2.04	−0.03	1738	−1.56	0.75	1506
	2	3.38	0.03	1593	−0.23	0.27	1612
	3	2.07	0.22	1826	−0.04	0.09	1686
	4	4.10	−0.28	1905	2.41	−0.13	1730

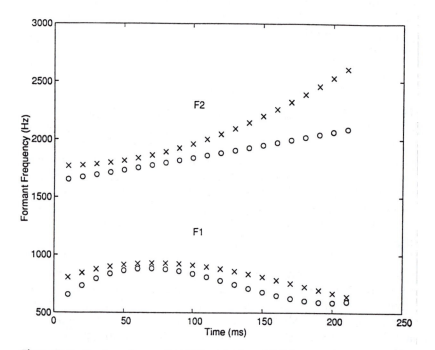

Figure 7–1. Tracing of mean first (F1) and second (F2) formant frequencies of (aɪ) in the production of "buying" by four matched pairs of stuttering (x) and nonstuttering (o) children.

Table 7–4. Energy (dB) of /b/ and /k/ in Utterance-Initial and Later Positions in Fluent Words of Four Matched Pairs of Stuttering (Ss) and Nonstuttering (Ns) Children.

Initial	Pair	Ss	Ns
/b/	1	61.26	57.09
	2	46.19	43.26
	3	55.70	64.27
	4	74.91	73.65
/k/	1	53.79	54.95
	2	68.52	71.76
	3	59.36	57.91
	4	43.47	50.24

Later	Pair	Ss	Ns
/b/	1	66.40	63.24
	2	55.02	55.05
	3	59.54	68.42
	4	71.12	71.24
/k/	1	59.69	60.56
	2	62.31	46.11
	3	45.83	60.55
	4	63.65	68.49

that the energy in both word-initial plosives and the remainder of the word might have been lower among stuttering children, these differences did not achieve statistical significance ($p > 0.05$).

DISCUSSION

The significant interaction found for the first formant frequencies of the vowels analyzed suggests that the vowel productions of some children who stutter may differ from those of their nonstuttering peers. Interestingly, the stuttering children's mean first formant for /æ/ closely approximates the values presented by Baken (1987) and Olive, Greenwood, and Coleman (1993) for the mid-vowel /ɛ/. This type of acoustic shift indicates a reduction or a centralization of /æ/, according to Shriberg and Kent (1995). In addition, the first and second formant frequency tracings of /aɪ/ depicted opposing trends in the transitions of these formants among the children who stuttered. The transition of the first formant

Table 7–5. Energy (dB) in the Word Segments Following Initial Plosives in Utterance-Initial and Later Positions Produced by Four Matched Pairs of Stuttering (Ss) and Nonstuttering (Ns) Children.

Initial	Pair	Ss	Ns
Bill	1	71.98	73.73
	2	63.09	53.06
	3	71.40	76.54
	4	80.23	78.41
Karen	1	72.06	65.81
	2	70.48	73.63
	3	68.80	69.52
	4	71.34	72.58

Later	Pair	Ss	Ns
Buying	1	69.78	70.89
	2	61.75	55.06
	3	63.77	71.19
	4	73.97	76.16
Candy	1	67.94	67.74
	2	50.60	50.68
	3	47.73	67.79
	4	70.47	74.49

was more linear, whereas that of the second formant was less linear. Moreover, the mean second formant frequency closely approximated (<11%) the frequency of centralized phonemes in Olive et al. (1993), which is consistent with the shift in production that was hypothesized for the vowel /æ/.

The perception of schwa vowels in the fluent speech of adults who stutter has been reported by Allen, Peters, and Williams (1975) and Freeman, Borden, and Dorman (1976). In contrast, the apparent shift towards a centralized vowel by these four stuttering children did not affect our perceptual identification of them as /æ/ phonemes. Consequently, the extent to which the acoustic differences found in this study are a precursor of those that may result in the perception of schwa vowels among stuttering adults cannot be determined. If such acoustic shifts are precursors of the findings reported for stuttering adults (Howell & Vause, 1986; Klich & May, 1982), they may be an early indicator of a child's risk for continuing to stutter as an adult. It is not readily apparent that any of the therapy techniques currently used with children who

Table 7–6. Energy (dB) Differences (Ss − Ns) of Word-Initial Plosives and Following Word Segments Fluently Produced in Initial and Later Utterance Positions of Four Matched Pairs of Children.

Pair	Position	Plosive	Word
		/b/	Bill
1	Initial	4.1757	−1.7517
2		2.9331	10.0325
3		−8.5751	−5.1411
4		1.2567	1.8187
		/k/	Karen
1		−1.1613	6.2420
2		−3.2310	−3.1533
3		1.4504	−0.7279
4		−6.7956	−1.2349
		/b/	buying
1	Later	3.1638	−1.1147
2		−0.0227	6.6853
3		−8.8843	−7.4192
4		−0.1230	−2.1879
		/k/	candy
1		−0.8698	0.2048
2		16.1941	−0.0745
3		−14.7157	−20.0585
4		−4.8378	−4.0221

stutter would be likely to result in acoustic records which appear to reflect restrictions in the excursions of articulatory gestures when producing vowels. It is possible, however, that such restrictions may be a compensatory speech production behavior that children who stutter commonly adopt.

The absence of between group, energy level differences in the utterance- and word-initial plosives of the two groups was not anticipated. Not only did none of the energy level comparisons distinguish the two groups, even the direction of the statistically nonsignificant differences found was contrary to expectation.

For the four children who stutter, intensity levels of both word-initial plosives in both utterance positions and the intensity levels of the remaining portions of words either approximated or fell below those of their nonstuttering peers. Because all of the children who stuttered were enrolled in therapy when these speech samples were recorded, their therapy procedures, which may have included slightly slower, more relaxed, smoother movements of utterance-initial syllables (see Gregory & Hill, 1993), may have affected all of these energy level measures.

Unlike similar studies with adults (e.g., Runyan & Adams, 1978, 1979; Wendahl & Cole, 1964; Young, 1984), listeners have been unable to distinguish between groups of stuttering and nonstuttering children when listening to recordings of their fluent speech (Colcord & Gregory, 1987; Krikorian & Runyan, 1983; Winkler & Ramig, 1986; Zebrowski et al., 1985). Although differences in speaking tasks, methods of observation, measures obtained, and data analysis, as well as the effects of maturation on speech production could account for the failure of children's studies to parallel those of adults, such failures may indicate that the stutter-free speech of children who stutter is normal and does not differ from that of nonstuttering peers. A study of the perceptually fluent speech of adolescents who stutter and nonstuttering controls by Brown and Colcord (1987) found that these two groups could be reliably distinguished by listeners, findings which are consistent with suggestions that the differences observed in adults' stutter-free speech results, at least in part, from years of stuttering and therapy.

Alternatively, if the linguistic and motor processes necessary for normally fluent speech are, in fact, less stable or are more susceptible to disruption among young children who begin to stutter, such differences might not be perceptible to listeners, even if reliable acoustic differences can be found. The spoken language of such children, especially those who continue to stutter as adults, may include more frequent and more apparent differences in their fluent speech as stuttering persists. In time their speech could come to evidence the compensatory habits and treatment residuals perceived in adults' speech after many years of stuttering and therapy. Because adults who stutter are a relatively small subset of the children who ever stutter, study samples of young children who stutter are likely to include many children who will stop stuttering whether or not they receive therapy. Such children's fluent speech may not contain sufficient cues to permit listeners to discriminate it from that of nonstuttering children. If so, it would not be surprising if listeners were unable to distinguish the fluent speech of groups of young children who do not stutter from groups containing only a few children who will continue to stutter as adults. The findings from Brown and Colcord's (1987) study of adolescents do not conflict with this explanation either.

None of the differences in stutterers' and nonstutterers' fluent speech discussed here have identified variables which have been shown to have a functional relationship to stuttering or its clinical management. Even those variables that reliably discriminate groups of stuttering children and adults from matched groups of nonstutterers (e.g., speech reaction time) have yet to demonstrate an etiological link to stuttering or a value in diagnosis or treatment. Empirical comparisons of stuttering and nonstuttering samples typically evidence overlap in the two groups' data. Such overlap indicates that the variables represented in these overlapping sets of data do not have either a necessary or a sufficient relationship with stuttering. The acquisition, use, and disruption of the communication behaviors of few animals are well understood. Perhaps it is naive, if not presumptuous, to believe that invariant, linear relationships are likely to account for the kinds of interruptions in spoken language which characterize stuttering (e.g., Smith & Kelly, 1997).

Stuttered and stutter-free speech are usually studied and discussed as if they are categorical variables. Indeed, stuttering research has focused on the most noticeable disruptions of spoken language as the critical events for study and largely ignored surrounding speech that is free of perceptible stutters. Curiously, even casual observations of stuttering speakers make it readily apparent that stutters vary in type, duration, frequency, apparent effort, and accompanying accessory behaviors across time and contexts, as if stuttered speech is not a categorical variable, but forms a continuum. Similarly, the brief pauses, phoneme extensions, atypical formant transitions, intensity perturbations, and other barely noticeable signs of less well-coordinated movements during stutter-free speech seem not to be heard, or are just ignored, as if speech free of stutters lacks any features or characteristics which reflect different degrees of fluency along a continuum. Although it seems highly unlikely to us that a better understanding of stuttering will emerge until there is a better understanding of speech production that is free of stuttering, the extent to which the study of stutter-free speech will contribute to a better understanding of stuttering or its clinical management will not be known until such contributions can be viewed from the perspective and with the wisdom that hindsight will provide.

It should be apparent that generalizing the findings obtained in this study to other children who stutter is not appropriate given the small number of children studied, the few acoustic characteristics analyzed, and the limited sample of speaking tasks and phonemes examined. Nevertheless, it is apparent that further study is needed if the relationship between the perceptually fluent speech of children and adults who stutter and the events perceived as stuttering is to be clarified. Ingham persuasively argues (e.g., Chapter 4, this volume) that studies of stutterers' speech behaviors at peripheral levels of observation are unlikely to advance understanding of the nature of stuttering or its treatment and that brain imaging studies are much more promising. Until that promise is confirmed, however, it seems premature to abandon research of peripheral phenomena whose promise has yet to receive a thorough exploration.

ACKNOWLEDGMENT: This chapter is based on a thesis project completed by the first author under the direction of the second and third authors in partial fulfillment of the requirements for the Master of Science degree awarded by the Department of Speech and Hearing Sciences at the University of Arizona in 1995.

REFERENCES

Allen, G. R., Peters, R., & Williams, C. (1975). *Spectrographic study of fluent and stuttered.* A paper presented at the annual convention of the American Speech and Hearing Association in Washington, DC.

Baken, R. J. (1987). *Clinical measurement of speech and voice* (pp. 352–393). Needham Heights, MA: Allyn & Bacon.

Bloodstein, O. (1987). *A handbook on stuttering* (4th ed.). Chicago: National Easter Seal Society.

Brown, S., & Colcord, R. (1987). Perceptual comparisons of adolescent stutterers' and nonstutterers' fluent speech. *Journal of Fluency Disorders, 12,* 419–427.

Colcord, R., & Gregory, H. (1987). Perceptual analysis of stuttering and nonstuttering children's fluent speech productions. *Journal of Fluency Disorders, 12,* 185–195.

Conture, E. G. (1984). Observing laryngeal movements of stutterers. In R. F. Curlee & W. H. Perkins (Eds.), *Nature and treatment of stuttering: New directions* (pp. 116–129). Needham Heights, MA: Allyn & Bacon.

Conture, E. G. (1997). Evaluating childhood stuttering. In R. F. Curlee & G. M. Siegel (Eds.), *Nature and treatment of stuttering: New directions* (2nd ed., pp. 239–256). Needham Heights, MA: Allyn & Bacon.

Few, L. R., & Lingwall, J. B. (1972). A further analysis of fluency within stuttered speech. *Journal of Speech and Hearing Research, 15,* 356–363.

Freeman, F. J. (1984). Laryngeal muscle activity of stutterers. In R. F. Curlee & W. H. Perkins (Eds.), *Nature and treatment of stuttering: New directions* (pp. 104–116). Needham Heights, MA: Allyn & Bacon.

Freeman, F. J., Borden, G., & Dorman, M. (1976, November). *Laryngeal stuttering: Combined physiological and acoustic studies.* A paper presented at the annual convention of the American Speech and Hearing Association in Houston, TX.

Gregory, H. H., & Hill, D. (1993). Differential evaluation—differential therapy for stuttering children. In R. F. Curlee (Ed.), *Stuttering and related disorders of fluency* (pp. 23–44). New York: Thieme Medical Publishers.

Gronhovd, K. D. (1977). A comparison of the fluent oral reading rates of stutterers and nonstutterers. *Journal of Fluency Disorders, 2,* 247–252.

Healey, E. C., & Gutkan, B. (1984). Analysis of stutterers' voice onset times and fundamental frequency contours during fluency. *Journal of Speech and Hearing Research, 27,* 219–225.

Hillman, R., & Gilbert, H. (1977). Voice onset times for voiceless stop consonants in the fluent readings of stutterers and nonstutterers. *Journal of the Acoustical Society of America, 61*, 610–611.

Howell, P., & Vause, L. (1986). Acoustic analysis and perception of vowels in stuttered speech. *Journal of the Acoustical Society of America, 79*, 1571–1579.

Klich, R. J., & May, G. M. (1982). Spectrographic study of vowels in stutterers' fluent speech. *Journal of Speech and Hearing Research, 25*, 364–370.

Krikorian, C. M., & Runyan, C. M. (1983). A perceptual comparison: Stuttering and nonstuttering children's nonstuttered speech. *Journal of Fluency Disorders, 8*, 283–290.

Love, L., & Jeffress, L. A. (1971). Identification of brief pauses in the fluent speech of stutterers and nonstutterers. *Journal of Speech and Hearing Research, 14*, 229–240.

Markel, J., & Gray, A. (1976). *Linear prediction of speech.* New York: Springer-Verlag.

Metz, D. E., Samar, V. J., & Sacco, P. R. (1983). Acoustic analysis of stutterers' fluent speech before and after therapy. *Journal of Speech and Hearing Research, 26*, 531–536.

Nemhauser, G. (1966). *Introduction to dynamic programming.* New York: John Wiley & Sons.

Ohashi, Y., Kenjo, M., & Ozawa, E. (1994). Acoustic analysis of fluent speech production in stuttering children and normally fluent peers. In C. W. Starkweather (Ed.), First World Congress on Fluency Disorders: Abstracts. *Journal of Fluency Disorders, 19*, 198.

Olive, J. P., Greenwood, A., & Coleman, J. (1993). *Acoustics of American English: A dynamic approach.* New York: Springer-Verlag.

Prosek, R. A., & Runyan, C. M. (1982). Temporal characteristics related to the discrimination of stutterers' and nonstutterers' speech samples. *Journal of Speech and Hearing Research, 25*, 29–33.

Qi, Y. (1990). Replacing tracheoesophageal voicing sources using LPC synthesis. *Journal of the Acoustical Society of America, 88*, 1228–1235.

Qi, Y. (1992). Time normalization in voice analysis. *Journal of the Acoustical Society of America, 92*, 2569–2576.

Qi, Y., & Hunt, B. (1993). Voiced-Unvoiced-Silence classifications of speech using hybrid features and a network classifier. *IEEE Transactions on Speech and Audio Processing, 1*, 250–255.

Rabiner, L., & Sambur, M. (1977). Application of an LPC distance measure to the Voiced-Unvoiced-Silence detection problem. *IEEE Transactions on Acoustics, Speech, and Signal Processing, 25*, 338–343.

Ramig, P. R., Krieger, S. M., & Adams, M. R. (1982). Vocal changes in stutterers and nonstutterers when speaking to children. *Journal of Fluency Disorders, 7*, 369–384.

Runyan, C. M., & Adams, M. R. (1978). Perceptual study of the speech of "successfully therapeutized" stutterers. *Journal of Fluency Disorders, 3*, 25–39.

Runyan, C. M., & Adams, M. R. (1979). Unsophisticated judges' perceptual evaluations of "successfully treated" stutterers. *Journal of Fluency Disorders, 4*, 29–38.

Samar, V. J., Metz, D. E., & Sacco, P. R. (1986). Changes in aerodynamic characteristics of stutterers' fluent speech associated with therapy. *Journal of Speech and Hearing Research, 29,* 106–113.

Shriberg, L. D., & Kent, R. D. (1995). *Clinical phonetics* (2nd ed., pp. 32–43). Needham Heights, MA: Allyn & Bacon.

Smith, A., & Kelly, E. (1997). Stuttering: A dynamic, multifactorial model. In R. F. Curlee & G. M. Siegel (Eds.), *Nature and treatment of stuttering: New directions* (2nd ed., pp. 204–217). Boston, MA: Allyn and Bacon.

Walker, M., Shine, R., & Hume, G. (1994). Spectrographic analysis of fluent speech in normally fluent and stuttering children. In C. W. Starkweather (Ed.), First World Congress on Fluency Disorders: Abstracts. *Journal of Fluency Disorders, 19,* 218–219.

Watson, B. C., & Alphonso, P. J. (1982). A comparison of LRT and VOT values between stutterers and nonstutterers. *Journal of Fluency Disorders, 7,* 219–241.

Wendahl, R. W., & Cole, J. (1964). Identification of stutterers from recorded samples of their "fluent" speech. *Journal of Speech and Hearing Research, 4,* 281–286.

Winkler, L. E., & Ramig, P. (1986). Temporal characteristics in fluent speech. *Journal of Fluency Disorders, 11,* 217–229.

Wong, D., Markel, J., & Gray, A. (1979). Least squares glottal inverse filtering from the acoustic speech waveform. *IEEE Transactions on Acoustics, Speech, and Signal Processing, 27,* 350–355.

Young, M. A. (1964). Identification of stutterers from recorded samples of their "fluent" speech. *Journal of Speech and Hearing Research, 7,* 302–303.

Young, M. A. (1984). Identification of stuttering and stutterers. In R. F. Curlee & W. H. Perkins (Eds.), *Nature and treatment of stuttering: New directions* (pp. 13–30). San Diego: College-Hill Press.

Young, M. A. (1993). Supplementary tests of statistical significance: Variation accounted for. *Journal of Speech and Hearing Research, 36,* 644–656.

Zebrowski, P. M., Conture, E. G., & Cudahy, E. A. (1985). Acoustic analysis of young stutterers' fluency: Preliminary observations. *Journal of Fluency Disorders, 10,* 173–192.

Zimmerman, G. N. (1980). Articulatory dynamics of fluent utterances of stutterers and nonstutterers. *Journal of Speech and Hearing Research, 23,* 95–107.

CHAPTER

Efficacy Research to Develop Treatment Programs for Preschool Children Who Stutter

BRUCE P. RYAN, Ph.D.

Establishing the efficacy of stuttering treatment means establishing that the treatment is effective and efficient using replicable, well-described procedures to permanently eliminate or reduce stuttering in a reasonable amount of time. For this chapter "effective" will be defined in terms of whether the treatment leads to a permanent reduction or elimination of stuttering. "Efficient" will be defined as the time taken to achieve such results. Such efficacy has been demonstrated for the Monterey Fluency Program (e.g., Ryan & Ryan, 1983, 1995; Ryan & Van Kirk, 1974a, 1974b, 1978) for school-age children and adults. The search for effective treatment programs for preschool children who stutter began in 1982 with the Genesis of Stuttering cross-sectional/longitudinal project (Ryan, 1984, 1990, 1993; Ryan & Marsh, 1985, 1987).

The first goal of this study was to identify the variables that made a contribution to the development of stuttering. This goal was to be accomplished by comparing children who stuttered to children who did not stutter on a wide variety of variables including speech, topography, conversational speech acts, interruption, and linguistic variables. The variables to be examined, such as number of statements made by children and the percentage of statements stuttered, were selected with the criteria that they must be observable and measurable, and possibly related to stuttering as suggested by the literature.

Second, these studies were designed to follow the stuttering children over time to determine the relationship(s) between these variables and stuttering (i.e., If the frequency of stuttering changed, did the frequency of one or more these variables also change?). Third, the possible contributing variables identified in phases one and two were to be studied in single-subject designs to further confirm their contribution and to develop intervention or treatment programs (collection of independent variables arranged in a logical sequence to install a desired behavior or eliminate an undesired behavior) based on these variables. After completing the first two phases of this study and reading the literature, the independent variables of conversational speech acts (e.g., questions and statements), interruption, linguistic complexity, and speaking rate were selected for further analysis. These variables have also been identified in literature reviews like those of Nippold (1990), Nippold and Rudzinski (1995), Bernstein Ratner (1992, 1993), Kelly (1993, 1994) and in articles on individual variables (e.g., interruption: Meyers & Freeman, 1985a; linguistic complexity: Bernstein Ratner & Sih, 1987; speaking rate: Meyers & Freeman, 1985b; Stephenson-Opsal & Bernstein Ratner, 1988; Zebrowski, Weiss, Savelkoul, & Hammer, 1996).

Since 1982, a total of 51 stuttering preschool children have been studied, some for over 10 years. For this chapter, samples were selected of 20 stuttering compared to 20 nonstuttering children evaluated on a variety of tests (e.g., Test of Language Development [TOLD], Newcomer & Hammill, 1982b) (Ryan, 1992), observed conversations with their mothers (Ryan, 1998), and a sample of 11 stuttering children for longitudinal analysis (Ryan, 1990, 1993). Finally, representative results based on 3 of the 12 single-subject design studies we have conducted within this project will be shown.

One organizing theme of this chapter is that a great number of single-subject design studies are needed to identify the contribution of each of the many independent variables that may be related to the development and treatment of stuttering. These single-subject analyses should be completed in addition to the extensive group research that is presently in progress (e.g., Yairi, Ambrose, Paden, & Throneburg, 1996). The issue of the relative merits of single-subject design versus group design in stuttering research was revisited recently by Ingham (1997) and Kalinkowsi, Stuart, and Armson (1997). This chapter presents both group and single-subject research data related to that issue, and there remains a need for additional single-subject design research as discussed in greater detail below. Also, it should be noted that if one studies a large enough number of single subjects, one can put the results together and also do a group, small sample inferential statistical analysis of that single-subject data (e.g., Ryan & Ryan, 1983, 1995).

Table 8–1. Selected Results of Cross-Sectional Studies Comparing 20 Stuttering with 20 Nonstuttering Preschool Children.

Variable (metric or average)	Stuttering		Nonstuttering		Significance
	M	SD	M	SD	
Age (months)	52.4	8.7	52.8	9.2	NSSD
Stuttered words per minute (SW/M)	12.0	6.0	2.2	1.2	$p < .01$
Conversational Speech Acts					
Statements	25.6	11.1	24.4	9.6	NSSD
Statement stuttered %	32.3	17.5	8.6	9.0	$p < .01$
Questions %	17.7	9.2	19.5	10.5	NSSD
Questions stuttered %	20.9	17.3	3.8	.8	$p < .0l$
Linguistic					
TOLD	92.2	10.9	100.8	10.2	$p < .01$
Grammatic Completion	6.6	2.7	10.3	3.1	$p < .01$
DSS	8.9	2.4	9.5	1.8	NSSD
DSS Stuttered	10.9	3.8	12.1	5.1	NSSD
Interruption %	19.2	11.3	22.1	16.3	NSSD
Syllables per minute (SPM)	202.6	37.9	205.6	24.8	NSSD

Sources: From Ryan, B. (1992). "Articulation, Language, Rate, and Fluency Characteristics of 20 Stuttering and Nonstuttering Preschool Children." *Journal of Speech and Hearing Research, 35,* 333–342; and Ryan, B. (1998). "Speaking Rate, Conversational Speech Acts, and Linguistic Complexity of 20 Preschool Stuttering and Nonstuttering Children and Their Mothers." Submitted for publication.

Note: TOLD is the Test of Language Development (Newcomer & Hammill,1982b); Grammatic Completion is a subtest of the TOLD; and DSS is Developmental Sentence Score (Lee, 1974).

PHASE I: CROSS-SECTIONAL STUDY RESULTS

A sample of the cross-sectional data for 20 (mean age = 4 years: 4 months) preschool stuttering and 20 nonstuttering preschool children is shown in Table 8–1 (individual data points from Ryan, 1992, 1998). The procedure of defining stuttering as whole-word repetitions, part-word repetitions, prolongation, and struggle (Ryan, 1974) resulted in identifying such behaviors, especially whole- and part-word repetitions, in the speech of nonstuttering children as well as in the speech of children who stuttered. These behaviors were counted in the speech of both groups of children, although the nonstuttering children were not thought of as "stutterers" by their parents probably because these behaviors occurred relatively infrequently and were of short duration. One other caveat is that the metric stuttered words per minute (SW/M) is used along with the metric syllables spoken per minute (SPM). The author started reporting research in SW/M (Ryan, 1971, 1974) and has observed that there is almost no difference between stuttered syllables per minute and SW/M except for the rare occurrence of stuttering on more than one syllable in a word. Most of the data reported here are with young children who, for the most part, do not use a high proportion of multisyllabic words, nor stutter more than once on a word. Stuttered words and stuttered syllables are, at least, comparable, if not the same.

These comparisons revealed relatively few significant differences between the stuttering and nonstuttering preschool children with the exception of differences in stuttering behavior and any variable which involved stuttering. There were no differences in conversational speech acts except those associated with stuttering. It was also noted that the five conversational speech acts which were most often stuttered by the children who stuttered were, in order, statements (29.0% of which were stuttered), corrections (25.5%), commands (22.3%), and questions (20.6%). Answers (11.6%) were also the most frequent act (37.5% of all conversational speech acts), followed by statements (24.8%) and questions (17.5%) (Ryan, 1998).

A few significant differences were observed in linguistic variables, such as the TOLD score and its Grammatic Completion subtest. Although the stuttering group scored significantly lower than the nonstuttering group on these linguistic measures, none of the stuttering children demonstrated a clinical language problem (Ryan, 1992). Most importantly, the Developmental Sentence Score (DSS; Lee, 1974) of the stuttering children was not significantly different from that of the nonstuttering children and was within the normal range for DSS scores. The DSS score best represents the children's normal use of language in conversation. There were some intragroup significant differences (e.g., both groups demonstrated more stuttering on more linguistically complex utterances). Interruption and speaking rates were not different between the two groups of children. A stepwise discriminant functional analysis (Dixon, 1983; Glass & Hopkins, 1984) revealed no distinguishing patterns between the two groups except for stuttering.

It appeared from these data that group comparisons between stuttering children and nonstuttering children demonstrated few differences between the two groups except, of course, for any measure which included stuttering. One may also infer the same thing from the extensive reviews of Nippold (1990) and Nippold and Rudzinski (1995). Both of these reviews concluded with recommendations for more, albeit better, group research. Two important alternatives, however, as discussed below, are longitudinal and single-subject design analyses.

PHASE II: LONGITUDINAL STUDY RESULTS

Preliminary longitudinal data are shown in Figure 8–1 for 11 stuttering children for 8 of the 12 variables shown in Table 8–1 for approximately a 1-year period (Ryan, 1984, 1990, 1993). None of these children received any treatment during this period, including parent counselling. The four test points were approximately 3–4 months apart. These data include both children who eventually outgrew the problem (natural or sponta-neous recovery) and children who did not. Conclusions drawn from these data are tentative and presented here only to make a simple point that most of the children (circa 67%) had both spontaneously decreased stuttering and had improved in almost all other measures. The children were approximately 4 years old during the first measure and 5 years old at the fourth measure, a year later.

The first measure shown in Figure 8–1 is stuttering rate. It can be seen that there was a decrease in stuttering for the group from 10.9 SW/M to 9.2 SW/M, which does not show some of the individual subjects who demonstrated extensive reduction. Additionally, these major im-provements were somewhat masked by the scores of the one subject who became worse. Only statements are shown in Figure 8–1, but both statements and questions increased and their percent stuttered de-creased. The TOLD score showed an increase up to over 100, well within normal range. This was a scaled score which controlled for age. There was a large increase between test period 1 (91.5) and test period 2 (101), a difference of 10.5 points, and another large change is seen between test period 3 (97.0) and test period 4 (105.0). Although this may suggest a test-retest reliability problem, the test-retest reliability (stability) of the TOLD total score is reported to be .99 (Newcomer & Hammill, 1982a, p. 21, 1982b). Next, the grammatic completion subtest demonstrated a dramatic increase from well below normal (5.5) to a mean 9.8 (10 is normal). The test-retest reliability of this test is re-ported to be .96. The changes in this score alone may have accounted for a large part of the change in the overall TOLD score. The DSS scores also indicate growth. These data suggest that any language problem, if it ever existed, disappeared by the second test period. The next measure is interruption, which also demonstrated an increase. As the children became more fluent, they and their parents interrupted each other more often. Finally, speaking rate demonstrated an increase, partly due to maturation and partly due to the reduction in stuttering. May one infer that any one or more of these variables caused the im-provement in stuttering? Or, were these changes simply reflective of growth and/or low test-retest reliability of some measures? It is not clear.

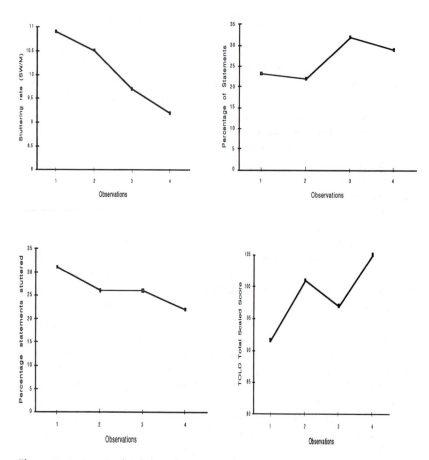

Figure 8–1. Longitudinal data (four quarterly observations) for eight variables for 11 subjects over a 1-year period, from Ryan (1984). *Continued on page 169*

One additional effort to determine a possible relationship between or among these variables and stuttering was completed in a group research format (Ryan, 1984). A multiple correlation (stepwise and all possible subsets regression) (Dixon, 1983; Glass & Hopkins, 1984) was performed to predict SW/M of the fourth test period. Predictor variables studied included scores from the first test period, including the 12 from Table 8–1 and topographical variables such as part-word repetition and phrase repetition (Johnson, 1961; Ryan, 1974).

As shown in Table 8–2, the first major predictor variable chosen was Grammatic Completion; this variable was also one of the 12 on which stuttering children had performed significantly worse than non-stuttering children (Table 8–1). The next three variables (two to four) were initial stuttering itself (SW/M) and two types of normal disfluency

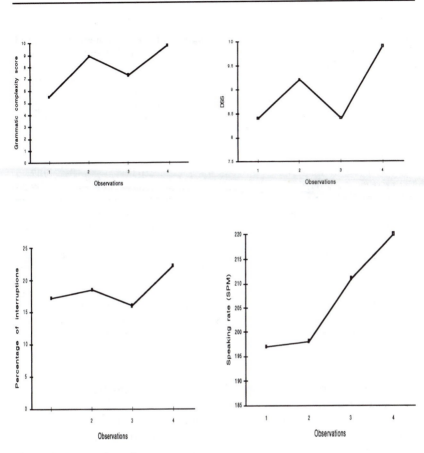

Figure 8–1. (*continued*)

(Revision and Incomplete Phrase). Finally, percentage of questions stuttered was added to take the predictive Multiple R to .997. These are of some interest, but hardly startling or definitive proof of a relationship between stuttering and any one or more of these variables. In fact the results were rather circular, because four of these five variables were stuttering itself or related behaviors.

The statistical procedure of Multiple R, additionally, has many limitations, such as that it may be only meaningful for the subset of scores used in the original computation and correlation does not mean causation. The formula shown in the note in Table 8–2 to predict SW/M in the fourth measurement period, while effective for children inside the initial set, demonstrated 40% error for child outside the initial set, hardly accurate enough to demonstrate real relationships between these variables

Table 8–2. Multiple Correlation (2-Step Regression) for 11 Stuttering Preschool Children Employing 46 Variables of First Test Period to Predict Stuttering (SW/M) in Fourth Test Period.

Variables	Partial Correlation	Multiple R
1. Grammatic completion (TOLD)	−.451	.635
2. Stuttered words per minute (SW/M)	.644	.851
3. Revisions	−.204	.945
4. Incomplete phrases	.163	.982
5. Questions stuttered %	−.287	.997

Source: From Ryan, B. (1984). "Stuttering in Preschool Children: A Comparison and Longitudinal Study." Paper presented at the annual convention of the American Speech-Language-Hearing Association, San Francisco, CA.

Note: The formula from the R: 15.2 −.451 (Grammatic Completion) + .644 (SW/M, test period 1) −.204 (Revisions) + .163 (Incomplete Phrase) −.287 (Questions stuttered %) = SW/M (test period 4) was applied to two selected subjects, one from within and one from without the set. The example from within the set indicated: Subject 1 15.2 −.451 (4) + .644 (10.9) −.204 (0) + .163 (12.5) − .287 (0) = 22.5 SW/M predicted with 22.8 observed for a difference of .3 SW/M less. The example for Subject 12 from outside the set predicted 10.7 SW/M while the observed was 5.8 SW/M, yielding a difference of 4.9 SW/M more.

and stuttering or to be clinically helpful in predicting who would outgrow stuttering and who would not.

In sum, group research using both difference and correlation statistical analysis provided little, if any, helpful, positive information concerning stuttering and any one or more of the 72 variables studied to this point. Multiple R studies designed to predict children's stuttering from mother behavior variables also did not result in meaningful conclusions, except that speaking rate surfaced as a predominant variable for both mothers and children (Ryan, 1998). This lack of findings appears to suggest that group research, even with relatively sophisticated design and inferential statistical analysis, could not reveal much clinically relevant information regarding a large number of variables which were suspected of being related to stuttering.

PHASE III: SINGLE-SUBJECT STUDIES RESULTS

The three areas of linguistic proficiency (as represented by conversational speech acts and DSS linguistic complexity), interruption, and speaking rate were selected for single-subject design study in Phase III. These variables had not shown much value or relationship to stuttering in group design (Phase I) or longitudinal (Phase II) investigations. Nevertheless, other researchers and clinicians were still writing about these variables, studying them, and speculating about their possible contribution to stuttering development and treatment (e.g., speaking rate: Kelly, 1993; interruption: Meyers & Freeman, 1985a; linguistic: Bernstein Ratner, 1993).

It seemed possible that single-subject design, with its inherent flexibility and experimental nature (Attanasio, 1994; Barlow, Hayes, & Nelson, 1984; Barlow & Hersen, 1984; Connell & Thompson, 1986; Kearns, 1986; McReynolds & Kearns, 1983; McReynolds & Thompson, 1986), might show a functional relationship between one or more of these variables and stuttering, if such a relationship existed.

Following single-subject design principles (Attanasio, 1994; Connell & Thompson, 1986, Barlow & Hersen, 1984; McReynolds & Kearns, 1983; McReynolds & Thompson, 1986) studies were designed to manipulate only one independent variable (e.g., interruption) and experimentally examine its functional relationship with stuttering; that is, would its presentation increase or decrease the frequency of the one dependent variable, stuttering, in simple ABA designs? If the contribution of these independent variables could be identified, they could then be controlled or used to develop appropriate treatment programs for stuttering, if they were of value.

The 12 single-subject studies conducted to date have used different single-subject designs and forms of the variables (e.g., three forms of interruption), or levels or types of the variables (e.g., various speaking rates). The designs may be characterized as extensions of the basic ABA formats, such as ABCDA with three different treatments or variations of an independent variable. A continual, per-session base rate (similar to generalization or multiple probes; Horner & Baer, 1978) was used to control for spontaneous or natural recovery between sessions, which might have influenced the stuttering of the child, and to detect generalization, if any occurred. Thus, some of the designs may be viewed as daily ABA or ACA or ADA formats. These designs may also be described as interrupted time series with continual, per-session base rate natural conversations between the clinician and/or mother with the children (Bordens & Abbott, 1996, pp. 167–168, 302–305; Hegde, 1994, pp. 197–210) concurrent with manipulation or manipulation conversations with mother or clinician-experimenter. These designs are representative of those suggested by McReynolds and Kearns (1983, Chapter 6) and the flexibility of single-subject research discussed by Connell and Thompson (1986), Kearns (1986), and McReynolds and Thompson (1986). These designs often did not include complete return to base rate or to premanipulation levels of the dependent variable (e.g., AAABBBAA-ACCCAAA), because it was desired to efficiently test many independent variables, observe the daily generalization from manipulation conversations to continuing base rate conversations with preschool stuttering children, and to avoid lengthy postmanipulation base rates in an effort to return to base rate levels. The limitation of interpretation due to not returning to base rate until the dependent variable resumes its premanipulation level in between treatments is recognized and conclusions were accordingly tempered.

Some may view some of the designs as Alternating Treatment Designs (ATD) (Barlow & Hersen, 1984, pp. 252–284) because of the daily "alternation" of manipulation and the continuing base rate conditions (e.g., ABABABA) of a session. The label of the design is not as important as the observations of the functional relationship between the dependent variable and the independent variable. A simple description of the arrangements is desired. Finally, to identify base rate conversations (no arranged manipulations or contingencies) as treatment conditions (arranged manipulations or contingencies) seems inconsistent.

The basic tenets of single-subject design were also followed: objective measurement, changing only one element per phase, at least three data points during each phase, appropriate reliability procedures, and the use of trend, level, and slope strategies of analysis (McReynolds & Kearns, 1983). Because of the space restrictions of this chapter and for other reasons, this chapter will present only minimal, representative results of these studies, to make the point that such studies are necessary and helpful. The complete data will be found in articles published elsewhere (e.g., Wood & Ryan, 1998).

One important facet of these single-subject designs was to use clinician-experimenter or mother and child conversation with no manipulanda (e.g., toys). A purely conversational format provided for more talking by the preschool child, consistently contained the most stuttering of all the many different measurements, and prevented the problems that might be associated with differences in behavior between "pure" conversation and "play" conversation with Legos (Allen, 1985). For these single-subject studies each of the conversations were 10 min in length. The first 120 turns (60 for each partner), about 2 min of child and mother or clinician- experimenter talk time (Ryan, 1974), were analyzed from each conversation which commonly yielded about 300 words or 333 syllables (Ryan, 1998) within the first 5–7 min of the 10-min conversation. This was consonant with previous cross-sectional research (Ryan, 1998) so comparisons could be made, if necessary. The entire 10 min of the manipulation session conversations were analyzed in order to observe experimental results.

The design of these studies also had to control for other factors including spontaneous or natural recovery. Observation of preschool stuttering children in the longitudinal study (Phase II) had shown that these children could spontaneously recover within as short a period as a week, although most took longer (mean = 3 years). To control for this and to measure generalization, each single-subject study incorporated at least three monthly premanipulation base rate and continual base rate (generalization or multiple probe) measures.

Second, in order to control for motivation and consequences, positive consequences were provided for desired behavior in the manipulation portions of a session or a combination of positive statements and inexpensive toys were provided after selected sessions. "Stop, speak fluently" or "Slow down" were used as forms of punishment delivered contingent on stuttering or some combination of both. Finally, because the children in these studies were very young, sessions were no more than 40 min in length and most commonly no more than 30 min, with some change of partner or activity from clinician-experimenter to mother, or from manipulation to base rate conversation, every 10 min.

Linguistic Proficiency:
Conversational Speech Acts and Linguistic Complexity

No preschool stuttering child, out of the 51 in the past 15 years in the Genesis of Stuttering project, has had a measurable clinical language problem (see Ryan, 1992). Still, it seemed desirable to test the possible contribution of language proficiency to stuttering, in part because more complex linguistic forms appeared to be accompanied by increased stuttering (Bernstein Ratner & Sih, 1987). However, nonstuttering children had also demonstrated the same phenomenon (see Table 8–1 with items from Ryan, 1998), which suggested that this phenomenon may be representative of preschool children's developing language ability rather than reflecting a connection between language proficiency and stuttering. It had also been observed that complex language forms were used relatively infrequently by preschool stuttering and nonstuttering children in conversations with their mothers (Ryan, 1995; Soyejima, 1993), so the point may be moot.

Despite these considerations, studies were designed to train the subject on language proficiency (independent variable) to see if increased language proficiency would reduce stuttering (dependent variable). Meyers and Freeman (1985b) had observed lowered performance by stuttering children on the Peabody Picture Vocabulary Test (Dunn & Dunn, 1981), as had Ryan (1992) on the Picture Vocabulary Test of the TOLD. Both of these findings suggested that reduced receptive vocabulary was a possible contributing linguistic factor. Ryan (1984, 1998) had also observed that stuttering children had difficulty in conversation in the use of irregular verbs (e.g., using "sawd" for the past tense of the verb, "to see").

The language training program used for this study had four parts. The first part, Program B–1, was to train the subject to correctly name selected Peabody Picture Language Development Kit vocabulary cards

Table 8–3. Representative Language Measures for Pretest, Post-Language Training (Post 1), and Post-Language/Fluency Training (Post 2) for One Subject.

Measures	Pretest	Post-Language Training	Post-Language/ Fluency Training
Conversation correct irregular verbs %	75	86	80
Peabody Picture Vocabulary Test	81	98	101
TOLD			
Total	91	104	99
Subtests			
Picture vocabulary	11	12	11
Sentence imitation	5	7	6
Grammatic completion	7	10	7

Sources: From McFadden, D. (1996). "The Experimental Manipulation of Stuttering Using Language Training and Consequences II." Unpublished master's thesis, California State University, Long Beach; and Butcher et al. (1998). "The Effects of Language Training on Stuttering." Manuscript in preparation.

Note: Peabody Picture Vocabulary Test and TOLD test total and subtest scores are scaled scores adjusted for age.

(Dunn & Smith, 1965) and correctly identify pictures of Boehm concepts (Boehm, 1969). The second part, Program B–2, was to train correct use of irregular verbs. The third part, Program B–3, used the five conversational speech acts in the reverse order of which they evoked stuttering: answers, statements, questions, commands, and corrections (Ryan, 1998). The fourth part, Program C (language/fluency training), was a repeat of Program B–3 with the contingency of "Stop, speak fluently," following each stuttered word and "Good" and tokens for fluent utterances. We measured stuttering both within training sessions and in accompanying continual base rate conversations with the clinician-experimenter and the mother. Training phase B was conducted the first semester and training phase C was conducted the second semester, twice weekly for 50 min over the two 3-month semester periods, respectively.

Representative data on the effects of the language training on language proficiency are shown in Table 8–3 for six language measures administered pre- and twice posttraining for one subject (Butcher, McFadden, Quinn, & Ryan, 1998; McFadden, 1996). Language improved on all six measures from the pretest to the first posttest after 3 months of language training (Program B). Language scores then slightly decreased after an additional 3 months of language/fluency training (Program C) which primarily focussed on improving fluency across five conversational speech acts by consequating stuttering and positively reinforcing fluency.

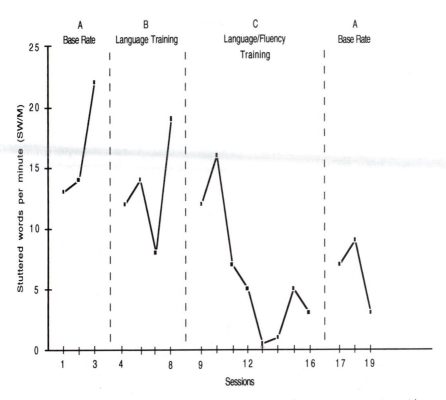

Figure 8–2. Stuttered words per minute (SW/M) for a subject in conversation with mother during continual base rate (generalization probes) while in language and language-fluency training, from McFadden (1996) and Butcher et al. (1998).

Second, representative data on the effects on stuttering frequency of language training (Program B) and language/fluency training (Program C) on stuttering frequency are shown in Figure 8–2 (from Butcher et al., 1998; McFadden, 1996). These data were drawn from the continual base rate conversations (generalization probes) with the mother that were held in each session along with the manipulation sessions with the clinician. The first base rate A represents three measures at 4-month intervals. The results shown in Figure 8–2 clearly demonstrate minimal or no effect on stuttering during the 3 months of pure language training (B). Only during Program C, with its contingencies for stuttering and fluency instituted, were there reductions in stuttering. The slight increase in stuttering in the second base rate A phase may not be a clear indication of the withdrawal effect of the training program, but it does suggest partial generalization of the improved fluency shown in the training phase to the A phase, which was a positive result for the child.

It appears from these data that language training did noticeably improve language proficiency as measured by the tests employed, but this improvement did not influence stuttering frequency. Stuttering was reduced only after contingencies for fluent and stuttered speech were added to the language program. Further, the observation that language proficiency was actually slightly diminished concurrent with the improvement in fluency (Table 8–3) suggests that the two behaviors, language proficiency and stuttering, may function independently of each other.

None of the data anywhere else in the literature (e.g., Bloodstein, 1987, 1995) are persuasive of the need for, or value of, language training for young stuttering children. The one consistent finding that more complex language evokes more stuttering is not a difficult issue, because most behavioral research has demonstrated effective treatment of stuttering with no special attention to linguistic complexity (e.g., Lincoln, Onslow, Lewis, & Wilson, 1996; Onslow, Andrews, & Lincoln, 1994; Ryan & Ryan, 1983, 1995).

This single-subject design research essentially demonstrated one more time, in one more way, that there is no important role of language proficiency in stuttering treatment. The GILCU Program (Ryan, 1974; Ryan & Ryan, 1983, 1995) does imply the existence of a linguistic component, but the essence of the GILCU program is a gradual increase in the number of words and a conversational speech act sequence (reading to monologue to conversation) with minimal specific control of true linguistic complexity, per se (e.g., DSS level). The minimal role of language in stuttering development and treatment is also confirmed by the observation that although stuttering children may show minor language deficiency, they do eventually, naturally overcome it (Figure 8–1). If language deficiency produces stuttering there should be a large number of children with bona fide clinical language problems who also stutter. There are not. Neither language proficiency as measured by tests of language (e.g., Ryan, 1992), nor linguistic complexity in conversation (e.g., DSS, Ryan, 1998), nor the pragmatic aspect of conversational speech acts (e.g., questions, Ryan, 1998), nor accompanying language training (Butcher et al., 1998; McFadden, 1996), seems to play much of a role in either stuttering development or treatment.

Interruption

Interruption is still viewed as possibly evoking stuttering (Gottwald & Starkweather, 1995; Ramig & Bennett, 1995) or at the very least, as evoked by stuttering, although empirical studies (e.g., Kelly & Conture,

1992; Meyers & Freeman, 1985a; Ryan, 1998; see Table 8–1) have failed to find differences in interruption behavior between children who stutter and those who do not. Again, the logic behind the following study was to test the contribution of interruption in a single-subject design format, with interruption as the independent variable and stuttering as the dependent variable.

Previous research (see Table 8–1, Ryan, 1998) had shown interruption to occur in about 20% of the mother-child conversational turns and that there were three major forms of interruption: the speaker as interrupter, the speaker as interruptee, and simultaneous start where two speakers start to speak at the same time. Therefore, the following conditions of interruption were tested: (a) the clinician-experimenter interrupted stuttered speech making the subject the interruptee, (b) the subject interrupted the clinician-experimenter, making the clinician-experimenter the interruptee, (c) the clinician-experimenter interrupted fluent speech making the subject, again, the interruptee, (d) simultaneous start, and (e) no interruption. Interruption was increased to 50% of the turns or more than twice as much interruption during manipulation sessions.

Representative data for the first two conditions for the subject from Livingston (1993) and Livingston, Flowers, Hodor, and Ryan (1998) are shown in Figure 8–3 as SW/M for the child during continual base rates with mother and clinician-experimenter and manipulation with the clinician-experimenter. There was a decreasing trend of stuttering in both phase B, clinician-experimenter interrupts child, and phase C, child interrupts clinician-experimenter. Stuttering rates from the continual base rates with mother and clinician-experimenter generally paralleled those of the manipulation sessions, although the actual levels varied with the child demonstrating more stuttering with mother than with the clinician-experimenter and more stuttering during manipulation than in continual base rate with the clinician-experimenter. Unfortunately, the postmanipulation base rate A data were obtained months after the conclusion of the study, and so are not meaningful. Of some interest, the child continued to speak more fluently and was more fluent with mother than with the clinician.

Of most interest is that increasing interruption did not increase stuttering beyond prestudy base rate A levels, although this child did stutter more with the clinician-experimenter when the clinician-experimenter was interrupting more often (50%) in both manipulation phases B and C than when the clinician-experimenter did in continual base rate (20%). Single-subject design research provided similar results to that of group design; that is, interruption plays only a small, if any, role in stuttering (the difference being 8 SW/M vs. 6 SW/M in phase B and 10.5 SW/M vs. 7.5 SW/M in phase C for the clinician-experimenter conversations).

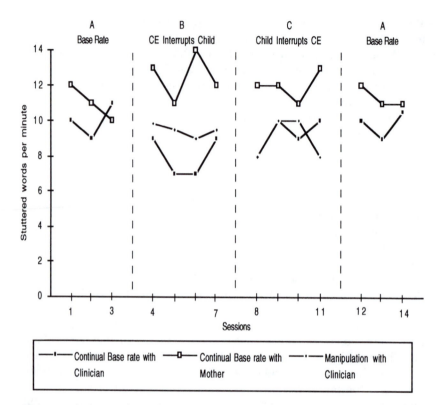

Figure 8–3. Stuttered words per minute (SW/M) for a subject in conversation during pre- and post-base rate, two continual base rates (generalization probes) with the clinician-experimenter and mother and two different manipulation of interruption conditions with the clinician-experimenter (CE), from Livingston (1993) and Livingston et al. (1998).

Hence, the attention to it as part of a clinical treatment program or as advice to parents of stuttering children (e.g., Gottwald & Starkweather, 1995; Ramig & Bennett, 1995) is not supported by these empirical data with the caveat that it was the clinician-experimenter, not the mother, who did the increased interruption in these studies.

Speaking Rate

The last variable examined in these studies was speaking rate. Subjects who had a high speaking rate and whose parents had a high speaking rate have been rarely encountered over the past 15 years (e.g., the subject in Wood & Ryan, 1998). There were certainly not enough of these children to suggest that stuttering children, as a group, demonstrated higher speaking rates than nonstuttering children (a finding also reported by Kelly & Conture, 1992 and by Ryan, 1992, 1998). Nor, for that matter, did the stuttering children show lower speaking rates as suggested by Meyers and Freeman (1985b). Mothers of children who stuttered did not speak faster than mothers of children who did not stutter (Kelly & Conture, 1992; Ryan, 1998). Surprisingly, there were few data on the effects of speaking rate on stuttering frequency, especially for children (for exceptions see Guitar, Schaefer, Donahue-Kilburg, & Bond, 1992; Johnson, 1980; Stephenson-Opsal & Bernstein Ratner, 1988; Zebrowski et al., 1996). There were also no reliable norms for nonstuttering fluent speakers, with the exception of those provided by Craven and Ryan (1985), for determining whether the speaking rate of a client or parent was abnormal. Although it may be argued that we do not need such norms because all that is necessary is the client's premanipulation base rate, such normative data for speaking rate could be clinically useful to (a) decide whether a particular client is speaking relatively fast and (b) provide appropriate clinical targets for fluent speech.

Slow speech was created by introducing pauses in between words (e.g., "I. . .want . . .you . . .to. . . talk. . .slow. . .ly") rather than prolonged speech (e.g., "IIIwaaantyouuutooootaaalkslooowlyyy"). Prolonged speech presents the problems of reduced normal prosody, the need for eventual elimination of it, and the difficulty some speech-language pathologists had in teaching it (Onslow & Ingham, 1989; Ryan & Ryan, 1983, 1995). For these reasons, paused speech (slow speech with pauses in between syllables not noticeably prolonged) was considered to be better than prolonged speech for these studies.

Wood and Ryan (1998) used slow, paused speech with a 9-year-old female and showed that increasing speaking rate had increased stuttering rate and vice versa. Further, gradually increasing speaking rate from a slow (100 SPM) to a normal, base rate of 250 SPM with consequences for stuttered and fluent speech, had resulted in normal fluency in a reasonable amount of time (3.5 hours) which had persisted over 3 years. The attendant problems of changes in prosody, difficulty in the resumption of normal rate, and difficulty in teaching this slow speech had not surfaced or were eliminated with this slow, paused speech strategy. It was also clear from this first study that the relationship between stuttering and speaking rate is not simple.

Because the results with this 9-year-old child seemed so similar to those achieved previously with prolonged speech (Ryan & Ryan, 1983, 1995; Ryan & Van Kirk, 1974a, 1974b, 1978), and therefore were not remarkable, the next step was to study the speaking rates of mother-child dyads. These investigations were designed to study that natural mother-child dyadic situation, and also to devise a program for mothers to alter their speech rate to change children's stuttering. Thus Jones (1994) and Jones and Ryan (1998) studied the effects of mother's slowed speech on the stuttering of the child. The mother was first asked to slow down her own speech rate, then the mother slowed the child's speech rate.

Representative data based on Jones (1994) and Jones and Ryan (1998) are shown in Figure 8–4. Speaking rate, SPM, was determined by counting syllables on the Stuttering Treatment Rating Recorder (STRR) (Fowler & Ingham, 1986) during talking time only (no pauses, see "talk time"; Ryan, 1974) and dividing the number of syllables by the actual on-line talking time. This is slightly different from "articulation rate" which excludes both pauses and any disfluencies. Both mother and child had demonstrated stability of response rate for stuttering and speaking rate across three monthly sessions during the premanipulation base rate A phase. During phases B and C, sessions were conducted twice weekly. During these phases, there were three 10-min conversations between mother and child per session: a 10-min premanipulation conversation (continuing base rate) just before manipulation, then 10 min of manipulation (slowing speaking rate), and finally 10 min more of normal conversation in a postmanipulation continuing base rate (postmanipulation generalization probe). Each manipulation session could therefore be characterized as either ABA or ACA.

For phase B (Mother Slow), the instructions to the mother were, "Please speak slowly," and she was calibrated to speak at under 100 SPM. As can be seen in Figure 8–4, the mother did slow down her speech rate and the child's stuttering rate also concurrently decreased although his speaking rate did not change. It appeared at that point that simply slowing the mother's speaking rate would decrease the child's stuttering, but the interpretation of this finding is limited in that there was no complete return to a base rate phase A other than the continuing base rate (not shown here) which did not show a change in the intersession measures, but did show generalization to the postmanipulation measures. In addition, casual observation of what was occurring during the manipulation session suggested that the child, too, was talking slowly, but the data on the child's averaged speaking rate did not reflect this change.

The relationship between stuttering rate and SPM is, indeed, not simple (Meyers & Freeman 1985b; Stephenson-Opsal & Bernstein Ratner, 1988). One may reduce a stuttering child's speaking rate which will decrease the stuttering, but concurrent with the decrease in stuttering, the child's overall speaking rate may increase because the child is not spending speaking time stuttering. If one averages the speaking rate for the whole session, there appears to be no change in speaking rate of the child because the slow speech rate utilized by the child to speak fluently

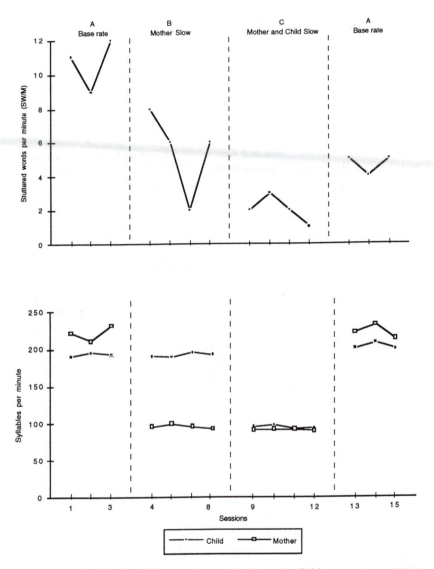

Figure 8–4. Stuttered words per minute (SW/M) and syllables per minute (SPM) for a subject and mother during base rate and two different manipulations of speaking rate, from Jones (1994) and Jones and Ryan (1998).

will be balanced by the increase in the child's speaking rate due to increased fluency. Without careful study of the within-session behavior of the subject, one will not detect that subtle interaction and averaging the whole session will mask it. The subject also had been talking slowly, but in streaks, not consistently. The subject's stuttering rate eventually increased (see session 8).

In phase C, the mother was instructed to reduce her speaking rate and to get the child to do likewise. The mother instructed the child to speak slowly and she consequated fast talking by telling the child, "Slow down, speak like I do." It can be seen that both the speaking and stuttering rates of the child decreased during this phase and remained at those low levels. In the poststudy base rate A phase, the child's speaking rate slightly exceeded that of the prestudy base rate A level, whereas the stuttering rate was less than that in the prestudy base rate A phase, suggesting that generalization had occurred. This inference that the reduced stuttering rate was related to phase C activities is limited by the fact that there was no full return to base rate between phases B and C, but is supported by the continual base rate data (not shown here) reported in Jones (1994) and Jones and Ryan (1998). The increased speaking rate was probably a function of reduced stuttering rate.

Both interruption rates and linguistic complexity levels (DSS scores) were measured for phase A base rate and manipulation sessions. No meaningful difference was observed. The DSS scores for the child were equal to or higher for the manipulation phases than for the prebase rate A. Mother's DSS, although variable, was not significantly different between the premanipulation base rate A and the manipulation phases. These results suggest that changing speaking rate did not significantly change linguistic complexity, but Bernstein Ratner (1992) had reported that both instructions to slow down and instructions to slow down and simplify linguistic complexity induced mothers to produce slower and less complex utterances. This difference between the two studies is even more dramatic, given that the mothers in our studies commonly lowered their speaking rates to less than 100 SPM (approximately 75 words per minute), whereas the mean in the Bernstein Ratner (1992) study for slow speech for 20 mothers was about 150 words spoken per minute. The major differences between these two studies were that Bernstein Ratner used normally fluent children and their mothers in a group research design with only two (pre and post) observations. Both of these factors could explain the differences in findings. Continued time-series observations, at least three per phase, in the single-subject design format, of stuttering children provided for a much different picture of the relationship between stuttering and speaking rate, and speaking rate and linguistic complexity, from that of two observations of normally fluent children and their mothers.

The subject continued to stutter at around 3.0 SW/M over the next 18 months during weekly maintenance sessions in which the mother spoke slowly and asked the child to speak slowly. Normally fluent speech was not achieved until we added the components of (a) mother had to accurately identify each stuttered word (90% or better), and (b) had to insist that the child did, indeed, slow down contingent on the mother's instructions to do so. Four months (12 sessions) of this produced normally fluent speech which the child has demonstrated for over 1 year now during gradually decreasing follow-up sessions.

Single-subject research had permitted observation of the important functional relationship between stuttering and speaking rate. The problem was not to be solved through group research trying to determine whether children who stuttered spoke faster or slower than children who did not; rate of speech itself was a major determinant of stuttering and varying that rate produced an effect. However, it was single-subject design that permitted us to tease out the relationship between speaking rate and stuttering and lead us to an effective treatment program.

Further Issues in Single-Subject Design

A recent study by Onslow, Packman, Stocker, van Doorn, and Siegel (1997) on the effects of time-out in an ABA single-subject design with three subjects is also relevant to this discussion. The study by Onslow et al. (1997) clearly demonstrated the relationship between stuttering and response-contingent stimulation, replicating some earlier research. It also replicated the findings of Ryan and Van Kirk (1974a) and Ryan and Ryan (1983). Onslow et al. (1997) observed that time-out (punishment), although effective in reducing stuttering in two of three subjects, did not produce the same effect for the third severe subject. This result is similar to those obtained with four subjects (Ryan & Ryan, 1983; Ryan & Van Kirk, 1974a) using a different form of punishment. This observation suggests that appropriate systematic replication is an important part of any research program.

Many questions remain unanswered such as those raised by the work of Onslow and colleagues (e.g., Lincoln et al., 1996). Do we really need only to control the consequences of stuttering and fluency, or must we also have some other component such as gradual increase in length of utterance or slowed speaking rate in order to produce efficacious treatment for young stuttering children? Although Lincoln et al. (1996) made the point that their subjects were at normal speaking rates after the conclusion of operant, consequence control, they did not share data about speaking rate during the process of achieving fluent speech. How did the subjects do that? Did they first slow down to become fluent, and then speed up as they became fluent? The relationship between speaking rate and stuttering is complex. Only further research will answer that question, but it appears that the control of speaking rate and consequences for fluency may provide one possible treatment of stuttering in preschool children, if parents can be informed about and trained in these procedures.

In the last 2 years during the process of attempting to publish single-subject studies (Livingston et al., 1998; Wood & Ryan, 1998), as exemplified by those presented above, I have run into colleagues serving as reviewers who apparently do not understand single-subject design research. I was able to document 97 different statements by reviewers and editors clearly demonstrating lack of knowledge of single-subject design which I incorporated in a letter to both the publication board and the journal's association president. The responses from both were polite, but the problem was not acknowledged and nothing changed.

A second, but different, illustration of reduced knowledge of single-subject research is the published research on mothers' and children's speaking rates by Bernstein Ratner (1992), Stephenson-Opsal and Bernstein Ratner (1988), and Zebrowski et al. (1996).

In addition to numerous other design problems (e.g., too few subjects for even small group research), these studies failed to cast their research and consequent reports in single-subject design format. Had they used the scientific strategies available in single-subject design research (Attanasio, 1994; Barlow, Hayes, & Nelson, 1984; Barlow & Hersen, 1984; Connell & Thompson, 1986; Kearns, 1986; McReynolds & Kearns, 1983; McReynolds & Thompson, 1986), they probably would have shown less variability in their results and produced more helpful, accurate information about the relationship between speaking rate and stuttering in mother-child dyads. One is left to infer that the researchers did not understand single-subject design well enough to employ it, or if they did understand single-subject design, they did not respect the power of single-subject design to answer such research questions as theirs. Instead, their studies demonstrated, again, that group research or quasi-case study research is not going to clearly demonstrate the true, functional relationship between any independent variable (e.g., speaking rate) and stuttering.

A third illustration is found in the otherwise comprehensive and accurate review of the research in the development of stuttering of Nippold and Rudzinski (1995), who recommended only more sophisticated cross-sectional group research to tease out the relationship between the variables they discussed and stuttering. They did not offer that single-subject design studies might also be very appropriate to determine these relationships.

A fourth illustration is found in Ingham and Cordes (1996) where they suggest and document that research in stuttering often demonstrates a lack of respect for, or understanding of, scientific treatment data. These same factors (lack of respect for and knowledge of science) may explain the problems of reduced knowledge and practice of single-subject design research discussed above. Finally, there is a paucity of single-subject research reported in our literature.

It appears that our profession may lack the knowledge, hence the will and/or ability, either to carryout single-subject design research or to evaluate the single-subject design research of others, much less understand the need for single-subject design research. I am concerned about the apparent low level of knowledge, in my opinion, of single-subject design demonstrated by many of the editors and reviewers of our major journals (read active researchers) and what that augurs for the future of our much needed single-subject research. This may help explain why there is such a need for single-subject design research at the present time. Only a few people are doing it, because only a few people understand it well enough to engage in such research or to recast their research questions into a form which may be solved by single-subject design research, and those who do single-subject research will find difficulty in the publication process. The resolution is for the field to increase the knowledge and practice of single-subject design research.

CONCLUSIONS

A major conclusion is that single-subject design research produced different results from group design research in the study of variables related to stuttering. In the case of *linguistic variables*, group research suggested some differences between stuttering and nonstuttering children, whereas single-subject design did not indicate a functional relationship. Proponents of the value of the study of linguistic variables in stuttering research have yet to demonstrate functional relationships in single-subject research, and probably will not, and yet are critical of those who do not control for linguistic complexity in their research.

In the case of *interruption*, both single-subject and group design indicated no differences or correlations and minimal functional relationships. However, it should be noted that some authorities (e.g., Gottwald & Starkweather, 1995) continue to recommend control of interruption as a clinical treatment process.

In the case of *speaking rate*, group designs indicated no difference, whereas single-subject research suggested critical, important functional relationships between stuttering and speaking rate which have major implications for clinical application. Two of our six children on speaking rate treatment programs are normally fluent, one has moved away, three have greatly reduced their stuttering, and we are optimistic about them achieving normal fluency in the near future.

Single-subject study of clinically employed independent variables can lead to identification of those which will make a difference in the client's speech (e.g., see the work of Onslow and colleagues). Organizing these variables into a program will produce an efficacious treatment procedure (e.g., speaking rate control) for young stuttering children (e.g., Jones & Ryan, 1998; Wood & Ryan, 1998). Single-subject design research can be used to answer the recent question raised by the work of Onslow and colleagues of whether both contingencies for stuttering and fluency and a procedure such as slow talk are necessary for effective treatment or only contingencies for stuttering and fluency. Single-subject research can demonstrate the important relationships between the independent variables we manipulate as clinicians and the problem which we wish to ameliorate, stuttering. We should increase our knowledge and practice of single-subject research.

ACKNOWLEDGMENTS: I wish to acknowledge the Communicative Disorders Department students of California State University, Long Beach for their contribution to the collection and analysis of the data reported in this chapter, especially Karen Allen, Linda Livingston, Pat Jones, Cheryl Marsh, Denis McFadden, Lisa Soyejima, and Mary Sorci Wood.

REFERENCES

Allen, K. (1985). *A comparison of conversations with and without Legos*. Unpublished manuscript, California State University–Long Beach.

Attanasio, J. (1994). Inferential statistics and treatment efficacy studies in communication disorders. *Journal of Speech and Hearing Research, 37*, 755–759.

Barlow, D., Hayes, S., & Nelson, R. (1984). *The scientist practitioner: Research in clinical and educational settings*. Boston: Allyn & Bacon.

Barlow, D., & Hersen, M. (1984). *Single case experimental designs. Strategies for studying behavior change* (2nd ed.). New York: Pergamon Press.

Bernstein Ratner, N. (1992). Measurable outcomes of instructions to modify normal parent-child verbal interactions: Implications for stuttering therapy. *Journal of Speech and Hearing Research, 35*, 14–20.

Bernstein Ratner, N. (1993). Parents, children, and stuttering. *Seminars in Speech and Language, 14*, 238–249.

Bernstein Ratner, N., & Sih, C. (1987). Effects of gradual increase in sentence length and complexity on children's disfluency. *Journal of Speech and Hearing Disorders, 52*, 278–287.

Bloodstein, O. (1987). *A handbook on stuttering* (4th ed.). Chicago, IL: The National Easter Seal Society.

Bloodstein, O. (1995). *A handbook on stuttering* (5th ed.). San Diego, CA: Singular Publishing Group.

Boehm, A. (1969). *Boehm Test of Basic Concepts*. New York: The Psychological Corporation.

Bordens, K., & Abbott, B. (1996). *Research design and methods: A process approach.* Mountain View, California: Mayfield Publishing Co.

Butcher, K., McFadden, D., Quinn, B., & Ryan, B. (1998). *The effects of language training on stuttering.* Manuscript in preparation.

Connell, P., & Thompson, C. (1986). Flexibility of single-subject designs. Part III: Using flexibility to design or modify experiments. *Journal of Speech and Hearing Disorders, 51,* 214–225.

Craven, D., & Ryan, B. (1985). *Disfluent behavior of normal speakers: Three tasks.* Paper presented at the annual convention of American Speech-Language-Hearing Association, Washington, DC.

Dixon, W. (Ed.) (1983). *BMDP Statistical Software.* Berkeley: University of California Press.

Dunn, L., & Dunn, L. (1981). *Peabody Picture Vocabulary Test* (Rev. ed.). Circle Pines, MN: American Guidance Service, Inc.

Dunn, L., & Smith, J. (1965). *Peabody Language Development Kit for Level P (Primary).* Circle Pines, MN: American Guidance Service, Inc.

Fowler, S., & Ingham, R. (1986). Stuttering Treatment Rating Recorder (Version 2.0)[Computer software]. Santa Barbara, CA: University of California, Santa Barbara.

Glass, G., & Hopkins, K. (1984). *Statistical methods in education and psychology* (2nd ed.). Englewood Cliffs, NJ: Prentice-Hall.

Gottwald, S., & Starkweather, C. (1995). Fluency intervention for preschoolers and their families in the public schools. *Language, Speech, and Hearing Services in Schools, 26,* 117–126.

Guitar, B., Schaefer, H., Donahue-Kilburg, G., & Bond, L. (1992). Parent verbal interactions and speech rate: A case study in stuttering. *Journal of Speech and Hearing Research, 35,* 742–754.

Hegde, M. (1994). *Clinical research in communicative disorders: Principles and strategies* (2nd ed.). Austin, TX: Pro-Ed.

Horner, D., & Baer, D. (1978). Multiple-probe technique: A variation of the multiple baseline. *Journal of Applied Behavior Analysis, 11,* 189–196.

Ingham, R. (1997). Valid distinctions between findings obtained from single-subject and group studies of stuttering: Some reflections on Kalinowski et al. (1995). *Journal of Fluency Disorders, 22,* 51–56.

Ingham, R., & Cordes, A. (1996). *On watching a discipline shoot itself in the foot: Some observations on current trends in stuttering treatment research.* Based on a paper read to the third Annual Leadership Conference of the American Speech-Language-Hearing Association's Special Interest Division 4, Monterey, California, May 2, 1996.

Johnson, L. (1980). Facilitating parental involvement in treatment of the disfluent child. *Seminars in Speech, Language and Hearing, 1,* 301–310.

Johnson, W. (1961). Measurements of oral reading and speaking rate and disfluency of adult male and female stutterers and nonstutterers. *Journal of Speech and Hearing Disorders, Monograph Supplement, 7,* 1–20.

Jones, P. (1994). *An experimental analysis of the relationship between speaking rate and stuttering rate during mother-child conversation.* Unpublished master's thesis, California State University, Long Beach.

Jones, P., & Ryan, B. (1998). *Experimental analysis of speaking rate and stuttering in a mother-child dyad I*. Submitted for publication.

Kalinowski, J., Stuart, A., Armson, J. (1997). Response to Ingham: Seeking the truthfulness of stuttering research data. *Journal of Fluency Disorders, 22,* 57–60.

Kearns, K. (1986). Flexibility of single-subject designs. Part II: Design selection and arrangement of experimental phases. *Journal of Speech and Hearing Disorders, 51,* 204–213.

Kelly, E. (1993). Speech rates and turn-taking behaviors of children who stutter and their parents. *Seminars in Speech and Language, 14,* 203–214.

Kelly, E. (1994). Speech rates and turn-taking behaviors of children who stutter and their fathers. *Journal of Speech and Hearing Research, 37,* 1284–1294.

Kelly, E., & Conture, E. (1992). Speaking rates, response time latencies, and interrupting behaviors of young stutterers, nonstutterers, and their mothers. *Journal of Speech and Hearing Research, 35,* 1256–1267.

Lee, L. (1974). *Development sentence analysis.* Evanston, IL: Northwestern University Press.

Lincoln, M., Onslow, M., Lewis, C., & Wilson, L. (1996). A clinical trial of an operant treatment for school-age children who stutter. *American Journal of Speech-Language Pathology, 5,* 73–85.

Livingston, L. (1993). *The experimental analysis of interruption during conversation of a mother-child stuttering dyad.* Unpublished master's thesis, California State University, Long Beach.

Livingston, L., Flowers, Y., Hodor, B. & Ryan, B. (1998). *The experimental analysis of interruption during conversation for three children who stutter.* Manuscript submitted for publication.

McFadden, D. (1996). *The experimental manipulation of stuttering using language training and consequences II.* Unpublished master's thesis, California State University, Long Beach.

McReynolds, L. & Kearns, K. (1983). *Single-child experimental designs in communicative disorders.* Baltimore, MD: University Park Press.

McReynolds, L. & Thompson, C. (1986). Flexibility of single-subject designs. Part I: Review of the basics of single-subject designs. *Journal of Speech and Hearing Disorders, 51,* 194–203.

Meyers, S., & Freeman, F. (1985a). Interruptions as a variable in stuttering and disfluency. *Journal of Speech and Hearing Research, 28,* 428–435.

Meyers, S., & Freeman, F. (1985b). Mother and child speech rates as a variable of stuttering and disfluency. *Journal of Speech and Hearing Research, 28,* 436–444.

Newcomer, P., & Hammill, D. (1982a). *Manual of construction and statistical characteristics of the TOLD.* Austin, TX: Pro-Ed.

Newcomer, P., & Hammill, D. (1982b). *Test of language development.* Austin, TX: Pro-Ed.

Nippold, M. (1990). Concomitant speech and language disorders in stuttering children: A critique of the literature. *Journal of Speech and Hearing Disorders, 55,* 51–60.

Nippold, M., & Rudzinski, M. (1995). Parent's speech and children's stuttering: A critique of the literature. *Journal of Speech and Hearing Research, 38,* 978–989.

Onslow, M., Andrews, C., & Lincoln, M. (1994). A control/experimental trial of an operant treatment for early stuttering. *Journal of Speech and Hearing Research, 37*, 1244–1259.

Onslow, M., & Ingham, R. (1989). Whither prolonged speech? The disquieting evolution of stuttering therapy procedure. *Australian Journal of Human Communication Disorders, 17*, 67–81.

Onslow, M., Packman, A., Stocker, S., van Doorn, J., & Siegel, G. (1997). Control of children's stuttering with response-contingent time-out: Behavioral, perceptual, and acoustic data. *Journal of Speech, Language, and Hearing Research, 40*, 121–133.

Ramig, P., & Bennett, E. (1995). Working with 7–12-year-old children who stutter: Ideas for intervention in the public schools. *Language, Speech, and Hearing Services in Schools, 26*, 138–150.

Ryan, B. (1971). Operant procedures applied to stuttering treatment for children. *Journal of Speech and Hearing Disorders, 36*, 264–280.

Ryan, B. (1974). *Programmed therapy for stuttering in children and adults.* Springfield, IL: Charles C. Thomas.

Ryan, B. (1984). *Stuttering in preschool children: A comparison and longitudinal study.* Paper presented at the annual convention of American Speech-Language-Hearing Association, San Francisco, CA.

Ryan, B. (1990, November). *Development of Stuttering: A Longitudinal Study, Progress Report 4.* American Speech-Language-Hearing Association, Seattle, WA.

Ryan, B. (1992). Articulation, language, rate, and fluency characteristics of 20 stuttering and nonstuttering preschool children. *Journal of Speech and Hearing Research, 35*, 333–342.

Ryan, B. (1993, November). *Development of stuttering: A longitudinal study, Progress Report 5.* American Speech-Language-Hearing Association, Anaheim, CA, 1993.

Ryan, B. (1995). Language of stuttering and nonstuttering preschool children in tests and conversation. *Stuttering: Proceedings of the First World Congress on Fluency Disorders.* Munich: Germany: The International Fluency Association, pp. 191–197.

Ryan, B. (1998). *Speaking rate, conversational speech acts, and linguistic complexity of 20 preschool stuttering and nonstuttering children and their mothers.* Submitted for publication.

Ryan, B., & Marsh, C. (1985, November). *Stuttering in preschool children: A longitudinal study, Report 2.* American Speech-Language-Hearing Association, Washington, DC.

Ryan, B., & Marsh, C. (1987, November). *Stuttering in preschool children: A longitudinal study, Report 3.* American Speech-Language-Hearing Association, New Orleans, LA.

Ryan, B., & Ryan, B. (1983). Programmed treatment for children: Comparison of four programs. *Journal of Fluency Disorders, 8*, 291–321.

Ryan, B., & Ryan, B. (1995). Programmed stuttering treatment for children: Comparison of two establishment programs, through transfer, maintenance, and follow-up. *Journal of Speech and Hearing Research, 38*, 61–75.

Ryan, B., & Van Kirk, B. (1974a). *Programmed stuttering treatment for children. Final report*. Office of Education Project 0-72-4422, U.S. Department of Health, Education and Welfare, Washington, DC.

Ryan, B., & Van Kirk, B. (1974b). The establishment, transfer, and maintenance of fluent speech in 50 stutterers using delayed auditory feedback and operant procedures. *Journal of Speech and Hearing Research, 39*, 3–10.

Ryan, B., & Van Kirk, B. (1978). *Monterey fluency program*. Monterey, CA: Monterey Learning Systems.

Soyejima, L. (1993). *Stuttering and nonstuttering preschoolers' productions as measured by the Language Assessment, Remediation, Screening Procedure (LARSP)*. Unpublished master's thesis, California State University, Long Beach.

Stephenson-Opsal, D., & Bernstein Ratner, N. (1988). Maternal speech rate modification and childhood stuttering. *Journal of Fluency Disorders, 13*, 49–56.

Wood, M., & Ryan, B. (1998). *Experimental analysis of the speaking and stuttering rate in a child who stutters*. Submitted for publication.

Yairi, E., Ambrose, N., Paden, E., & Throneburg, R. (1996). Predictive factors of persistence and recovery: Pathways of children stuttering. *Journal of Communicative Disorders, 29*, 51–71.

Zebrowski, P., Weiss, A., Savelkoul, E., & Hammer, S. (1996). The effect of maternal rate reduction on the stuttering, speech rates and linguistic productions of children who stutter: Evidence from individual dyads. *Clinical Linguistics and Phonetics, 10*, 189–206.

CHAPTER

Control of Stuttering with Prolonged Speech: Preliminary Outcome of a One-Day Instatement Program

ELISABETH HARRISON, M.A.,
MARK ONSLOW, Ph.D.,
CHERYL ANDREWS, M.A.,
ANN PACKMAN, Ph.D.,
and MARGARET WEBBER, M.A.

For cases of early stuttering, control of stuttered speech is a necessary—even sufficient—treatment goal (Onslow & Packman, in press). Obviously, that would be an extreme position for management of advanced stuttering. However, this chapter presents research that is predicated on the assumption that, for a substantial portion of cases of advanced stuttering, such a treatment goal is appropriate. Some years ago, Roger Ingham elicited a discussion from Don Baer on the role of the client's complaint in the design of treatments for stuttering (Baer, 1988, 1990). It was argued that if the client's main difficulty with having the disorder relates to continuous speech perturbations that disrupt communication, then control of those perturbations might be an appropriate treatment goal.

The persuasiveness of that argument led the authors and colleagues to more closely relate to clients for the express purpose of exploring what was bothering them. Indeed, the needs of some of them did not involve the control of stuttered speech. Some of them, for example, were simply affected by speech anxiety that could be treated independently of stuttered speech. Others simply had nothing to gain by the control of stuttered speech, because they were excellent communicators despite stuttering. But the problems of many indeed focused on the distress associated with the effects of stuttered speech on daily life. For those clients, learning to speak without stuttering, and doing so for long periods of their lives, was well worth the considerable effort involved. It is beyond the scope of this chapter to discuss the portion of those who stutter for whom this is the case. No doubt, there would be disparate views on what that number would be, but it certainly is sufficiently large to justify a program of research designed to refine means by which those who have this disorder can speak without the overt signs of its disruptive effects.

Variants of Goldiamond's (1965) procedure, referred to generically as "prolonged speech" (PS) in this chapter, is an extremely popular way of controlling stuttered speech, if not the most popular way among clinicians worldwide. The intensive treatment format seems to be a favored mode of service delivery for these treatments, with established programs available around the world (see Onslow, 1996, for a review). Goldiamond is generally credited with the development of this technique, but it clearly has existed in some form from at least the early part of the 18th century (see Ingham, 1984, for a review). Goldiamond's contribution was the first systematic clinical experimentation with the procedure. Research to date has shown that recurring problems with the treatment are a significant relapse rate and unnatural sounding speech posttreatment (for reviews, see Ingham, 1984; Onslow, 1996; Onslow, Costa, Andrews, Harrison, & Packman, 1996). Nonetheless, it is possible for adults and adolescents to control stuttered speech for clinically significant periods with the PS technique, although the mechanisms of that control are not clear at present.

At the time of this writing, the last published report of PS treatment for chronic stuttering in adults was by the authors and colleagues (Onslow et al., 1996). This report was a clinical trial of a 2-week intensive PS treatment developed by Roger Ingham (Ingham, 1981, 1987). The treatment is described in a number of places (Onslow, 1996; Onslow et al., 1996). It consists of residential and nonresidential components. During residential components, clients live in the treatment setting while they undertake performance contingent, programmed speech tasks to establish and generalize stutter-free, natural sounding speech. The program imposes no target speech rates, but uses an ordinal scale (Martin, Haroldson, & Triden, 1984) to target speech naturalness and to shape clients' speech toward that target (Ingham & Onslow, 1985). During the latter part of the residential phase of treatment, clients complete a performance contingent self-evaluation phase. During a postresidential phase, clients complete a further performance contingent self-evaluation phase and a 126-week performance contingent maintenance phase.

The Onslow et al. report showed that clients were able to achieve near-zero stuttering, in everyday speaking situations, for clinically significant periods, and that they were able to do so without resorting to unusually slow speech rates, and that their speech probably sounded reasonably normal. Figure 9–1 shows the results for two of the clients in this report that had excellent outcomes. These results are encouraging; however, there is a problem remaining with the Onslow et al. (1996) treatment that relates to outcome. Treatment efficacy is one aspect of treatment outcome, but another aspect is treatment efficiency, and this treatment is inefficient to the extent that it requires many clinical hours.

A conservative estimate of the clinician hours consumed by each client in the Ingham (1987) program is 130: Four clinicians, working in two overlapping shifts, treat six clients for an average of fourteen 12-hr days, followed by an average of 18 hr per client required during the maintenance phase of treatment. That estimate is conservative, because the treatment is conducted in a residential setting which requires considerable personnel infrastructure. Further, the estimate of 130 clinical hours per client does not take into account that many clients will experience significant posttreatment relapse at some stage and will consequently require further clinician training to re-establish their treatment gains.

For many reasons, it is unsatisfactory that this number of clinician hours were used to bring stuttered speech under control in the Onslow et al. (1996) report. Most obviously, clinic hours translate to cost, and the health care dollar is being scrutinized throughout the world. Consequently, it is difficult to defend so many resources being devoted to the control of stuttered speech in adults, especially when there is a considerable chance of those clients relapsing and re-entering treatment at some future time. Long treatment times for adults are especially problematic considering that data for the Lidcombe Program of early stuttering intervention showed a median treatment time of 10.5 clinician hours for preschool-age children to achieve near-zero stuttering levels (Onslow, Andrews, & Lincoln, 1994; Onslow, Costa, & Rue, 1990). Perhaps the most onerous sign of the need to respond to this problem is the recent closure in Sydney of the PS treatment program of Gavin Andrews and colleagues (Neilson & Andrews, 1993). This was one of the most comprehensively researched programs in the world (see Onslow, 1996, for a review), and functioned also as a prominent service provision facility in Australia. Ostensibly, the reason for its closure was the problem in justifying such a cost ineffective treatment.

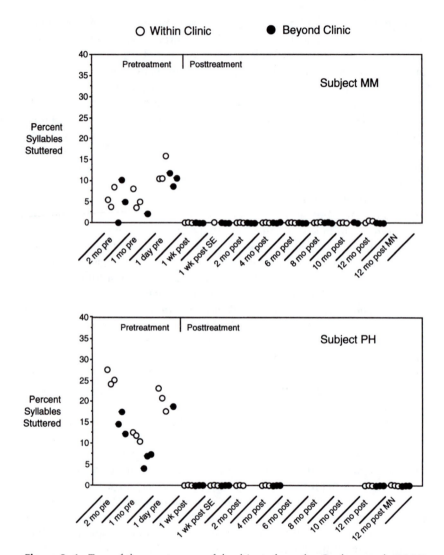

Figure 9–1. Two of the most successful subjects from the Onslow et al. (1996) report. (Adapted from Onslow, M., Costa, L., Andrews, C., Harrison, E., & Packman, A. 1996. Speech outcomes of a prolonged-speech treatment for stuttering. *Journal of Speech and Hearing Research, 39,* 734–749. Reprinted with permission of the American Speech-Language-Hearing Association.)

The origins of this problem appear to be in the durations of the two major components in the Onslow et al. (1996) treatment, the Instatement and Transfer Phases, each of which required 5–7 days for clients to complete. Yet the durations of those components seem largely to be arbitrary—more an artifact of the original experimental methods to research this treatment than any intrinsic clinical need (Onslow & Ingham, 1989). There are certainly no data to indicate that these treatment components of intensive PS require such long periods.[1] Further, there are no data to justify a Transfer component of the kind outlined by Ingham (1987), where clients systematically introduce their newly learned stutter-free speech into real speaking situations. It certainly makes clinical sense to follow such a "sequential modification" (Stokes & Baer, 1977) technique, but there are no data to show that such a procedure is, in fact, beneficial to treatment outcome when it is included in an intensive PS program.

Considering the serious implications of the cost ineffectiveness of the Onslow et al. (1996) treatment, and the absence of any data to support the retention of the program in the form in which it was reported by Onslow et al., it would be of interest to know how radical modifications would influence treatment effectiveness. In short, what would happen if the Instatement Phase was reduced to a single, 12-hr day, and the Transfer Phase was dispensed with altogether? Would the treatment become virtually useless, or would it retain some clinical benefits? And if it retained some clinical benefits, would those be sufficient to argue a productive trade-off between increased efficiency and decreased effectiveness? The data presented here describe the effects of such a radical modification to the Ingham (1987) program, in order to determine whether a search for such a trade-off might be profitable.

METHOD

The Adapted PS Intensive Program

The adaptation of the Ingham program in the present study consists of two phases: A 1-day Instatement Phase and a 12-month Maintenance Phase. During the Instatement Phase, clients spend a 12-hr day in the clinic completing a programmed, performance contingent schedule of monologue speaking tasks intended to establish stutter-free, natural sounding speech. The day begins with clients learning the PS pattern, which incorporates consonant production with "soft contacts" and vowel production with "gentle onsets" and "continuous vocalization."

---

[1] James, Ricciardelli, Hunter, and Rogers (1989), however, showed that a PS treatment comprised of 32 clinical hours was equally effective for a 6-month period regardless of whether the treatment format was intensive or nonintensive.

Subsequently, clients complete a performance contingent schedule that incorporates the following syllables per minute (SPM) speech rate targets, plus or minus 20 SPM: 40 SPM, 70 SPM, and 100 SPM. At each of these speech rate targets, clients are required to complete three consecutive, stutter-free monologues with PS. At 40 SPM the monologues are 300 syllables in duration, at 70 SPM they are 500 syllables in duration, and at 100 SPM they are 700 syllables in duration.

Clients then complete three further steps that target various levels of clinician-judged speech naturalness, using a 9-point scale: Na, Nb, and Nc. This procedure was described by Ingham (1987) and Onslow et al. (1996). During each of these three final Instatement Phase steps, clients are again required to complete three consecutive stutter-free monologues, and these are 900, 1,100, and then 1,300 syllables in duration. However, in place of speech rate criteria, clients are required to meet speech naturalness targets. During these three stages, clients may exaggerate or minimize features of PS to the extent they wish, providing they remain stutter-free and maintain their target level of speech naturalness. During the monologues, clinicians score the client's naturalness each 60 s and the speech naturalness score for the entire monologue is based on the average of those scores. The speech naturalness criteria targeted for Na is two scale values below the mean clinician-judged speech naturalness measures attained by the client during the 100 SPM monologues. Then, during Stages Nb and Nc, the naturalness of stutter-free speech is reduced in two further steps down to a score of 2 on the naturalness scale, or as close to this level as the individual client can achieve.

The Maintenance Phase begins on the day following the Instatement Phase. During this phase clients complete a 44-step performance contingent schedule, which involves 12 clinic visits. At each visit, clients are required to complete within-clinic conversations and to present tape recorded conversations from beyond the clinic, which are recorded during the week prior to the maintenance visit. Details of this maintenance schedule are presented in Figure 9–2. During the first and second week after the Instatement Phase, clients visit the clinic on six occasions. Subsequently, clients begin a weekly visit schedule, which eventually incorporates a visit each 8 weeks. During Section One of the Maintenance Phase (see Figure 9–2), clients are not required to have zero stuttering during within-clinic conversations; however, zero stuttering is required in all subsequent parts of maintenance. During Section One, clients are required to evaluate their beyond-clinic recordings for naturalness and stuttering, but their progression through the schedule is not dependent on correct evaluation. However, any discrepancies between clinician and client evaluations are discussed. For the first two visits of Section Two of the Maintenance Phase, clients are required to match the clinician's evaluation of stuttering and speech naturalness on the

		WITHIN CLINIC TASKS		BEYOND CLINIC TASKS	
	Weeks 1 & 2	1300-syllable conversations: • 1 Clinician • 1 Phone		10-minute taped conversations: • 1 Family • 1 Friend • 1 Phone	
SECTION 1	Tuesday	"		"	Client evaluates
	Wednesday	"		"	tapes for stutters
	Friday	"		"	and speech naturalness, and
	Monday	"		"	these are compared with clinician
	Wednesday	"		"	evaluation. Progress
	Thursday	"		"	to Section two occurs regardless of results
			PROGRESS IF:		**PROGRESS IF:**
	Week 3	"	0%SS	"	Clinician and Client Evaluations Match:
	Week 4	"	"	"	Stutters ±5% Naturalness ±1
SECTION 2	Week 5	"	"	"	0%SS
	Week 6	"	"	"	"
	Week 7	"	"	"	"
	Week 8	"	"	"	"
				10-minute taped conversations: • 2 Family • 2 Friend • 2 Phone	
	Week 9			"	"
SECTION 3	Week 10			"	"
	Week 12			"	"
	Week 14			"	"
	Week 18	"	"	"	"
	Week 22			"	"
SECTION 4	Week 30			"	"
	Week 38			"	"
	Week 44	"	"	"	"

Figure 9–2. Details of the client maintenance schedule used in the present report.

beyond-clinic recorded conversations. The match must be for the number of stutters on tapes, ± 5%, and ± one naturalness scale value. Subsequently, the criteria for progression through Maintenance are that beyond-clinic recordings contain zero stutterings. During Sections Three and Four of the Maintenance Phase, the client visits the clinic on Weeks 18 and 44 only, but mails beyond-clinic recordings to the clinic for assessment at Weeks 9, 10, 12, 14, 22, 30, and 38.

This abbreviated treatment is conducted by two clinicians who work in two overlapping shifts, with Clinician One present from 7:30 A.M. to 2:30 P.M., and Clinician Two present from 1:00 P.M. to 8:00 P.M. There are 24 total treatment hours for the abbreviated treatment (two clinicians, two clients, one 12-hr day, twelve 1-hr maintenance visits). The clients begin learning prolonged speech at 8:00 A.M., and continue monologues throughout the day. There are two breaks of at least 30 min for meals, and at least three group conversations during the day, during

Table 9–1. Subject Details: The Pretreatment Percent Syllables Stuttered (%SS) Data Are Means of Pretreatment Assessments (see Outcome Evaluation Methodology).

Subject	Sex	Age (years)	Treatment history	Pretreatment Mean %SS
TW	male	14	Unsuccessful PS program ("smooth speech") 2 years previously	5.5
DM	male	31	Two previous intensive PS treatments, at ages 19 years and 21 years, with posttreatment relapse	9.2
MO	female	28	PS intensive ("smooth speech") at 17 years, followed by "relaxation therapy" at 19 years, both with short-term effects	4.6
SW	female	13	History of varied and unsuccessful treatments since 9 years, including PS ("smooth motion technique"), visits to psychologist, and ELU	5.0
NM	female	16	History of treatment since 12 years involving combined ELU and TO; successful outcome followed by relapse	12.5
CC	male	32	No previous treatment	2.4

which a clinician and both clients meet for 10 min. At other times the clients are in separate rooms and work individually with a clinician.

Subjects

Six adult stuttering clients from the Stuttering Unit waiting list, who were due to commence treatment, were recruited for this study. Details of these subjects are presented in Table 9–1.

Outcome Evaluation Methodology

Speech Measures

The primary dependent measure in this study was Percent Syllables Stuttered (%SS). This measure—based on a count of stuttered syllables and nonstuttered syllables—is not free of problems, the most notable of which concerns reliability (see Cordes & Ingham, 1994). However, for outcome research this measure is acceptable because large differences are of interest (considerable stuttering before treatment and virtually none after treatment). If more subtle effects were of interest, for example, a difference as small as 1 %SS between two experimental groups, a %SS measure might be problematic. Added to the primary dependent measure of %SS is a measure of speech rate in SPM. Both these measures are obtained on-line from audiotape recordings using a button-press timing and counting device. Separate buttons are used to count stuttered and nonstuttered syllables. The timing mechanism of the device is triggered each time a button is pressed.

One of the major weaknesses in stuttering treatment outcome research to date is the absence of a measure of speech naturalness (see Onslow, 1996; Onslow et al., 1996, for reviews). Prolonged speech treatment involves an unusual speech pattern, yet existing PS outcome research has generally failed to incorporate methods to assess the extent to which clients achieve natural sounding speech. This shortcoming could mean that existing outcome research is simply misleading to its consumers; it might convey control of stuttered speech with an associated assumption that the person's speech was reasonably normal. It is clear that a speaker can control stuttering and concurrently sound extremely unnatural. And if that is an outcome of a PS treatment, then it is important for consumers of outcome research to be so informed. To address this issue, this and other studies have used speech naturalness (NAT) measures, collected on-line using a 9-point, nonstandardized ordinal scale, where "1" = "highly natural" and "9" = "highly unnatural" (Martin et al., 1984). NAT ratings are assigned by a listener at the end of each minute of tape recorded speech, and these ratings are averaged to give a single mean score for each recording of a subject. The NAT scale has been used in previous PS research, and much of that research has demonstrated its validity and reliability (Ingham, Gow, & Costello, 1985; Ingham & Onslow, 1985; Kalinowski, Noble, Armson, & Steward, 1994; Martin & Haroldson, 1992; Martin et al., 1984; Metz, Schiavetti, & Sacco, 1990; Onslow et al., 1996; Onslow, Hayes, Hutchins, & Newman, 1992; Runyan, Bell, & Prosek, 1990). For the present study, on-line NAT measures were reported only for posttreatment samples[2], and for only five of the six subjects. The reason for this is that one subject spoke Cantonese as a first language and spoke English with an accent. Nonnative accents

---

[2] We considered that it would be pointless to attempt comparison of pretreatment with posttreatment speech naturalness because of the confounding effects of pretreatment stuttering on perceived speech naturalness.

are a potential confound in the use of the speech naturalness scale with English-speaking subjects and judges (see Onslow, Adams, & Ingham, 1992), so NAT scores were not reported for this subject.

Speech Sampling

Speech samples were based on 10-min recordings of conversational speech, and at each assessment occasion three were collected, each from a different speaking situation: with family, with friends, and speaking on the telephone. Each assessment occasion was based on a total of 30 min of speech. Subjects used portable audiotape recorders to record their beyond-clinic speech. During the pretreatment phase of the study, an additional 30 min of speech samples were collected within the clinic at each assessment occasion, comprising a conversation with a clinician, with a stranger, and a telephone conversation. The reason for this additional speech sampling during the pretreatment period was to be sure that there were no systematic data trends occurring for any subject during the pretreatment period. No such data trends were detected, and the treatment was introduced for each client after the 2-month pretreatment period.

Many assessment occasions occurred during the period in which the subjects were studied, in a fashion similar to that described by Onslow et al. (1996). *Pretreatment* assessments occurred at 2 months, 1 month, and 1 day. *Posttreatment* assessments occurred at 1 week post the intensive phase, then 2 months post, 4 months post, 6 months post, 8 months post, 10 months post, and 12 months post. The posttreatment assessments occurred during the 44-week maintenance program.

This methodology is rigorous and quite labor intensive but is justified for at least two reasons. First, it enables detection of any clinically significant posttreatment trends in patients which would be of interest to consumers of outcome research. Certainly, clinically significant posttreatment trends are apparent in recent PS outcome reports. For example, 69% of Boberg and Kully's (1994) subjects showed an increase of %SS from the immediate posttreatment assessment to the final posttreatment assessment. In fact, of subjects for whom three or four posttreatment assessments were available, 33% showed a stepwise increase in %SS scores over each assessment. Figure 9–3 presents data from two of the one-quarter of the Onslow et al. subjects for whom clinically significant posttreatment trends were detected.

The other benefit of repeated speech assessments during the posttreatment period relates to the notorious reactivity of stuttering to measurement. It simply is not convincing to present only one or two measurements during a long posttreatment period. There is a likelihood with such methodology that the subject will, for the purposes of the assess-

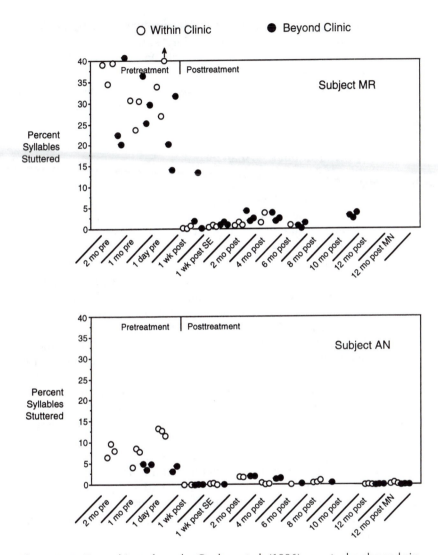

Figure 9–3. Two subjects from the Onslow et al. (1996) report who showed significant posttreatment regression trends. (Adapted from Onslow, M., Costa, L., Andrews, C., Harrison, E., & Packman, A. 1996. Speech outcomes of a prolonged-speech treatment for stuttering. *Journal of Speech and Hearing Research, 39,* 734–749. Reprinted with permission of the American Speech-Language-Hearing Association.)

ment, produce speech that is atypical. This problem is compounded if the assessment comprises only one speaking situation, as occurs more often than not in PS outcome research (see Onslow et al., 1996, for a review). Repeated assessment during the posttreatment period does not overcome this problem altogether, but outcome data so generated are at least more credible when the client routinely makes a series of tape recordings in everyday speaking situations.

Post Hoc Speech Naturalness Analysis

In addition to the on-line NAT measures described above, subjects' post-treatment speech naturalness was perceptually studied in relation to matched, normal speakers. Five subjects were included in this analysis, deleting the subject mentioned above who spoke with an accent. For each subject, a control subject was selected, matched for age (to within 6 months), sex, and educational level.

For experimental subjects, two 30-s speech samples were dubbed from posttreatment tape recordings: one from the 1-week postinten-sive assessment recordings, and one from the 6-months postintensive assessment recordings. These were conversational samples, but they were dubbed so that the recordings entirely consisted of the subject's speech. The samples contained speech that was perceptually stutter-free, according to all the authors. For each control subject, a conversa-tional speech sample was recorded, and two 30-s samples were assem-bled. The speech of control subjects was recorded using the same tape recorders used by experimental subjects to record their posttreatment speech samples.

The 20 samples (5 subjects × 2 samples per subject × 2 groups) were placed in random order on a listening tape. Ten unsophisticated listeners were recruited to listen to the tape and assign a speech natu-ralness score to each sample. Listeners were given the standard in-structions for the use of the 9-point scale of speech naturalness (Martin et al., 1984).

Covert Speech Measures

As indicated previously, stuttering is notoriously reactive to measure-ment. Consequently, there are many examples of discrepancies between overt and covert data (for example, Ingham, 1980). However, based on the present researchers' experiences with outcome studies (Lincoln, Onslow, Wilson, & Lewis, 1996; Onslow, Andrews, & Lincoln, 1994; Ons-low et al., 1996), it seems that overt and covert posttreatment assess-ments give results that are generally not too discrepant. However, they are included in the present report because they continue to provide useful information about whether assessment methodology is providing trustworthy information about subjects' everyday posttreatment speech. Sometimes, covert assessment confirms that beyond-clinic measures are valid, and sometimes covert assessment gives reason to question whether that is the case. The covert assessment procedure is an extremely rigorous test, because it occurs by means of telephone conversation with a stranger (see below), which is likely to be a troublesome speaking situation for many who stutter.

The procedure for covert assessment was that a staff member, who was unknown to the subjects, telephoned each of them at some time during the posttreatment period. The staff member posed as a public relations officer for the hospital in which the treatment was conducted. The caller conducted a telephone "survey" of patient satisfaction, while claiming to have no knowledge of the condition for which the subject received treatment. Covert tape recording of telephone conversations is illegal in Australia, so the staff member used the button-press counting and timing device to measure %SS and SPM during these "surveys."

Reliability of Speech Measures

Ten percent of the assessment recordings were selected for intrajudge reliability analysis; three pretreatment recordings from each subject and three posttreatment recordings from each subject. These recordings were re-presented in random order to the independent clinician 6 months after the clinician collected the original data. The clinician was instructed to collect %SS, SPM, and NAT scores in an identical manner to the original data collection. To assess interjudge reliability, the recordings selected for reliability analysis were presented in random order to a Stuttering Unit clinician who was not a program clinician. The clinician was instructed to collect %SS, SPM, and NAT scores in an identical manner to the clinician who originally gathered those data.

RESULTS

Clinical Progress

There was no subject attrition, with all six clients completing the 1-day Instatement Phase and the subsequent Maintenance Phase.

Percent Syllables Stuttered

Figure 9–4 shows the %SS scores for each client over the pretreatment and posttreatment phases of the study. There were a total of 92

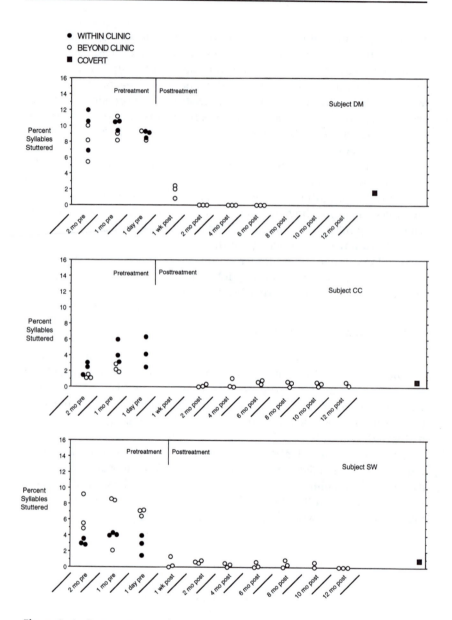

Figure 9–4. Pretreatment and posttreatment percent syllables stuttered (%SS) levels for six subjects. *Continued on p. 205.*

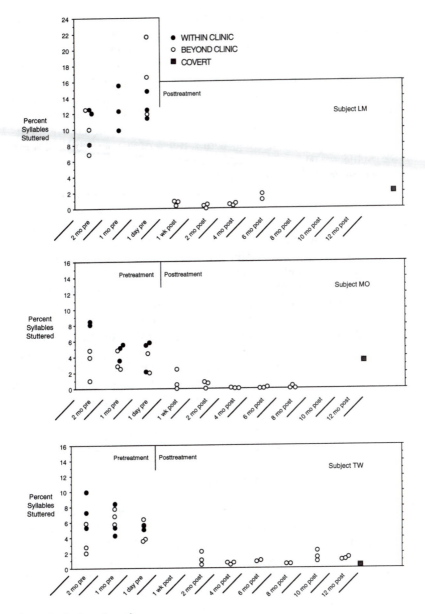

Figure 9–4. (*continued*)

posttreatment %SS scores representing the clients' stuttering severity in everyday situations (excluding the covert assessments). Of these, 80 (87.0%) were in the range 0–1.0 %SS, 8 (8.6%) were in the range 1.1–2.0 %SS, and 4 (4.4%) were in the range 2.1–3.0 %SS. There was no posttreatment %SS score greater than 3.0 recorded for any client. The mean post-treatment %SS score for all clients was 0.41 %SS, with a range of subject means from 0.24 %SS (Subject MO) to 0.76 %SS (Subject TW). In terms of beyond-clinic %SS scores, subjects showed a mean posttreatment reduction of 93.8% of their stuttering, with a range of 86.2% (Subject TW) to 97.3% (Subject DM).

A covert %SS measure was recorded for all subjects. For three subjects (SW, CC, TW), the covert %SS measure was representative of the overt %SS measures. However, for Subject DM, the mean posttreatment %SS measure was 0.25 and the covert %SS measure was 1.3, and for Subject NM the mean posttreatment %SS measure was 0.56 and the covert %SS measure was 2.1. For Subject MO, the mean posttreatment %SS measure was 0.24 and the covert %SS measure was 3.6.

Intrajudge reliability of %SS scores was satisfactory. In total, 28/35 (74.3%) of the clinician's second scores differed from the first score by 1.0 %SS or less, 32/35 (91.4%) differed by 2.0 %SS or less, and 35/35 (100%) differed by 3.0 %SS or less. Interjudge reliability of the %SS scores in the study was also satisfactory and comparable with previous studies. In total, 22/34 (64.7%) of the clinicians' scores differed by 1.0 %SS or less, 27/34 (79.4%) differed by 2.0 %SS or less, 30/34 (88.2%) differed by 3.0 %SS or less, 33/34 (97.1%) differed by 6.0 %SS or less, and 34/34 (100%) differed by 7.0 %SS or less. These levels of inter- and intrajudge reliability of %SS scores are satisfactory and comparable to those in other recent PS outcome reports (for example, Boberg & Kully, 1994; Onslow et al., 1996).

Syllables Per Minute

Intrajudge reliability of SPM scores was unsatisfactory. In total, 10/25 (40%) of score differences were less than or equal to 10 SPM, 15/25 (60%) of score differences were less than or equal to 20 SPM, 20/25 (80%) of score differences were less than or equal to 30 SPM, 22/25 (88%) of score differences were less than or equal to 40 SPM, and 25/25 (100%) of score differences were less than 50 SPM. Because of these unsatisfactory reliability results, SPM scores are not reported.

Speech Naturalness

Mean NAT scores gathered by the experimenter for beyond-clinic assessments (during the posttreatment period) are presented for each subject in Figure 9–5. For each beyond-clinic assessment, NAT scores for

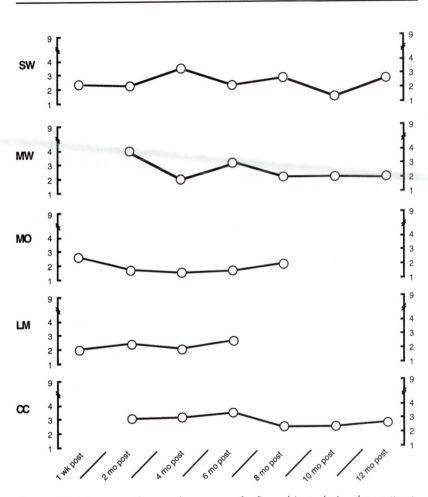

Figure 9–5. Mean speech naturalness scores for five subjects during the posttreatment period, assigned by one listener. Data points represent the mean of NAT judgments, assigned by the listener each 60 s, for all posttreatment recordings. One subject was deleted from the analysis because he spoke with an accent.

individual recordings were obtained from the mean of each of the experimenter's 60-second naturalness ratings while listening to the recordings. The actual naturalness scores assigned to the listeners are of limited significance because the naturalness scale is subjective and the data in Figure 9–5 are generated by one listener only. However, the value of these data is in demonstrating that the clinician's naturalness scores show no sign of systematic increases over the posttreatment period. In other words, in everyday speaking situations and for clinically significant periods, the subjects seem not to have used a more exaggerated speech pattern than the one they were using at the time of their discharge from the intensive component of treatment. However, with the possible exception of Subject MW, it also appears that subjects did not improve their perceived levels of speech naturalness during the post-treatment period.

Intrajudge reliability of NAT scores for posttreatment speech samples was satisfactory. In total, 14/17 (82.4%) of scores differed by less than one value on the naturalness scale, and 17/17 (100%) of scores differed by less than two scale values. Interjudge reliability of NAT scores also was satisfactory. In total, 9/17 (52.9%) of scores differed by less than one value on the naturalness scale, 14/17 (82.4%) of scores differed by less than two scale values, and 17/17 (100%) of scores differed by less than three scale values.

Post Hoc Speech Naturalness Analysis

Figure 9–6 presents the speech naturalness scores for experimental and control subjects. Determining the intrajudge reliability of the data in Figure 9–6 was problematic because there were few speech samples, and the listeners may have recalled their scores on a repeat listening. To get around this problem, a listener was deemed to have unsatisfactory reliability if the NAT scores for the two samples from any control subject differed by more than one scale value. Because the two samples for each control subject were collected from the same recorded conversation, they were almost certainly equivalent in speech naturalness. Therefore, if a listener's scores did not reflect that similarity, that listener was considered to have unsatisfactory intrajudge reliability. Five judges showed unsatisfactory intrajudge reliability according to this criterion and consequently were removed from the analysis. The interjudge reliability of the remaining five judges was that 53% of their NAT scores were within two scale values.

Figure 9–6 shows that two subjects attracted mean NAT scores from the unsophisticated listeners that were in the range of the mean scores given to the control subjects. This suggests that those two speakers achieved stutter-free speech that was equivalent to the controls in terms of perceived speech naturalness. One subject achieved mean NAT scores that were just beyond the range of the control scores, and the mean NAT scores of two control subjects was clearly beyond the range of the controls' scores. However, the present methodology does not allow any further statements about the extent to which these two subjects' speech resembled that of normal speakers. The subject whose data point has a cross within it is the only subject who showed a change of more than one NAT scale value across the two assessment occasions.

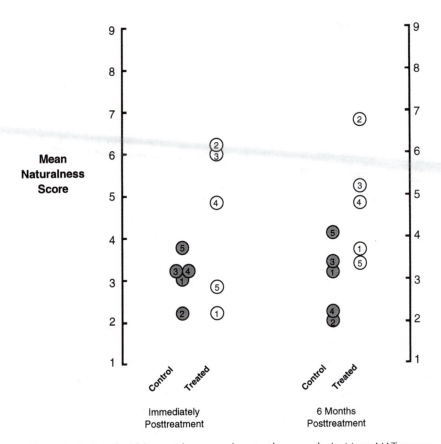

Figure 9–6. Results of the post hoc speech naturalness analysis. Mean NAT scores assigned by the listeners to control and experimental subjects at two occasions. The numbers identify the subjects.

CONCLUSIONS AND DISCUSSION

The present outcome data show that the majority of measures of everyday posttreatment stuttering were in the range 0–1.0 %SS, without posttreatment regression, and that some subjects achieved speech naturalness scores in the normal range. Some clients did noticeably worse than others, with occasional %SS measures above 2.0, and covert assessment of some clients showed slightly higher %SS scores than overt assessment. This summary of results is essentially the same as for Onslow et al. (1996). The mean beyond-clinic stuttering rate posttreatment in the present study was .41 %SS, and in the Onslow et al. report this value was

0.38 %SS. The difference between the two values is not clinically significant. In the present study, 88.1% of beyond clinic posttreatment scores were in the range 0–1.0 %SS, and in the original study the figure was 88.7%. Again, this difference is not clinically significant. In the present study, the mean improvement in posttreatment stuttering rates was 93.8%, and in the original study the value was 96.5%. Arguably, this difference is clinically significant, but it is a small difference and the only noticeable one between the two studies. Procedures for collection of speech samples and dependent measures were similar in the two studies, hence these comparisons seem valid.

The finding of an overall similarity of the findings between this and the Onslow et al. (1996) study is surprising, considering that the instatement phase was shortened to a single 12-hour day, the "transfer" phase was deleted, and the postresidential phase was shortened from 18 visits to 12 visits. Each client in the adapted program consumed 24 clinician hours compared to 130 clinician hours in the original. In effect, then, the adapted program represents a reduction of treatment costs to less than one fifth of the original program.

These results suggest that there may be aspects of the original treatment that may not contribute to its outcome. In the first instance, the present results raise a suggestion that the substantial duration of the 1987 version of the Ingham PS treatment program may not be critical to its effectiveness. Further, these results raise a question about the value of the common "transfer" procedure that is based on sequential modification (Stokes & Baer, 1977). Although such a procedure is accepted practice in PS programs throughout the world, and although it is intuitively correct from a clinical viewpoint, its value must be challenged because removing the procedure from the treatment appeared to have little impact on treatment outcome. Further research will be necessary to resolve this issue, because it may have been the case that the beyond-clinic tape recordings made by clients during the Maintenance Phase functioned, in effect, as a "transfer" procedure.

Provocative as the present outcome data for the adaptation of the Onslow et al. (1996) program may be, they are nonetheless preliminary. The present report contains a few subjects who have been followed only for the medium-term posttreatment. It may be that a 2-week intensive PS treatment provides more durable treatment effects in the long term. Nonetheless, these results are sufficient to suggest that there is much development yet to occur with the Onslow et al. (1996) program in order to provide the most efficient service provision for clients. A comprehensive series of controlled experimental investigations is under way with substantial subject numbers. Among other variables, these studies are investigating the role of programmed instruction in achieving satisfactory PS outcome. It is also planned to add to Ingham's (1980) data about the value of programmed maintenance. Finally, it is planned to investigate the value of a preintensive clinical regime during which clients are taught the PS pattern. It may be that the intensive phase of treatment is of more value to clients if they have mastered the basics of their new speech pattern some time previously. Ideally, the outcome of this program of research will be that the present results can be systematically replicated, and perhaps even that treatment times can be further reduced; then control of stuttered speech with the PS technique may be a justifiable use of healthcare resources.

REFERENCES

Baer, D. (1988). If you know why you're changing a behavior, you'll know when you've changed it enough. *Behavioral Assessment, 10,* 219–223.

Baer, D. (1990). The critical issue in treatment efficacy is knowing why treatment was applied: A student's response to Roger Ingham. In C. Olswang, C. K. Thompson, S. Warren, N. Minghetti (Eds.), *Treatment efficacy research in communication disorders* (pp. 31–39). Rockville, MD: American Speech-Language-Hearing Foundation.

Boberg, E., & Kully, D. (1994). Long-term results of an intensive treatment program for adults and adolescents who stutter. *Journal of Speech and Hearing Research, 37,* 1050–1059.

Cordes, A., & Ingham, R. J. (1994). The reliability of observational data. II: Issues in the identification and measurement of stuttering events. *Journal of Speech and Hearing Research, 37,* 279–294.

Goldiamond, I. (1965). Stuttering and fluency as manipulatable operant response classes. In L. Krasner & L. P. Ullman (Eds.), *Research in behavior modification* (pp. 106–156). New York: Holt, Rinehart & Winston.

Ingham, R. J. (1980). Modification of maintenance and generalization during stuttering treatment. *Journal of Speech and Hearing Research, 23,* 732–745.

Ingham, R. (1981). *Stuttering therapy manual: A hierarchy control schedule.* Sydney, Australia, Cumberland College of Health Sciences.

Ingham, R. J. (1984). *Stuttering and behavior therapy: Current status and experimental foundations.* San Diego, CA: College-Hill Press.

Ingham, R. (1987). *Residential prolonged speech stuttering therapy manual.* Santa Barbara, CA: Department of Speech and Hearing Sciences, University of California–Santa Barbara.

Ingham, R. J., Gow, M., & Costello, J. M. (1985). Stuttering and speech naturalness: Some additional data. *Journal of Speech and Hearing Disorders, 50,* 217–219.

Ingham, R. J. & Onslow, M. (1985). Measurement and modification of speech naturalness during stuttering therapy. *Journal of Speech and Hearing Disorders, 50,* 261–281.

James, J., Ricciardelli, L., Hunter, C., & Rogers, P. (1989). Relative efficacy of intensive and spaced behavioral treatment of stuttering. *Behavior Modification, 13,* 376–395.

Kalinowski, J., Noble, S., Armson, J., & Stuart, A. (1994). Pretreatment and post-treatment speech naturalness ratings of adults with mild and severe stuttering. *American Journal of Speech-Language Pathology, 3*, 61–66.

Lincoln, M., Onslow, M., Wilson, L., & Lewis, C. (1996). A clinical trial of an operant treatment for school-age stuttering children. *American Journal of Speech-Language Pathology, 5*, 73–85.

Martin, R. R., & Haroldson, S. K. (1992). Stuttering and speech naturalness: Audio and audiovisual judgments. *Journal of Speech and Hearing Research, 35*, 521–528.

Martin, R. R., Haroldson, S. K., & Triden, K. A. (1984). Stuttering and speech naturalness. *Journal of Speech and Hearing Disorders, 49*, 53–58.

Metz, D. E., Schiavetti, N., & Sacco, P. R. (1990). Acoustic and psychophysical dimensions of the perceived speech naturalness of nonstutterers and post-treatment stutterers. *Journal of Speech and Hearing Disorders, 55*, 516–525.

Neilson, M., & Andrews, G. (1993). Intensive fluency training of chronic stutterers. In R. F. Curlee (Ed.), *Stuttering and related disorders of fluency* (pp. 139–165). New York: Thieme Medical Publishers.

Onslow, M. (1996). *Behavioral management of stuttering.* San Diego, CA: Singular Publishing Group.

Onslow, M., Adams, R., & Ingham, R. J. (1992). Reliability of speech naturalness ratings of stutterers' speech during therapy. *Journal of Speech and Hearing Research, 35*, 994–1001.

Onslow, M., Andrews, C., & Lincoln, M. (1994). A control/experimental trial of an operant treatment for early stuttering. *Journal of Speech and Hearing Research, 37*, 1244–1259.

Onslow, M., Costa, L., Andrews, C., Harrison, E., & Packman, A. (1996). Speech outcomes of a prolonged-speech treatment for stuttering. *Journal of Speech and Hearing Research, 39*, 734–749.

Onslow, M., Costa, L., & Rue, S. (1990). Direct early intervention with stuttering: Some preliminary data. *Journal of Speech and Hearing Disorders, 55*, 405–416.

Onslow, M., Hayes, B., Hutchins, L., & Newman, D. (1992). Speech naturalness and prolonged-speech treatments for stuttering: Further variables and data. *Journal of Speech and Hearing Research, 35*, 274–282.

Onslow, M., & R. Ingham (1989). Whither prolonged speech? The disquieting evolution of a stuttering therapy procedure. *Australian Journal of Human Communication Disorders, 17*, 67–81.

Onslow, M., & Packman, A. (in press). The Lidcombe Program of Early Stuttering Intervention. In N. Bernstein Ratner & E. C. Healey (Eds.), *Treatment and research: Bridging the gap.* Mahwah, NJ: Laurence Erlbaum Associates.

Runyan, C. M., Bell, J. N., & Prosek, R. A. (1990). Speech naturalness ratings of treated stutterers. *Journal of Speech and Hearing Disorders, 55*, 434–438.

Stokes, T. F., & Baer, D. M. (1977). An implicit technology of generalization. *Journal of Applied Behavior Analysis, 10*, 349–367.

CHAPTER

10

Treatment Outcomes in Stuttering: Finding Value in Clinical Data

J. SCOTT YARUSS, Ph.D

When reviewing existing literature on the outcomes of treatment for adults who stutter, it rapidly becomes apparent that certain types of treatments have been quite well documented, while other approaches have been less thoroughly examined (see reviews in Andrews, Guitar, & Howie, 1980; Bloodstein, 1995; Cordes, Chapter 6; St. Louis & Westbrook, 1987). Specifically, there are numerous reports demonstrating that treatments based on behavioral principles can reduce stuttering, but comparatively less research that demonstrates the efficacy of so-called integrated or "eclectic" approaches (i.e., treatments that emphasize both speech changes and counseling to address clients' reactions to stuttering). Indeed, of the 15 adult-treatment studies conducted between 1980 and 1986 that were reviewed by St. Louis and Westbrook (1987, pp. 245–247), only a small number were reported to include a counseling component.[1] As noted by Cordes (Chapter 6), however, many of the treatment approaches that have been less thoroughly researched are also those that are frequently recommended to practicing clinicians in books and articles about stuttering.

---

[1] It is important to note that many of the studies reviewed by St. Louis and Westbrook (1987) that were not reported to include counseling most certainly incorporated some type of discussion about stuttering and therapeutic interaction that could be labeled counseling; however, the nature and focus of that counseling is somewhat less clear.

THE NEED FOR TREATMENT OUTCOMES RESEARCH

The fact that some treatments are frequently recommended, seemingly in the absence of unequivocal demonstration that they are effective in helping individuals who stutter, poses something of a problem (Cordes, Chapter 6; Ingham & Cordes, in press). At the very least, it does not seem appropriate for scientific practitioners to promote a treatment program without making some attempt to verify its efficacy.

There are three potential responses to this situation. The first option is to simply accept the fact that there have always been, and probably always will be, many different perspectives on the nature and treatment of stuttering (e.g., Bloodstein, 1995; Gregory, 1979). According to this view, it seems unlikely that clinical researchers in stuttering will ever arrive at a consensus regarding which treatment approaches are most appropriate or most effective. Although based on a realistic view of the vast differences of opinion that exist in our field, this option does not account for the changes facing the field of speech-language pathology (as well as the broader field of health-related professions), as clinicians come under increasing pressure to demonstrate that the treatments they recommend are effective (e.g., Frattali, 1998).

A second option, more mindful of current and future changes in healthcare policy, is to recommend that treatment be restricted only to approaches that have been proven to be effective, through scientifically valid research methodologies. Although perhaps more satisfying to insurance companies and other third-party payers, this option seems quite unrealistic, given the aforementioned disagreement across the field about how to best treat stuttering. Such an approach might also be unnecessarily restrictive, since the treatments that are frequently recommended for treating stuttering were presumably developed for some reason—most likely because they do indeed help people with their stuttering. Although the history of this field is replete with examples of individuals who stutter receiving less than ideal treatment, it is also clear that many have received appropriate and helpful treatment. Thus, the problem may be more the *documentation* that is lacking, rather than the actual efficacy of the treatments.

This possibility leads to a third option. Given the increasing requirements for accountability, combined with the broad range of options for treating stuttering, it would seem appropriate for proponents of less thoroughly evaluated treatment approaches to begin to more carefully document the outcomes of their treatments. Of the three options presented here, this may be the most viable, because it allows for differences of opinion across the field, while still recognizing and preparing for the coming changes in documentation requirements.

It is toward this third option that this chapter is directed. Specifically, this chapter presents preliminary results from the first phase of a treatment outcomes project that involves a series of ongoing studies designed to evaluate the adult stuttering treatment program that has been developed and used at Northwestern University (NU) by Gregory and colleagues for the past 30 years. Aside from being used at the NU Speech and Language Clinics, this approach has been described and recommended in books on stuttering treatment (e.g., Gregory, 1968, 1972, 1986, in press) and is currently taught throughout the United States and around the world in workshops such as the yearly "Stuttering Specialist Workshop," jointly sponsored by NU and the Stuttering Foundation of America (SFA). Because of the far-reaching impact of this program, it seems particularly important that its utility for treating stuttering be clearly demonstrated.

The first attempt to document the outcome of this program was conducted by Gregory (1972), who reported that 16 subjects experienced statistically significant reductions in their stuttering severity, as well as general improvements in speech attitudes, following treatment. Although these early results were quite promising, there have a been a number of substantive changes to the treatment approach that have occurred during the past 25 years. Thus, there is a clear need for additional data regarding the results of this treatment. Unfortunately, however, there are a number of roadblocks that complicate the process of evaluating the efficacy of this treatment approach. Because of these roadblocks, which will be discussed in more detail below, the present analysis focuses primarily on ways to support future outcomes research by examining the clinical records of clients who have participated in the treatment in the past 25 years.

Defining Success: The Nature
of the Client's Complaint

Before presenting the data from this study, it is appropriate to consider the rationale for this treatment approach. Central to this topic is the question of how "success" should be defined. This chapter will utilize the broad definition of success offered by Baer (1988, 1990), who suggested that an effective treatment is one that addresses "the client's complaint" (see also Ingham & Cordes, 1997). Although seemingly straightforward, this definition does not answer all questions regarding the definition of successful treatment, for there is considerable disagreement among clinical researchers about the nature of the complaint presented by adults who stutter.

The Complaint as the Stuttering Events

Some treatment programs apparently view the client's complaint to be stuttering *events* (i.e., the frequent disruptions in speech fluency that are often characterized by audible and visible features such as physical tension and struggle). Accordingly, the definition of success for these treatment programs is the reduction (or elimination) of stuttering events. These are the types of programs that have received the most attention in prior treatment outcomes studies (review Cordes, Chapter 6).

The Complaint as the Stuttering Disorder

Other treatment programs, however, view the client's complaint to be the stuttering *disorder*, including not only the speech disruptions, but also the complex mix of negative feelings and emotions that often accompany the production of stuttering events (e.g., Conture, 1990; Culatta & Goldberg, 1995; Gregory, 1972; Manning, 1996; Peters & Guitar, 1991). For these treatment approaches, the goal is not just to reduce the frequency of stuttering events, but also to help the client improve attitudes toward speaking and stuttering, and adjust to the fact that he or she is likely to continue stuttering to some degree even following treatment. Accordingly, these treatments do not define success in terms of the elimination of stuttering events, but rather in terms of a combination of reduced stuttering, decreased struggle and avoidance, and improved attitudes and self-concepts.

The Need for a Unifying Framework

Because of the diversity of opinions regarding the nature of the client's complaint, combined with the considerable differences in treatment approaches used to address these complaints, it would seem quite useful to have a unifying framework for categorizing different types of stuttering treatment. Such a framework could help guide the process of evaluating treatment efficacy by providing a common language that clinicians and researchers could use to describe their understanding of the client's complaint, as well as the nature of their treatments and the definition of success used in their programs.

One such framework that accomplishes this goal is the World Health Organization's (WHO, 1980) three-part classification scheme for describing the consequences of disorders. Known as the *International Classification of Impairments, Disabilities, and Handicaps*, or ICIDH, this framework states that the consequences of a disorder such as stuttering can be viewed at three separate but related levels, or "planes of experience" (WHO, 1980):

Impairment: . . . any loss or abnormality of psychological, physiological, or anatomical structure or function.

Disability: . . . any restriction or lack (resulting from an impairment) of ability to perform an activity in the manner or within the range considered normal for a human being.

Handicap: . . . a disadvantage for a given individual, resulting from an impairment or a disability, that limits or prevents the fulfillment of a role that is normal (depending on age, sex, and social and cultural factors) for that individual. (pp. 25–29)

The ICIDH has been applied to stuttering by a number of authors (Conture, 1996; Curlee, 1993; McClean, 1990; Prins, 1991); however, as the present author has argued elsewhere (Yaruss, 1998), the definitions of *impairment, disability,* and *handicap* used in the stuttering literature to date are not consistent with the definitions proposed by the WHO in the ICIDH. Specifically, previous authors have used *impairment* to refer to the underlying etiology associated with stuttering and *disability* to refer to the stuttering events themselves. According to researchers at the WHO Collaborating Center (WCC) for the ICIDH, however, the ICIDH is seen as quite distinct from the WHO's classification of the *etiology* of disorders described in the *International Classification of Diseases*, now in its tenth edition (ICD-10; WHO, 1992): "ICD covers causes and underlying conditions and ICIDH covers the consequences" (de Kleijn-de Vrankrijker, 1995, p. 109; see also Chamie, 1990; Halbertsma, 1995; Thuriaux, 1995). Thus, when using the ICIDH for describing stuttering, the term *impairment* is not used to refer to the underlying causes of stuttering. Instead, *impairment* refers to the stuttering itself. Similarly, *disability* refers not to the stuttering behaviors, but to the reductions in an individual's ability to perform certain tasks that may be associated with stuttering.

The ICIDH Classifications for Stuttering

To better understand how the ICIDH can provide a useful framework for understanding the nature of various stuttering treatments, it is instructive to examine the ICIDH in detail to determine how stuttering (and the consequences of the stuttering disorder) should be classified relative to the terms impairment, disability, and handicap (Yaruss, 1998).

Impairment

A review of the detailed summary of impairments found in the ICIDH reveals that stuttering is listed as an "impairment of speech form," under section 37.0, "Impairment of speech fluency: stammering, stuttering." Thus, according to the ICIDH, stuttering is, in and of itself, an impairment. It is important to note that individuals who stutter may experience a number of other impairments associated with their stuttering, such as an "Impairment of Emotion, Affect, or Mood" (WHO, 1980, Section 26.0, p. 63), seen when the client exhibits a high degree of anxiety associated with stuttering. In general, the presence of these "secondary" impairments will be dictated by the individual's reactions to stuttering.

Disability

The most common disability associated with stuttering is the reduction in the individual's ability to perform daily tasks, such as talking with others ("disability in talking . . . loss or restriction of the ability to produce audible verbal messages and to convey meaning through speech," WHO, 1980, Section 21, p. 154). Other disabilities may include "occupational role disability . . . disabilities in work performance" (WHO, 1980, Section 18.4, p. 152), involving difficulty using the telephone to complete tasks associated with a job. An individual who avoids speaking in certain situations, on the other hand, may exhibit a "disability relating to situational behavior," such as a "situation coping disability . . . disturbance in the ability to perform everyday activities in specific situations, such as outside the home" (WHO, 1980, Section 14.2, p. 150). As with the secondary impairments described above, the occurrence of disabilities is governed to a great extent by the individual's reactions to stuttering.

Handicap

The handicaps associated with stuttering involve the disadvantages experienced by an individual because of the stuttering impairment and associated disabilities in talking or interacting with others. One example of a handicap that an individual who stutters might experience is "curtailed occupation" (§4.2), which describes "individuals who are unable to participate in all the activities associated with their customary occupation" (WHO, 1980, p. 197). Another example of handicap involves an "economic self-sufficiency handicap," which describes "individuals who, although economically self-sufficient, have suffered a reduction in economic well-being when compared with . . . that expected if the individual were not impaired or disabled" (WHO, 1980, Section 6.3, p. 203). As with secondary impairments and disabilities, the occurrence of handicaps will be affected by the individual's reactions to stuttering. Furthermore, handicaps are often defined in terms of expected social roles, so the speaker's environment also plays an important role in determining whether any disadvantages will occur.

The Role of Reactions

As noted above, the occurrence of many impairments, disabilities, and handicaps is mediated, to a great extent, by the individual's reactions to stuttering. These reactions are often discussed in terms of affective, behavioral, and cognitive responses, the so-called "ABCs" of stuttering. Thus, even though an individual stutters, perhaps even severely, he or she will not experience any disabilities or handicaps unless there are reductions in the ability to perform tasks or disadvantages in fulfilling expected roles. In an attempt to more specifically reduce the disability or handicap of stuttering, then, many treatment approaches also attempt to address the individual's ABC reactions.

The ICIDH as a Framework for Evaluating Stuttering Treatment

Based on these definitions, it seems that the ICIDH can provide a useful framework for answering questions regarding the nature of the client's complaint and the definition of success in different types of stuttering treatment. Specifically, as noted above, some treatments for stuttering view the nature of the client's complaint as the stuttering impairment itself. Accordingly, these impairment-based treatment programs focus on reducing the production of stuttered disfluencies, either through prolonged speech or some other fluency shaping procedure, as noted above (e.g., Boberg & Kully, 1994; Ingham, 1984; Neilson & Andrews, 1993; Onslow & Packman, 1997; Ryan, 1979; Webster, 1980). Other programs view the nature of the client's complaint as the entire stuttering disorder, and therefore attempt to address multiple factors, including the impairment, the ABC reactions, and, to varying degrees, the resulting disabilities and handicaps. Accordingly, these broad-based treatments involve multiple components to achieve their goals (e.g., Conture, 1990; Culatta & Goldberg, 1995; Gregory, 1998; Peters & Guitar, 1991; Van Riper, 1982). To address the stuttering impairment, these programs typically incorporate some type of speech change that may be similar to prolonged speech (or using some form of easier onsets, which reduce speaking rate and tension at the beginning of words, phrases, or utterances). To address the client's ABC reactions, as well as the resulting disabilities and handicaps, the programs incorporate some type of desensitization training and counseling to reduce feelings such as anxiety, shame, and embarrassment.

By examining the components of various stuttering treatments using this framework, it is possible to identify the reasons that a clinician might use or recommend a treatment approach that has not been clearly demonstrated to be effective. If the clinician views the nature of the client's complaint to involve aspects of his ABC reactions, the disability, or the handicap of stuttering in addition to the basic stuttering impairment itself, then the clinician will not be willing to adopt a treatment approach that focuses primarily on stuttering, even though there are data suggesting that these programs do in fact reduce the frequency of stuttering. Instead, the clinician will focus his or her treatment on multiple levels of the client's experience of the stuttering disorder. *It would seem that the rationale for the treatment is clear; however, in many cases, the supporting data are not yet available.* Thus, it is incumbent upon clinical researchers who promote these broad-based treatment approaches to begin to document the outcomes of their treatments.

A Plan for Documenting Treatment Outcomes

Elsewhere (Yaruss, 1997b), the present author has proposed a plan for remedying the situation described above, in which the outcomes of frequently recommended treatment programs are not fully documented. This approach is not dissimilar from those offered by other authors (e.g., Bloodstein, 1995; Ingham, 1984, 1990; Ingham & Costello, 1985); however, this particular plan is offered here as a guide to the process of documentation being undertaken in the treatment outcomes project described below. Specifically, the plan involves the following five-step process:

1. **Describe**, in detail, the nature of the treatment program. Ideally, this should include more than just general statements about whether the program uses "fluency shaping" or "stuttering modification" procedures. Instead, the description should provide information about the frequency and duration of treatment sessions, including the total number of hours of client contact, as well as the specific sequence and nature of the treatment techniques that are involved. Variations on commonly utilized techniques (such as cancellation or easy onsets) should be carefully described so that clinicians and other researchers will be able to thoroughly review the treatment program and compare the processes and results across programs.
2. **Define** success clearly. As noted above, the definition of success may vary greatly from one program to the other. Accordingly, treatment programs should be careful to specifically de-

fine what is meant by successful treatment. For some programs (particularly the impairment-based programs above), this may mean the elimination of stuttering during conversational speech. For other programs (particularly the broad-based programs), this will mean a combination of reduced (but not necessarily eliminated) stuttering, combined with improved speech attitudes and an increased ability to function in social and occupational settings.

3. **Operationalize** the clinical decision-making process, so that treatment goals are stated in a form that facilitates measurement. This step represents one of the major challenges for broad-based programs that focus on reducing stuttering and improving attitudes, since the goals are not often clearly stated in a measurable way. Thus, a preliminary step to evaluating the outcomes of these types of treatments may involve a detailed evaluation of how the treatment is conducted, in real-world settings, in order to identify, define, and, ultimately, operationalize the treatment procedures.

4. **Measure** the outcomes of the treatment. Once the previous three steps have been taken, the process of measuring outcomes should be relatively straightforward (though not necessarily simple). It is important that these measures be taken *before treatment* to document baseline behaviors, *during treatment* in order to inform the clinical decision-making process and to document changes over time, and *after treatment* to demonstrate that changes have occurred. A crucial aspect of measurement after treatment for stuttering is the establishment of *long-term* treatment outcomes by keeping in contact with clients for an extended period of time following the termination of treatment.

5. **Report** all changes (both positive and negative) objectively. Again, this is a step that represents something of a challenge in our field. Unfortunately, it is all too tempting for practitioners to emphasize findings that highlight the benefits of their programs while minimizing less-than-satisfactory results. A pitfall of this approach is that the objective analysis of treatment outcomes may be blurred by dogma and strong opinions. In order to help clinical researchers better understand the stuttering disorder, however, it is crucial that treatment outcomes research be approached from a more objective perspective. This will allow other clinicians and researchers the opportunity to evaluate the treatments and determine which aspects of treatment may be most appropriate for their own clients.

In sum, there is much work to be done in terms of documenting the outcome of stuttering treatments. As noted above, there are some types of treatment approaches that are further along in this process, but it is important that such data become available for a variety of treatment approaches from across the field.

The Value of Clinical Data

The remainder of this chapter attempts to follow the plan outlined above for describing a treatment program that is focused on addressing aspects of the stuttering impairment, reactions, disability, and, to a certain extent, handicap. Although this treatment program has been widely disseminated through books and chapters on stuttering, many of the treatment variables have not been sufficiently operationalized to allow comprehensive measurement of treatment outcomes. Furthermore, the lack of clear definitions makes it difficult to determine whether or not clients achieve their goals as a result of treatment. An appropriate first step toward remedying this situation, then, is to document, in as much detail as possible, the practices and procedures that have been utilized with this treatment approach. This will also help to more thoroughly define the relevant treatment variables. Accordingly, the present analysis is based on a retrospective, clinical analysis of treatment effectiveness, as defined below.

Retrospective, Clinical Analysis

In the scientific evaluation of treatment efficacy, one of the most important goals is to demonstrate that a treatment results in a specific, measurable change that would not have occurred (or would not have occurred to the same extent) if the treatment had not been introduced. It is important to note at the outset, then, that the study presented in this chapter cannot meet this goal, because this research design (specifically, a retrospective analysis of clinical data) cannot demonstrate a cause-and-effect relationship between the treatment and the outcome. Furthermore, the use of clinical data in this fashion has a number of other potential problems, including difficulties establishing the reliability of data that were collected by a number of different clinicians over a 25-year period (see below).

It would seem reasonable to ask, then, why a researcher would select this design to study treatment outcomes. The answer is related to the process of operationalizing the clinical decision-making process that was described above. In particular, even though this treatment program has been described in general terms in the stuttering literature, specific aspects of the treatment process, including the nature of the expected changes in fluency, attitudes, and other reactions, have not been thoroughly documented. Thus, one appropriate starting place for operationalizing the treatment process is to carefully observe and document the changes that have occurred during the course of treatment for clients who have previously undergone treatment.

Treatment Effectiveness Versus Treatment Efficacy

Because the data analyzed in this study were collected in a real-world setting, as opposed to under controlled conditions, it is properly referred to as a study of *treatment effectiveness*, rather than of *treatment efficacy*. According to the Agency for Health Care Policy and Research (1994), studies of treatment efficacy examine the extent to which a treatment can be shown to be beneficial under optimal (or ideal) conditions. Such studies typically involve careful selection of subjects and precise control of treatment parameters to establish that the treatment is actually responsible for the changes that are observed. Studies of treatment effectiveness, on the other hand, evaluate the extent to which treatment is shown to be beneficial under typical conditions. These studies demonstrate the results of the treatment as it is actually administered by practicing clinicians in the real world; as such, they are often affected by a variety of factors that may not be related to the treatment itself. For the purposes of the present study, and for the goals of this early phase of the broader treatment outcomes project, it is important to document the changes that occurred during treatment, to support the process of refining treatment goals and operationalizing clinical procedures so that specific measures of treatment outcomes can be made in future, prospective studies.

Summary

There is a great need to document the outcomes of treatments for stuttering. Nowhere is this need greater than for those treatments that view the nature of the client's complaint as the entire stuttering disorder, encompassing aspects of the stuttering impairment, as well as the client's reactions to stuttering and the associated disabilities and handicaps that may result. Rather than suggesting that the use of such treatments should be restricted because of the lack of outcome data, it seems appropriate to engage in a rigorous course of study to evaluate the outcome of these types of treatment. In an attempt to accomplish this important goal, the next section of this chapter will present preliminary results from an ongoing clinical study of treatment effectiveness for the NU Adult Stuttering Treatment Program.

PRELIMINARY RESULTS OF A STUDY
OF TREATMENT EFFECTIVENESS

The Treatment Outcomes Project

The purpose of the Treatment Outcomes Project described below is to document the effectiveness and efficacy of stuttering treatment programs, such as the one that has been developed and used at NU for the past 30 years. When completed, the first phase of this project will involve a retrospective analysis of the results of treatment for all clients who enrolled in the NU Adult Stuttering Treatment Program since approximately 1975, combined with long-term follow-up data collected via questionnaire and direct interviews for those subjects who can be contacted. Based on the results collected during phase one, additional studies will be planned that incorporate prospective analyses of changes that occur during the course of treatment, as well as a series of experimental studies designed to determine the changes associated with specific components of the treatment program. Future studies will differ from the present analysis in that the data will be collected in a more carefully controlled manner than in typical clinical settings. Also, studies will be designed to demonstrate a causal relationship between the treatment and improvements in the client's speech and related behaviors. Nevertheless, in order to demonstrate the potential value of using retrospective, clinical data as a starting point for the studies outlined in the project as a whole, this chapter will present results collected to date for a subset of the clients who have participated in the NU Adult Stuttering Treatment Program.

Description of Treatment

In keeping with the five-point plan for documenting treatment outcomes outlined above, this report will begin with a description of the treatment program. Because the data presented in this study actually begin at the time of diagnostic testing, this description will start with a brief summary of the data collected during the diagnostic evaluation.

Diagnostic Evaluation

Clients enter treatment following a comprehensive diagnostic evaluation designed to evaluate the severity and nature of the client's stuttering disorder. This diagnostic evaluation involves a detailed interview, designed to obtain information regarding the client's history of stuttering and prior speech treatment, as well as detailed information about the client's reactions to stuttering and feelings about his or her speaking abilities in general. To establish the client's fluency prior to treatment, the client is audio-video recorded while talking in a variety of standard speaking tasks and situations (reading, conversational speech, monologue, picture description), and the frequency and types of speech disfluencies produced during these situations are analyzed according to the procedures of the *Systematic Disfluency Analysis* (SDA; Campbell & Hill, 1987), or one of its predecessors, as described below. After the basic speech samples are collected, the client's general speech and language abilities (e.g., reading, receptive and expressive language, etc.) are evaluated using a number of standard tests, combined with an informal analysis of the conversational speech sample. Finally, in addition to this detailed speech and language testing, the client also completes a number of standard personality inventories, administered by a licensed psychologist in order to determine whether there are any concerns in addition to stuttering that may adversely affect the client's progress in treatment. (These psychological data will not be utilized in the treatment outcomes project, so they will not be further detailed here.)

SDA

The SDA is a detailed transcription system designed to examine the production of speech disfluencies in the context of the speaker's conveyed message (see Yaruss, 1997a). With this system, the clinician first prepares a verbatim transcription of 200 syllables of the client's speech from an audio-video recording. While preparing this transcription, the clinician identifies all instances of speech disfluencies, as well as audible and visible characteristics of those disfluencies. The clinician then categorizes these disfluencies as "more typical" of normal speakers (e.g., repetitions of multisyllabic words and phrases, interjections, hesitations and pauses, revisions) or "less typical" of normal speakers and more characteristic of individuals who stutter (e.g., repetitions of sounds, syllables, or monosyllabic words; prolongations; blocks; or any other type of disfluency produced with visible or audible tension) as described by Gregory and colleagues (Gregory, 1986; Gregory & Hill, 1993; see also Yaruss, 1997a). Next, the frequency of more typical and less typical disfluencies is calculated based on the number of each type of disfluency that occurs in the 200-syllable speech sample.[2] This procedure

---

[2]The SDA has recently been expanded to include a detailed severity analysis, based on a weighted-point system that is calculated based on the nature of the disfluencies produced (Campbell, Hill, & Driscoll, 1991). The vast majority of the clients who participated in the treatment program were seen before the development of this system, so the severity scores were not analyzed in this study.

is repeated for each of the four to five speaking situations that are recorded during the diagnostic evaluation.

Treatment Structure

The treatment program involves an extended program of intervention lasting 18 weeks (two academic quarters of approximately 9 weeks each, separated by a break of 3 to 4 weeks; total duration of intervention between 22–24 weeks). Clients meet in the clinic two times per week in both individual and small group sessions (four to five clients per group), each lasting approximately 1 hr. In addition, clients and clinicians meet for an informal gathering every other week in a setting other than the clinic, such as a local restaurant, to promote generalization and transfer of fluency skills. Thus, the total number of treatment sessions is approximately 54 sessions, with a total amount of treatment contact time of approximately 108 hr.

In the individual sessions, clients meet with a student-clinician (typically 2nd-year M.A. students enrolled in the NU Speech-Language Pathology program), under the direct supervision of a licensed and ASHA-certified speech-language pathologist. In the group sessions, clients meet with the supervising clinician and all of the student-clinicians. Specific aspects of the treatment procedures will be described below. In general, individual treatment sessions are primarily focused on developing clients' ability to employ fluency facilitating strategies, as well as stuttering management techniques. Group sessions are primarily focused on practicing treatment techniques, combined with counseling aimed at desensitizing the clients to their stuttering and reducing the interference of tension and struggle during speech as well as during stuttering.

Following their participation in the formal treatment program, clients also have the option of attending an ongoing monthly maintenance program. This continuation group has focused on reviewing treatment techniques, as well as supporting clients' progress with problem-solving and using modifications in real-world settings. The number of clients who attend these continuation group meetings on a regular basis has traditionally been relatively low; however, this group is offered as a free service to help clients maintain and expand their fluency following treatment.

Modification Techniques

The specific treatment procedures used in this treatment program combine stuttering modification techniques ("stutter more fluently" approaches) as well as speech modification techniques ("speak more fluently" approaches). These techniques are introduced to clients in an order and at a pace that the supervising clinician judges to be appropriate for the specific clients in each group.

The purpose of the stuttering modifications is to reduce the physical tension and struggle associated with stuttering and speaking, as well as to desensitize the client to the production of speech disfluencies. In order to reduce tension that may exist during speaking tasks in general, clients are taught a form of systematic relaxation designed to help them identify and, ultimately, release physical tension in their speech musculature and throughout the body. In order to modify tension specifically associated with moments of stuttering, clients are taught to use cancellations and pull-outs (e.g., Van Riper, 1973). Tension reduction is also addressed through negative practice of tense stuttering moments, in which the client intentionally produces a very tense disfluency, then repeats the stuttering while consciously modifying the tension. (This technique is similar to cancellation, in that the stuttered word is repeated with reduced tension; however, it is viewed as a set practice activity that does not occur in conjunction with conversational speech. In recent years, this has been introduced as a preliminary to the use of cancellation in conversational speech.) Further desensitization is accomplished though the use of voluntary disfluencies and, occasionally, voluntary stuttering, in which the client intentionally produces easy disfluencies during conversational speech.

The purpose of the speech modifications is to improve the client's speech fluency. The specific speech modification is called "Easy Relaxed Approach-Smooth Movement" (ERA-SM; e.g., Gregory, 1986). Essentially, this technique requires that clients slightly slow their articulatory speaking rate and reduce their degree of physical tension while producing the first sounds of the first words of phrases. Thus, the technique is generally similar to easy onsets or light contacts used in other treatment approaches, except that the modification is limited to the beginnings of phrases. Furthermore, there is considerable emphasis placed on the clients' visualization of more physically relaxed forward movement of speech, both in the approach to the first sound in a word, and in the movement from the first sound to the second sound. The remainder of the phrase is then produced at a normal rate, without obvious modification.

In the early stages of treatment, clients may be taught to increase the use of pausing and phrasing in order to provide additional opportunities to utilize ERA-SM and to slow the pace of communication. This use of increased pausing, both between words (pausing) and at the beginnings of phrases (delaying response), also facilitates the client's desensitization to time pressures. The ultimate goal of the speech changes, however, is that the clients' speech will sound natural, with normal phrasing and intonation.

Definition of Success

The goals for this treatment program are similar to those reported elsewhere for "integrated" treatment programs (e.g., Peters & Guitar, 1991). Specifically, treatment is aimed at helping the clients achieve the following three-part objective:

1. **Improved fluency**, while modifying speech using a combination of speech changes (ERA-SM) and stuttering changes (cancellation, pull-out, etc.).
2. An increased degree of **automated fluency**, that is, fluency without the constant need for modification (as in the remainder of phrases following ERA-SM, or when tension and struggle are reduced).
3. **Improved attitudes** toward speaking and stuttering, including acceptance of disfluencies that remain when the person is not using modification techniques to attain fluent speech.

It is important to note that the specific goals have changed somewhat during the past 25 years. It would seem fair to say that throughout most of the history of this treatment program, there had been considerable emphasis on achieving normal fluency (through speech modifications such as ERA-SM), with other aspects of treatment used to support the process of improving speech fluency. In more recent years, however, it is this author's impression that there has been a shift in emphasis toward achieving more of a balance between addressing attitudes and feelings in conjunction with addressing speech fluency itself.

As noted above, one of the issues that complicates the process of evaluating treatment outcomes for these types of treatment programs is the fact that treatment goals are often not stated in terms that facilitate measurement. The same is true of the goals presented here, since they are framed in terms of *improved* fluency or attitudes, rather than in terms of a specific target frequency of stuttering. The benefit to this approach is that the treatment can remain flexible enough to account for the considerable individual differences in clients' ability to achieve such goals, as well as in the client's personal goals in seeking treatment. To enhance researchers' ability to conduct outcome studies with this type of treatment, however, it is important for these types of goals to be restated in more measurable terms. This is, in part, the rationale for conducting a retrospective, clinical study of the sort presented in this chapter, since it is difficult to know, at the outset, how much improved fluency should be required to say that a client has been successful. By analyzing the results for clients who previously completed the program, and determining whether their treatment should be deemed "successful," it should be possible to more adequately operationalize the treatment goals in terms of the ultimate outcomes of treatment.

Methods

Subjects

Subjects involved in this study include adult clients (age ranges from 18 to 65 years) who were enrolled in the NU Adult Stuttering Treatment Program between 1975 and 1996. As noted above, the first phase of the Treatment Outcomes Project will ultimately include an analysis of the results of treatment for all such clients; the present chapter presents a subset of the data. The number of subjects included in each of the analyses will be reported below.

Data Collection

The data used in this preliminary study were obtained through two sources: (a) a detailed review of the clients' files developed while the clients were enrolled in treatment, and (b) a follow-up questionnaire mailed to clients in 1996.

The clinical files include information from diagnostic reports, quarterly progress reports, and, to the extent possible, treatment logs. These data were recorded on up to five different occasions: (a) at the time of the initial diagnostic evaluation, (b) at the onset of treatment, (c) at the end of the first treatment period, (d) at the beginning of the second treatment period, and (e) at the end of treatment. Not all clinical files have data available at all of these data collection points; however, at the minimum, data were collected at the beginning and end of treatment. From these clinical files, it was possible to collect information regarding (a) the observable characteristics of stuttering, (b) clients' use of modification techniques, (c) situational factors affecting the clients' stuttering, and (d) clients' affective/cognitive reactions to stuttering. Data regarding the observable characteristics of stuttering were taken from SDAs collected in up to four different speaking situations. Data regarding clients' use of modification techniques were drawn from clinicians' judgments during treatment sessions in structured conversational settings. Data regarding situational factors and clients' reactions to stuttering were based on clients' self-reports and statements made during treatment sessions.

To assess long-term treatment outcomes, all clients who had enrolled in the program between 1975 and 1996 were sent a detailed follow-up questionnaire that requested information about speech fluency, reactions to stuttering, success with modification techniques, satisfaction with the treatment, and occurrence of relapse since their dismissal from treatment. The time elapsed between the conclusion of treatment and the time that the clients completed the follow-up questionnaire ranged from 6 months to 20 years, but most of the clients who responded to the questionnaire completed the questionnaires within 4 to 5 years posttreatment. (It was often difficult to verify mailing addresses for clients who had attended treatment more than 8 to 10 years previously.)[3]

Measurement Reliability

As noted above, one of the problems with retrospective studies is that it is often difficult, if not impossible, to adequately assess the reliability of the measures that were made by multiple clinicians over a period of many years. For the purposes of the present study, however, a number of steps have been taken to ensure sufficient reliability of measurement. First, the student-clinicians who collected measures of speech fluency and prepared the diagnostic and treatment reports analyzed in this retrospective study had undergone detailed training regarding the identification of speech disfluencies (Campbell, Hill, Yaruss, & Gregory, 1996). Furthermore, many of the SDAs were reviewed by the authors of the SDA technique (June Campbell and Diane Hill) before data were included in the clinical files. Although reliability for the SDA procedure has not been published, two preliminary analyses (Yaruss, 1997c; Yaruss, Max, Newman, & Campbell, 1998) indicate that SDA data are sufficiently reliable for the purposes of the study. Specifically, the mean difference in the frequency of disfluencies obtained from original and re-scored SDAs is approximately 0.11% ($SD = 1.5\%$), and the Pearson correlation between original and re-scored samples is greater than .90 ($p > .01$). Although these results suggest that the reliability of the frequency measures made in this study is sufficient for defining treatment procedures, it is clear that considerably more work is needed to determine whether these clinical measures are sufficiently reliable to demonstrate that the changes observed are specifically related to the treatment procedures.

Results

Four results from this preliminary analysis will be presented, encompassing (a) changes in clients' frequency of disfluency, (b) clients' use of

---

[3] Future portions of this phase of the Treatment Outcomes Project will involve face-to-face interviews with those clients who returned the questionnaire so that clients' self-reports can be supplemented with data from direct observations of the clients' speech.

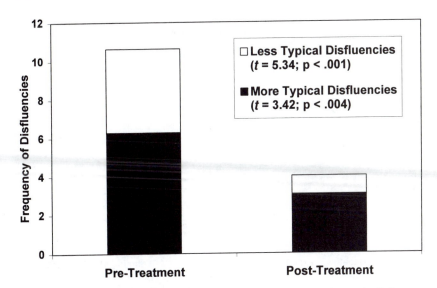

Figure 10–1. Average frequency of more typical and less typical speech disfluencies at the beginning vs. the end of treatment (averaged across subjects; $n = 15$). Paired t-tests revealed a significant reduction in the frequency of these types of speech disfluencies from the beginning to end of treatment.

modification techniques at the conclusion of treatment, (c) clinicians' reports of changes in affective and cognitive reactions to stuttering at the conclusion of treatment, and (d) clients' self-rating of their reactions to stuttering and use of modification techniques reported in the follow-up questionnaire.

Changes in Speech Fluency

Figure 10–1 shows the *average* frequency of more typical and less typical disfluency types at the beginning versus the end of treatment for 15 subjects. Paired t-tests revealed that clients exhibited a significant reduction in their frequency of speech disfluencies at the conclusion of treatment (less typical disfluencies: $t = 5.34$, $p < .001$; more typical disfluencies: $t = 3.42$; $p = .004$). In general, clients' production of less typical disfluency types was reduced to approximately 1%, while their production of more typical disfluency types was reduced to approximately 3%, suggesting that clients completed the program with speech that could be judged as within normal limits.

Figure 10–2 shows the changes in the frequency of speech disfluencies exhibited by a *single* subject (Subject #1). This client shows a

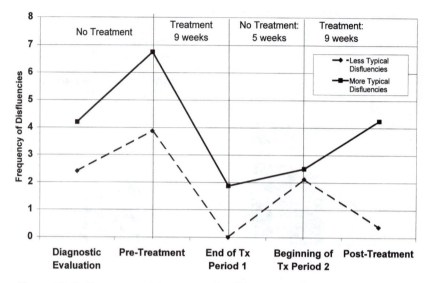

Figure 10–2. Frequency of more typical and less typical speech disfluencies for one subject (subject 1) at the time of initial diagnostic testing, at the onset of treatment, at the end of the first treatment period, at the beginning of the second treatment period, and at the conclusion of treatment.

considerable reduction in the production of both more typical and less typical disfluencies following the onset of treatment.

Client's Use of Modifications

Figure 10–3 summarizes the percentages of clients who were judged by clinicians to be able to use the various modification techniques taught during treatment ($N = 13$). It is difficult to determine exactly how clinicians made the determination that a client had mastered a given technique; however, it appears from the clinical reports that clinicians used a criterion level of modification in at least 80% of opportunities during structured conversational tasks in the clinical setting. All clients exhibited a mastery of the ERA-SM technique at the conclusion of treatment. Approximately two-thirds of the subjects exhibited mastery of delayed response, cancellation, and/or voluntary disfluency. Only one-third of clients exhibited mastery of pull-out at the conclusion of treatment, indicating that this technique may not have been sufficiently trained.

Changes in Affective/Cognitive Reactions

Information regarding changes in clients' affective and cognitive reactions to stuttering could be found in 15 of the clinical files analyzed. In

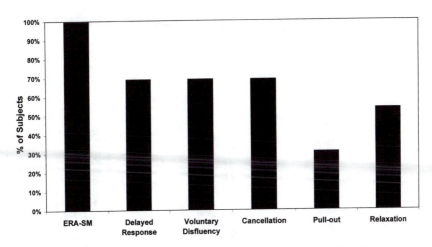

Figure 10–3. Percent of subjects (out of 15) who were judged by clinicians to exhibit mastery of various modification techniques in structured conversational settings at the conclusion of treatment.

general, two-thirds of these files indicated that clients achieved some improvement in cognitive/affective reactions, such as reduced fear or anxiety about speaking or improved attitudes about speaking and increased self-esteem. A major concern regarding this section of the reports, however, is that no specific measures of attitudes were utilized. Instead, these data seem to be based on verbal reports of clients during treatment, as well as the opinions of the clinicians.

Follow-up Data

Figure 10–4 summarizes data from the follow-up questionnaire, available for 15 subjects thus far, related to clients' self-reports of overall fluency, attitudes toward stuttering, and avoidance of speaking situations. Results indicate that subjects judged their fluency to improve dramatically following treatment, with continued but slower improvement between the conclusion of treatment and the time of the follow-up questionnaire. Similarly, clients judged their attitudes about speech and stuttering to considerably improve immediately following treatment, with residual long-term improvements. Finally, clients judged their avoidance of speaking situations to decrease immediately following treatment as well as in the long term.

Another interesting finding from the follow-up data is shown in Figure 10–5, which summarizes clients' reports about their use of modification techniques at the time they completed the follow-up

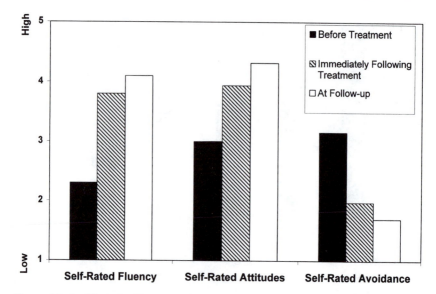

Figure 10–4. Clients' self-ratings of speech fluency, speech attitudes, and avoidance of situations before treatment, immediately following treatment, and at the time of the follow-up questionnaire (*n* = 15).

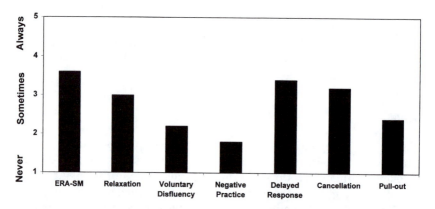

Figure 10–5. Clients' self-rating of the use of modification techniques at the time of the follow-up questionnaire (*n* = 15).

questionnaire. In general, clients tended to report that they used their modification techniques only some of the time. The most frequently used modifications were ERA-SM and delaying response (i.e., increasing pause time before producing an utterance). Interestingly, however, voluntary disfluency—the technique that is most clearly focused on desensitization—was used relatively infrequently, as were negative practice and pull-out—the techniques shown in previous analyses to have been mastered by fewer subjects at the conclusion of treatment.

Interpretation of Treatment Outcomes

Because of the preliminary nature of the data analyzed in this chapter, interpretations will be kept to a minimum. Again, the goal of presenting these data here is to support the argument being put forth in this chapter that there is value in documenting existing clinical practice as a first step in the process of determining the outcomes of stuttering treatments that have not previously been sufficiently studied.

Changes in Speech Fluency

Perhaps one of the most important aspects of stuttering treatment that can be assessed in any outcome study is the changes in the observable characteristics of stuttering that the client experiences following treatment. Data from the present analysis indicate that subjects did experience a reduction in their production of both more typical and less typical types of speech disfluencies following treatment. Speech disfluencies or stuttering were not eliminated, however, and this is consistent with the goals of this particular approach to stuttering therapy. Interestingly, the frequency of more typical types of speech disfluencies (i.e., nonstuttered disfluencies) did not change as dramatically or as consistently as the frequency of less typical disfluencies. This is not surprising, however, since one of the stuttering modifications that is taught in treatment (voluntary disfluency) actually requires the client to intentionally produce disfluencies in order to foster desensitization and to reduce anxiety about stuttering. Furthermore, some authors (e.g., Manning, 1996) have suggested that progress in treatment may actually result in an *increase* in the production of speech disfluencies if a client is working on reducing avoidance of speaking situations or of stuttering itself. Thus, as the goals for this type of treatment approach are refined and operationalized, it will be important that the definition of success allows increases in the frequency of speech disfluencies. Perhaps more appropriately, the goals related to fluency changes might specifically focus on reductions in stuttered types of speech disfluencies, while leaving open the frequency of more typical disfluency types. Such an approach would actually be quite consistent with the goals found in many behavioral treatments, which specify reductions in the frequency of stuttered types of disfluencies only and do not mention more typical disfluencies at all.

Use of Modification Techniques

Data from this study indicate that subjects were able to master many, but not all, of the modification techniques trained during treatment. This portion of the analysis is complicated by the fact that the criterion level used by clinicians to identify mastery was not fully specified. Thus, this analysis has identified another area where additional detail regarding clinical procedures will be needed to support future outcomes analysis. Based on the data presented here, it appears that the definition of successful treatment should allow for the fact that clients may achieve mastery of some, but not necessarily all, of the techniques.

Changes in Affective and Cognitive Reactions

Because of the lack of specific data relating to changes in clients' affective and cognitive reactions to stuttering, it is difficult to identify any real findings in this area. Nevertheless, feelings, thoughts, and emotions play a central role in this treatment approach, so it will be important for future attempts to document treatment outcomes to incorporate specific testing of client's affective and cognitive reactions to stuttering. There are a number of testing instruments available for achieving this goal (e.g., Andrews & Cutler, 1974; Ornstein & Manning, 1985; Watson, 1988), and it would be appropriate to incorporate these types of more formal measures into the clinical procedures so that clinicians will have a clearer understanding of how clients' feelings and thoughts about stuttering change during the course of treatment.

Follow-Up Data

In general, the follow-up data analyzed thus far indicate that those clients who responded to the questionnaire have achieved the goals associated with their treatment and maintained them over the long term. Based on self-reports, clients perceived improvements in speech fluency and related attitudes, and a decrease in avoidance behaviors. Of course, this type of sample is highly self-selected, so it is difficult to know the long-term results for other clients who did not respond to the questionnaire. The most interesting aspect of the follow-up data that are available, however, is the apparent finding that clients report that these improvements in their communication abilities even though they do not appear to use their modification techniques as frequently as they did following treatment. Indeed, all clients reported that they only used their modifications "sometimes," if at all. There are a number of ways to interpret this finding. One plausible explanation may be that clients have achieved a sufficient degree of automated fluency that they no longer feel the need to modify. Another explanation may be that clients have achieved a sufficient degree of acceptance of their stuttering that they no longer feel the need to use techniques in order to be more fluent. Finally, another possible explanation that is worthy of further consideration may be that clients' increased fluency is most directly related to the improvements in their attitudes that occurred during the course of treatment. In this interpretation, the modification techniques, and the fluency that accompanied their use, may only be necessary for giving clients the confidence to face their stuttering in a way they had been unable to do prior to treatment. Regardless of which interpretation is selected, it is clear that additional research on the outcomes of stuttering treatment, and the nature of the changes that occur during and after treatment, will be necessary to identify the precise agent of change for clients undergoing treatment.

An Additional Benefit: Improving Clinical Procedures

Aside from providing information to guide the process of evaluating treatment outcomes, data from this study also provide information about changes in clinical procedures that might improve the treatment itself. For example, as noted above, it is clear that more rigorous analyses of clients' affective and cognitive reactions to stuttering are needed. Also, this study has highlighted the need for clearer definitions of mastery for each modification technique. Not only would such definitions help standardize the clinical decision-making process and facilitate future comparisons between subjects and over time, but they will also help make the treatment more responsive to individual differences in clients. Such changes are currently being incorporated into the existing treatment structure, not only to improve the prospects for future outcome measures, but also to improve the level of service provided to clients who enroll in this program.

SUMMARY AND CONCLUSIONS

The purpose of this chapter was to suggest that there is a need for better documentation of the outcomes of stuttering treatments that incorporate both speech changes to reduce stuttering and counseling to help clients accept their stuttering. The rationale for this type of treatment was presented in terms of a unifying framework for viewing different types of stuttering treatment based upon the perceived nature of the client's complaint and the clinician's role in helping the client address that complaint. The WHO framework for describing the consequences of disorders in terms of impairment, disability, and handicap served as a way of conceptualizing and justifying differences in various approaches to stuttering treatment, particularly for those treatments that have not previously been demonstrated to be effective. Furthermore, a five-point plan for improving the documentation of treatment outcomes was introduced to provide a framework for the ongoing outcomes project currently being conducted at Northwestern University. One of the most challenging components of that plan, though, requires that the clinical decision-making process be operationalized so that specific measures of treatment outcomes can be reliably made. This step is difficult, in part, because the goals of many of these types of broad-based treatment approaches are not sufficiently defined to support this type of refinement and specification. A first step toward accomplishing the necessary documentation is to describe, in detail, exactly what clinicians and clients do during the course of treatment, and what types of changes have been seen in previous clients who have completed the treatment. Accordingly, this chapter presented data from an ongoing clinical study designed to document the changes seen in clients who have enrolled in the NU Adult Stuttering Treatment Program.

Although quite preliminary in nature, these data suggest that clients who participate in this treatment achieve the three-part goal that defines the program: Clients experience improved fluency when using modifications; an increased degree of automatic or effortless fluency that does not require modification; and acceptance of the remaining disfluencies, combined with improved speech attitudes overall. More importantly, the present analysis also provides information that can be used to guide future analyses of the outcomes of this treatment approach. Specifically, future phases of the Treatment Outcomes Project will employ more frequent measures of speech fluency, combined with specific definitions of criterion levels for determining that a client has mastered a given modification technique, and more formal testing of affective and cognitive reactions to stuttering. Changes along these lines are already being incorporated into the clinical procedures being used in the NU clinic, and such changes will continue as the ongoing analysis uncovers other areas where documentation practices can be strengthened to support future outcomes research.

In summary, retrospective clinical data such as those used in the present preliminary study certainly have their problems. Nevertheless, it is clear that the documentation of clinical practice, involving analysis of clients who have previously participated in treatment, can provide useful information to guide the analysis of the outcomes of treatments that have not previously been sufficiently analyzed. This chapter presents just one example of the value of using clinical data in this way; it is hoped that other clinical researchers will also begin to document more rigorously the outcomes of their treatments so that practicing clinicians will not need to wonder whether the treatments they select are effective in helping people who stutter.

ACKNOWLEDGMENT: The author is grateful to Dr. Anne K. Cordes for hosting the 1997 State-of-the-Art Conference at the University of Georgia, Athens, Georgia, at which portions of this paper were presented. Portions of this paper were also presented at the 1997 Leadership Conference of the American Speech-Language-Hearing Association's Division 4 on Fluency and Fluency Disorders, Tucson, Arizona. This manuscript was completed while the author was affiliated with Northwestern University. The author also wishes to express his gratitude to Dr. Hugo H. Gregory, June H. Campbell, Diane Hill, and Amy Soifer for frequent and substantive discussions about the nature of this approach to stuttering therapy.

REFERENCES

Agency for Health Care Policy and Research. (1994). *Distinguishing between efficacy and effectiveness.* Rockville, MD: Agency for Health Care Policy and Research.

Andrews, G., & Cutler, J. (1974). Stuttering therapy: The relation between changes in symptom level and attitudes. *Journal of Speech and Hearing Research, 39,* 312–319.

Andrews, G., Guitar, B., & Howie, P. (1980). Meta-analysis of stuttering treatment. *Journal of Speech and Hearing Disorders, 45,* 287–307.

Baer, D. M. (1988). If you know why you're changing a behavior, you'll know when you've changed it enough. *Behavioral Assessment, 10,* 219–223.

Baer, D. M. (1990). The critical issue in treatment efficacy is knowing why treatment was applied: A student's response to Roger Ingham. In L. B. Olswang, C. K. Thompson, S. F. Warren, & N. Minghetti (Eds.), *Treatment efficacy research in communication disorders* (pp. 31–39). Rockville, MD: American Speech-Language-Hearing Foundation.

Bloodstein, O. (1995). *A handbook on stuttering* (5th ed.). San Diego, CA: Singular Publishing Group, Inc.

Boberg, E., & Kully, D. (1994). Long-term results of an intensive treatment program for adults and adolescents who stutter. *Journal of Speech and Hearing Research, 37,* 1050–1059.

Campbell, J., & Hill, D. (1987, November). *Systematic disfluency analysis: Accountability for differential evaluation and treatment.* Miniseminar presented to the Annual Convention of the American Speech-Language-Hearing Association. New Orleans, LA.

Campbell, J., Hill, D., & Driscoll, M. (1991, November). *Systematic disfluency analysis: Using SDA to determine stuttering severity.* Poster presented to the Annual Convention of the American Speech-Language-Hearing Association. Anaheim, CA.

Campbell, J. H., Hill, D. G., Yaruss, J. S., & Gregory, H. H. (1996, November). *Integrating academic and clinical education in fluency disorders*. Invited seminar presented at the Annual Convention of the American Speech-Language-Hearing Association, Seattle, WA.

Chamie, M. (1990). The status and use of the International Classification of Impairments, Disabilities and Handicaps (ICIDH). *World Health Statistics Quarterly—Rapport Trimestriel de Statistiques Sanitaires Mondiales. 43*(4), 273–280.

Conture, E. G. (1990). *Stuttering* (2nd ed.). Englewood Cliffs, NJ: Prentice-Hall.

Conture, E. G. (1996). Treatment efficacy: Stuttering. *Journal of Speech and Hearing Research, 39*, S18–S26.

Cordes, A. K. (1998). Current status of the stuttering treatment literature. In A. K. Cordes, & R. J. Ingham (Eds.), *Treatment efficacy for stuttering: A search for empirical bases* (pp. 117–144). San Diego, CA: Singular Publishing Group.

Culatta, R., & Goldberg, S. (1995). *Stuttering treatment: An integrated approach to theory and practice*. Needham Heights, MA: Allyn & Bacon.

Curlee, R. F. (1993). Evaluating treatment efficacy for adults: Assessment of stuttering disability. *Journal of Fluency Disorders, 18*, 319–332.

de Kleijn-de Vrankrijker, M. W. (1995). The International Classification of Impairments, Disabilities, and Handicaps (ICIDH): Perspectives and developments (Part I). *Disability & Rehabilitation, 17*(3–4), 109–111.

Frattali, C. (1998). Outcome measurement: Definitions, dimensions, and perspectives. In C. Frattali (Ed.), *Outcome measurement in speech-language pathology* (pp. 1–27). New York: Thieme Medical Publishers.

Gregory, H. H. (1968). *Learning theory and stuttering therapy*. Evanston, IL: Northwestern University Press.

Gregory, H. H. (1972). An assessment of the results of stuttering therapy. *Journal of Communication Disorders, 5*, 320–334.

Gregory, H. H. (Ed.). (1979). *Controversies about stuttering therapy*. Baltimore, MD: University Park Press.

Gregory, H. H. (1986). *Stuttering: Differential evaluation and therapy*. Austin, TX: Pro-Ed.

Gregory, H. H. (Ed.). (1998). *Stuttering treatment: Rationale and procedures*. San Diego, CA: Singular Publishing Group.

Gregory, H. H., & Hill, D. (1993). Differential evaluation—Differential therapy for stuttering children. In R. F. Curlee (Ed.), *Stuttering and related disorders of fluency* (pp. 23–44). New York: Thieme Medical Publishers.

Halbertsma, J. (1995). The ICIDH: Health problems in a medical and social perspective. *Disability and Rehabilitation, 17*(3–4), 128–134.

Ingham, R. J. (1984). *Stuttering and behavior therapy: Current status and experimental foundations*. San Diego: College-Hill Press.

Ingham, R. J. (1990). Research on stuttering treatment for adults and adolescents: A perspective on how to overcome a malaise. In J. Cooper (Ed.), *Research needs in stuttering: Roadblocks and future directions* (*ASHA Reports, 18*, 91–95). Rockville, MD: American Speech-Language-Hearing Association.

Ingham, R. J., & Cordes, A. K. (1997). Self-measurement and evaluating stuttering treatment efficacy. In R. F. Curlee & G. M. Siegel (Eds.), *Nature and treatment of stuttering: New directions* (2nd ed., pp. 413–437). Needham Heights: MA: Allyn & Bacon.

Ingham, R. J., & Cordes, A. K. (in press). On watching a discipline shoot itself in the foot: Some observations on current trends in stuttering treatment research. In E. C. Healey and N. B. Ratner (Eds.), *Stuttering treatment efficacy*. New York: Lawrence Erlbaum.

Ingham, R. J., & Costello, J. C. (1985). Stuttering treatment outcome evaluation. In J. M. Costello (Ed.), *Speech disorders in adults: Recent advances* (pp. 189–223). San Diego: College-Hill Press.

Manning, W. (1996). *Clinical decision making in the diagnosis and treatment of fluency disorders*. Albany, NY: Delmar Publishers.

McClean, M. D. (1990). Neuromotor aspects of stuttering: Levels of impairment and disability. In J. Cooper (Ed.), *Research needs in stuttering: Roadblocks and future directions (ASHA Reports, 18*, 64–71). Rockville, MD: American Speech-Language-Hearing Association.

Neilson, M., & Andrews, G. (1993). Intensive fluency training of chronic stutterers. In R. Curlee (Ed.), *Stuttering and related disorders of fluency* (pp. 139–165). New York: Thieme-Stratton.

Onslow, M., & Packman, A. (1997). Designing and implementing a strategy to control stuttered speech in adults. In R. F. Curlee & G. M. Siegel (Eds.), *Nature and treatment of stuttering: New directions* (2nd ed., pp. 356–376). Needham Heights: MA: Allyn & Bacon.

Ornstein, A., & Manning, W. (1985). Self-efficacy scaling by adult stutterers. *Journal of Communication Disorders, 18*, 313–320.

Peters, T., & Guitar, B. (1991). *Stuttering: An integrated approach to its nature and treatment*. Baltimore, MD: Williams & Wilkins.

Prins, D. (1991). Theories of stuttering as event and disorder: Implications for speech production processes. In H. F. M. Peters, W. Hulstijn, & C. W. Starkweather (Eds.), *Speech motor control and stuttering* (pp. 571–580). Amsterdam: Elsevier Sciences Publishers.

Ryan, B. (1979). Stuttering therapy in a framework of operant conditioning and programmed learning. In H. Gregory (Ed.), *Controversies about stuttering therapy* (pp. 129–174). Baltimore, MD: University Park Press.

St. Louis, K., & Westbrook, J. (1987). The effectiveness of treatment for stuttering. In L. Rustin, D. Rowley, & H. Purser (Eds.), *Progress in the treatment of fluency disorders* (pp. 235–257). London: Taylor and Francis.

Thuriaux, M. C. (1995). The ICIDH: Evolution, status, and prospects. *Disability & Rehabilitation, 17*(3–4), 112–118.

Van Riper, C. (1973). *The treatment of stuttering*. Englewood Cliffs: Prentice-Hall.

Van Riper, C. G. (1982). *The Nature of stuttering* (2nd ed.). Englewood Cliffs, NJ: Prentice-Hall.

Watson, J. B. (1988). A comparison of stutterers' and nonstutterers' affective, cognitive, and behavioral self-reports. *Journal of Speech and Hearing Research, 31*, 377–385.

Webster, R. L. (1980). Evolution of a target-based behavioral therapy for stutter-ing. *Journal of Fluency Disorders, 5*, 303–320.

World Health Organization. (1980). *International classification of impair-ments, disabilities, and handicaps: A manual of classification relating to the consequences of disease.* Geneva: World Health Organization.

World Health Organization. (1992). *International statistical classification of diseases and related health problems* (ICD-10). Geneva: World Health Organization.

Yaruss, J. S. (1997a). Clinical measurement of stuttering behaviors. *Contempo-rary Issues in Communication Science and Disorders, 24*, 33–44.

Yaruss, J. S. (1997b, May). *A framework for discussing outcome measures in stuttering.* Invited presentation to the Fourth Annual Leadership Conference of the American Speech-Language-Hearing Association's Division 4 on Flu-ency and Fluency Disorders, Tucson, AZ.

Yaruss, J. S. (1997c). Clinical implications of situational variability in preschool children who stutter. *Journal of Fluency Disorders, 22*, 187–203.

Yaruss, J. S. (1998). Describing the consequences of disorders: Stuttering and the International Classification of Impairments, Disabilities, and Handicaps. *Journal of Speech, Language, and Hearing Research, 41*, 249–257.

Yaruss, J. S., Max, M., Newman, R., & Campbell, J. (1998). Comparing real-time and transcript-based techniques for measuring stuttering. *Journal of Fluency Disorders, 23*, 137–151.

CHAPTER

Theoretical and Pragmatic Considerations for Extraclinical Generalization

JAMES W. HILLIS, Ph.D.,
and
JEANNE McHUGH, M.S.

It has now been 20 years since Stokes and Baer (1977) reviewed some 270 studies of applied behavior analysis in an attempt to classify techniques for assessment and programming of behavior generalization. Before that time, according to those authors, many theorists had considered generalization to be a passive phenomenon—a natural outcome of behavior change and not requiring special attention. Only 2 years later, a major conference on client maintenance of treatment gains in speech fluency was held in Banff, Alberta, Canada, and the proceedings were published in 1981 (Boberg, 1981). Although the theme of the conference was *maintenance*, most of the strategies discussed at that meeting were applicable as well to the *generalization* of speech fluency. Generalization of clinically acquired speech fluency to situations outside the clinical setting continues to be a matter of major concern (Culatta & Goldberg, 1995).

While the topic of generalization does not occupy a large proportion of page space in the literature on treatment of speech fluency disorders, clinically useful and insightful deliberations continue to surface. In the last 5 years alone, several theoretical, descriptive, and evaluative papers have considered the issue. Among these are theoretical discussions

(R. Ingham, 1993a; Martin, 1993; Prins, 1993, 1997), suggestions of clinical procedures (Culatta & Goldberg, 1995; R. Ingham, 1993b), combined theoretical and clinical reviews (Onslow & Packman, 1997), and the mention of generalization procedures in clinical efficacy studies (Boberg & Kully, 1994[1]; Craig et al., 1996 [see Footnote 1]; Onslow, Andrews, & Lincoln, 1994; Onslow, Costa, Andrews, Harrison, & Packman, 1996 [see Footnote 1]; Ryan & Ryan, 1995 [see Footnote 1]).

The purpose of this chapter is to consider a number of factors that might lead to improved generalization of speech fluency from the clinic to a variety of situations removed from the clinic. The discussions will pertain to management of stuttering in adolescents and adults, although some of the procedures suggested would be applicable to children as well. Several features pertaining to fluency generalization will be treated in the order listed below.

1. Review of some relevant theoretical concepts applicable to generalization:
   (a) operationism and reliability
   (b) generalization and traditional learning theory
   (c) social cognitive and self-efficacy theory
2. Consideration of behavioral and attitudinal properties that might be generalized in the management of speech fluency disorders:
   (a) fluency-modifying motor speech patterns
   (b) "can-do" attitude
3. Suggestions for operationalizing the self-monitoring process as a clinical procedure for:
   (a) reliable self-identification of presumed fluency-enhancing motor speech patterns
   (b) self-monitoring of speech output to assess the extent to which presumed fluency-enhancing motor-speech patterns are present
   (c) monitoring the self-monitoring process
4. Procedures for tracking client progress and elevating efficacy expectations
5. Operational criteria for treatment withdrawal
6. Clinical illustrations of theoretical concepts and procedures.

---

[1] Generalization procedures were undertaken in these studies but not described in depth. In each case, readers were referred to previously documented descriptions.

SOME RELEVANT THEORETICAL CONCEPTS

Attention to certain theoretical concepts in behavioral management—some well established, some relatively new and untested—may serve well in the design of clinical generalization strategies for the management of stuttering. First, some of these concepts will be reviewed. Then succeeding sections of this chapter will follow with procedures and examples illustrating the applicability of the reviewed principles. Theoretical concepts to be discussed are *operationism, generalization* as viewed from the perspective of traditional learning theory, and the more recent *social cognitive theory of self-regulation*, which includes *self-efficacy theory.*

Operationism and Reliability

In science, the definition of what is to be observed and measured has always received attention, but the importance of definitional statements was brought into sharper focus in 1927 with Bridgman's discussion of "operationalism" and its contribution to the *physical* sciences. A scientific concept ". . . involves nothing more than the set of operations by which [it] is determined" (Bridgman, 1927, p. 5). In the *behavioral* sciences a few years later, Stevens (1935), using a shortened form of the term, stated: "Operationism consists simply in referring any concept for its definition to the concrete operations by which knowledge of the thing in question is had" (p. 323).

Even more simply, operationism pertains to the utilization of *operational definitions*, where an operational definition is "one which specifies the meaning of [a] *concept* [emphasis added] by denoting the measuring operations" (Underwood, 1957, p. 52). It is probably an understatement to declare, as Underwood did, that operationism makes better scientists—for without it there can be no science. *What may be less well understood is that operationism makes better clinicians by encouraging them to describe more precisely the concepts employed in clinical goal setting and treatment.*

To resurrect a quote from F. N. Kerlinger (1964), "A *concept* is a word that expresses an abstraction formed by generalization from particulars" (p. 31). For example, "speech fluency" may be considered a concept because the term is taken to represent a generalization concerning how fluent an individual's speech is perceived by that individual and listeners in the environment. A concept may be more precisely specified, but less generally, by defining it operationally, thus allowing it to function as a *construct*. A construct is a concept with the added meaning of having been deliberately and consciously invented or adopted and operationally defined for a special purpose. To paraphrase Kerlinger, "speech fluency," if allowed to function as a *construct*, must be so defined that it can be observed and measured to serve scientific or technical purposes. An operational definition allows a concept to function as a construct by specifying the activities or "operations" necessary to measure the phenomenon under consideration. "Observational" or "behavioral" definitions created by those who study human or animal behavior are a form of operational definition. "Speech fluency" may be operationally defined in terms of structured assessments, measures, scales, or tests of whatever fluency features are of interest. For example, one can make observations about speech fluency, as a construct, in a given client by administering a set of agreed-upon fluency evaluation procedures.

To quote Kerlinger again:

> Scientific investigators [and clinical professionals] must sooner or later face the necessity of measuring the variables . . . they are studying . . . . The importance of operational definitions cannot be overemphasized. They are indispensable . . . because they are bridges between the theory-hypothesis-construct level and the level of observation . . . observations are impossible without clear and specific instructions on what to observe. Operational definitions are such instructions. (Kerlinger, 1964, p. 35)

One must recognize, of course, that operational definitions, especially those of restricted dimensionality, have rather severe limitations in defining the "real" meaning of the concepts under consideration (cf. Siegel, 1987). Awareness of this shortcoming is registered in the ever present concern for the relevance or *validity* of measurement designs. That is, does a measurement plan designed to operationalize a concept of speech fluency *really* define the relevant properties of the concept under consideration? It is not uncommon for highly esteemed clinicians and scientists to view the validity of some measurement plans as flawed because the plans are noncomprehensive (e.g., Cooper, 1986; Perkins, 1983, 1990; Quesal, 1989; Sheehan, 1983; Starkweather, 1980). Nevertheless, no measurement system can be more comprehensive or *valid* than it is *reliable*.

Specifically, an observation can hardly be considered either comprehensive or valid if it is not even in agreement with other independent observations of the same phenomenon. Operational definitions are the *rules* of observation that lead to interobserver agreement and *reliability*, and reliability is the *first* requisite of validity. A discussion of the mechanics of assessing interobservation reliability will be presented in a subsequent section of this chapter under the heading "Operationalizing the Self-Monitoring Process."

Generalization and Traditional Learning Theory

The previously mentioned description by Stokes and Baer (1977) of techniques for assessment or programming of behavior generalization was based on common sense analysis and classification of methods then in use. Nevertheless, most of those clinical procedures have their roots in laboratory experimentation and the consequent evolution of learning theory dating back to the early years of this century.[2] Stokes and Baer defined generalization as "the occurrence of relevant behavior under different nontraining conditions (i.e., across subjects, settings, people, behaviors and/or time) without the scheduling of the *same* [emphasis added] events in those conditions as had been scheduled in the training conditions" (p. 150). Among the many phenomena included in traditional learning theory, *stimulus generalization* and *response generalization* are of particular interest in the generalization of speech fluency.

Stimulus Generalization

As early as 1937 Hovland (1937) noted that when a human subject is conditioned to produce a galvanic skin response to a given stimulus tone, other tones of higher or lower frequency will act as stimuli to produce the same response. That is, the galvanic skin response generalizes to other *similar* stimuli without additional conditioning. The closer a new stimulus tone is in frequency to the original stimulus tone, the greater will be the strength of that generalization. This phenomenon, termed "stimulus generalization," has been studied in depth throughout the succeeding decades and has been shown to have broad application to animal and human behavior. Stimulus generalization is one process that can facilitate transfer of behavior from one stimulus setting to another.

A special case of stimulus generalization is *associative shifting*, in which "To any new situation man responds as he would to some situation like it, *or like some element of it* [emphasis added] . . . The connection of [response] X with [stimulus] B, by virtue of connecting it first with [stimuli] A + B and then omitting [stimulus] A, is the simplest case of associative shifting" (Thorndike, 1937, p. 150). In this way a new

---

[2] See Garrett (1958) for reviews of experiments by Pavlov in classical conditioning and Thorndike in instrumental conditioning. See also Yates (1970) for a concise review of contributions from other early experimentalists (e.g., Bekhterev, Hovland, Hull, Spence).

stimulus set could be considered "similar" to an original stimulus set insofar as the new set includes elements of the stimulus field in which the original response was acquired. Thus, if a client acquires fluent speech in a clinic room with a clinician and family member, and then transfers that fluency with the same family member at home, stimulus generalization in the form of associative shift may have occurred. In this case, a significant element of the stimulus set to which the fluency response was acquired remained unchanged and the client generalized fluency to a new but similar stimulus field. "Shifting of response from one stimulus to another, or from the total situation to some part of it, enormously expands the animal's range of responses" (Garrett, 1958, p. 54).

This phenomenon was experimentally demonstrated in the modification of stuttering by Martin and Siegel (1966). They provided verbal stimuli "good" after each 30 seconds of fluent speech and "not good" after each occurrence of stuttering. Stuttering rates decreased during this condition of response-contingent verbal stimuli and increased again when the verbal stimuli were not applied. Associative shift was demonstrated in instances where a nylon strap had been fastened to the subject's wrist during the condition of response-contingent verbal stimuli. When the response-contingent verbal stimuli were withdrawn, reduced stuttering rates continued in the presence of the wrist strap alone.

Onslow and Packman (1997) have described clinical applications of this form of stimulus generalization. They require that a substantial part of treatment should occur in the presence of family and friends. These individuals become a part of the stimulus set in which original learning takes place, and their presence facilitates stimulus generalization to other situations where they are also present. Other elements of the stimulus set can become devices for associative shifting as well. For example, Onslow and Packman use an instrument for counting syllables and stuttering online. They found that the mere sight of that device may trigger stutter-free speech in the case of relapse.

Response Generalization

The principle of stimulus generalization, just described, allows a new stimulus to elicit a response that was previously acquired in the presence of another similar stimulus. Conversely, a new but similar response may arise in the presence of the same stimulus to which the response had previously been emitted in its original form. This latter phenomenon is termed "response generalization." Bekhterev (1932) reported an early experimental outcome fitting the general description of response generalization. In this case, a dog that was conditioned to lift a paw in response to a stimulus, lifted the other paw in response to the same stimulus when the previously conditioned paw was restrained.

In the succeeding years, a wide variety of behavior patterns have been interpreted as response generalization—for example the extension of communicative behavior in autistic children (Koegel & Koegel, 1988). Clinician-scientists working with speech fluency disorders have attempted to explain behavior change in terms of response generalization. Costello (1983, p. 275) described response generalization as occurring "when the effects of learning a particular behavior during treatment spread to other behaviors of the learner." Later, (J. Ingham, 1989), she described a previous experiment she and a colleague had conducted in which treatment only to one form of stuttering, say *tremor disfluencies*, also affected *repetitions*, another form of stuttering, presumably through response generalization. J. Ingham also described generalization of fluency responses from short utterances to long utterances and from monologue to reading to conversation as examples of response generalization. These latter forms of generalization seem to be the same or similar responses occurring across slightly altered stimuli and might therefore be classified, according to the preceding definitions, as *stimulus* generalization. Differences in opinion regarding the classification of these examples may be only a matter of interpretation, but in this context it is of interest to consider an interpretation of response generalization that may account for a negative form of generalization and consequent relapse of speech fluency.

If a client has succeeded in generalizing a clinically acquired, fluency enhancing motor speech pattern to some extraclinical situation, that speech pattern may be maintained as a result of reinforcement from the consequent speech fluency. However, through response generalization, the previously acquired motor speech pattern may deviate slightly over time. This generalized off-target response may be close enough to the original response to result in intermittent reinforcement by fluent speech. Intermittent reinforcement is known to condition responses that are difficult to extinguish, and consequently the off-target response is quite likely to stabilize. As the off-target response continues to be partially reinforced, the response may drift further from the original target until ultimately the frequency of stuttering is no longer satisfactory to the client. This kind of response generalization is undesirable and may be responsible for failures in generalization and maintenance.

Belief in this hypothesis has led some clinician-scientists (e.g., Webster, 1979) to recommend reliably measurable operational constructs as goals for treatment in place of such uncertain concepts as "fluent," "smooth," "prolonged," or "easy" speech. The utilization of operational constructs in this regard allows reliable assessment of drift from specified targets and provides a system for rather precise monitoring of generalization and maintenance. Devices for measuring and feeding back client accuracy in producing speech targets, or highly trained clinicians who could render reliable speech judgments, would be fundamental to the inhibition of this undesirable form of response generalization. For effective generalization, even clients might be trained to identify fluency enhancing speech patterns reliably and to monitor the occurrence of these motor speech behaviors in life situations (cf. R. Ingham & Cordes, 1997).

Parenthetically, the choice and definition of fluency enhancing speech patterns for modification and generalization through self-monitoring is a matter yet to be resolved.

> Therapy programs that use fluency initiation gestures, smooth motion speech, easy speech, and so on now rely on perceptually judged behaviors that have never been . . . shown to be necessary for the production of normally fluent speech . . . . The most overlooked issue, it seems to me, is whether in the midst of these treatments there actually is a fundamentally important variable, or set of variables, that is critical to stuttering treatment. (R. Ingham, 1993a, p. 65)

Consideration of behavioral and attitudinal properties that might be operationalized and monitored in the management of speech fluency disorders is indeed a neglected but also a pivotal issue. Although it will not be resolved in this chapter, the matter of developing and selecting constructs for generalization will be considered further in a section to follow under the heading "What to Generalize."

The basic concepts regarding traditional learning theory outlined up to this point date back more than 60 years. They are well established and widely accepted. Less well established is the notion of generalizing *cognitive processes* from clinical to life settings. A more contemporary social cognitive theory of self-regulation has recently attracted attention in the management of speech fluency disorders. This theory will be discussed next.

Social Cognitive and Self-Efficacy Theory

Albert Bandura and his colleagues have conducted research into treatment of phobias, skills, habits, social interaction, and the like. These investigations have led to Social Cognitive and Self-Efficacy Theories (SCSE) which attempt to provide conceptual models for treatment efficacy and generalization to life situations. The causal agency for behavior change in these theories is believed to reside in deliberate forethought and in self-regulatory mechanisms for translating treatment goals into reality (Bandura, 1977, 1986, 1991).

SOCIAL COGNITIVE THEORY OF SELF-REGULATION
Modified from Bandura (1991)

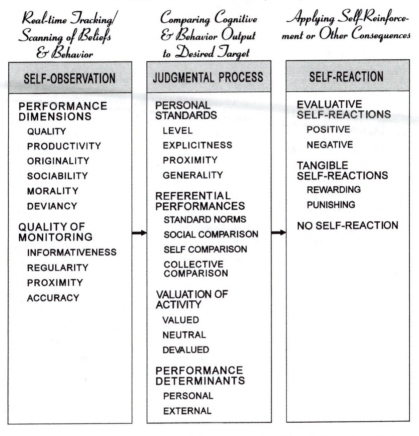

Real-time Tracking/
Scanning of Beliefs
& Behavior

Comparing Cognitive
& Behavior Output
to Desired Target

Applying Self-Reinforce-
ment or Other Consequences

SELF-OBSERVATION	JUDGMENTAL PROCESS	SELF-REACTION
PERFORMANCE DIMENSIONS	PERSONAL STANDARDS	EVALUATIVE SELF-REACTIONS
QUALITY	LEVEL	POSITIVE
PRODUCTIVITY	EXPLICITNESS	NEGATIVE
ORIGINALITY	PROXIMITY	
SOCIABILITY	GENERALITY	TANGIBLE SELF-REACTIONS
MORALITY		REWARDING
DEVIANCY	REFERENTIAL PERFORMANCES	PUNISHING
	STANDARD NORMS	
QUALITY OF MONITORING	SOCIAL COMPARISON	NO SELF-REACTION
INFORMATIVENESS	SELF COMPARISON	
REGULARITY	COLLECTIVE COMPARISON	
PROXIMITY		
ACCURACY	VALUATION OF ACTIVITY	
	VALUED	
	NEUTRAL	
	DEVALUED	
	PERFORMANCE DETERMINANTS	
	PERSONAL	
	EXTERNAL	

Figure 11–1. Bandura's structure of the system of self-regulation of motivation and action through internal standards and self-reactive influences. (From "Social Cognitive Theory of Self-Regulation," by Albert Bandura, 1991, *Organizational Behavior and Human Decision Processes, 50*, p. 24. Copyright 1991 by Academic Press, Inc. Adapted with permission.)

Self-Monitoring

Self-regulatory mechanisms in SCSE operate through what have been termed "psychological subfunctions" that must be mobilized for self-directed change. These subfunctions, displayed in Figure 11–1 (as modified from Bandura, 1991), may be viewed as the basic elements of *self-monitoring.* They are: (1) self-observation—the real-time tracking or scanning of beliefs as well as behavior output, (2) symbolization and judgment—comparing cognitive structures and behavior output to a desired target, and (3) self-reaction—applying self-reinforcement or other consequences. Interpretation of these subfunctions, as they might apply to the management of speech fluency disorders, appear in script above the respective panels.

In the Figure 11–1 panel concerned with self-observation, six *performance dimensions* as well as elements of the *quality of monitoring* are considered. It is not intended that self-observation would be simply a mechanical audit of physical performance. Cognitive structures, self-beliefs, and mood states are believed to influence both self-observation and consequent behavior patterns. However, interpretation of this notion, as it would apply to speech or other high-frequency motor behavior, suggests that self-observation of performance in those areas should not ordinarily be confounded with simultaneous self-observation of cognitive beliefs or emotional states. It would seem that self-observation of these latter conditions should instead be considered as *preparatory* to self-observation of newly acquired motor skills as they would be generalized to different discriminative stimuli.

In the center panel of Figure 11–1 where judgmental processes are outlined, four standards for comparison are named. These are *personal standards* (the perspective from which the individual makes observations), *reference standards*, (the benchmarks against which self-observed performance would be compared), *valuation standards* (a level of value assigned by the individual to the activity), and *performance determinants* (the extent to which the performance may be evaluated externally as opposed to personally).

The last panel summarizes how consequences may be self-applied on the basis of the judgmental process in the preceding panel. Self-applied consequences, if administered, may be either *evaluative* or *tangible* and either *positive* or *negative* depending on the judgment decision outlined in the previous panel.

An individual's *self-efficacy*—that is, belief in the ability to perform a task successfully—is thought to influence the operation of each of the three subfunctions just discussed. This concept will be described next.

Self-Efficacy

Bandura (1977) cites four sources, displayed in Figure 11–2, from which efficacy expectations may arise: (1) performance accomplishments, (2) vicarious experience, (3) verbal persuasion, and (4) emotional arousal. Note that each of these sources of efficacy expectation derives from clinical activities (on the right), termed "modes of induction." These con-

SELF-EFFICACY THEORY
Modified from Bandura (1977)

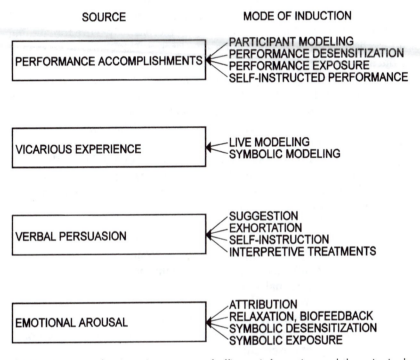

SOURCES AND MODES OF INDUCTION FOR EFFICACY EXPECTATIONS

SOURCE   MODE OF INDUCTION

PERFORMANCE ACCOMPLISHMENTS
- PARTICIPANT MODELING
- PERFORMANCE DESENSITIZATION
- PERFORMANCE EXPOSURE
- SELF-INSTRUCTED PERFORMANCE

VICARIOUS EXPERIENCE
- LIVE MODELING
- SYMBOLIC MODELING

VERBAL PERSUASION
- SUGGESTION
- EXHORTATION
- SELF-INSTRUCTION
- INTERPRETIVE TREATMENTS

EMOTIONAL AROUSAL
- ATTRIBUTION
- RELAXATION, BIOFEEDBACK
- SYMBOLIC DESENSITIZATION
- SYMBOLIC EXPOSURE

Figure 11–2. Bandura's major sources of efficacy information and the principal sources through which different modes of treatment operate. (From "Self-efficacy: Toward a Unifying Theory of Behavioral Change," by Albert Bandura, 1977, *Psychological Review, 84,* p. 195. Copyright 1977 by the American Psychological Association. Adapted with permission.)

sist of such well-known treatment activities as client modeling (role playing), desensitization, client performance, and clinician modeling. Note that even suggestion and exhortation may serve as modes of induction, as may attribution (i.e., leading clients to believe that previous fears associated with a given stimulus are no longer operational). It should be noted, however, that modes of induction based on such activities as suggestion, exhortation, and attribution "without arranging conditions to facilitate effective performance will most likely lead to failures that discredit the persuaders and further undermine the recipient's perceived self-efficacy" (Bandura, 1977, p. 198). Bandura cited two reviews (Lick & Bootzin, 1975; Paul, 1966) to support this contention.

To evaluate client percepts of self-efficacy in a given task, a technique termed "self-efficacy scaling" has been developed. This type of scaling is exemplified in a metric designed by Bandura, Adams, and Beyer (1977) to assess chronic snake phobia. Subjects were provided with a list of 29 performances describing increasingly more threatening interactions with a red-tailed boa constrictor. The client tasks ranged from approaching the cage to allowing the snake to crawl on the client's lap. Clients rated their ability and willingness to participate in these situations on a 100-point probability scale ranging in 10-point intervals from complete uncertainty (0) to complete certitude (100).

To summarize, in SCSE therapy the clinician employs various modes of induction (Figure 11–2) to convince the client that by correctly invoking the three self-monitoring subfunctions (Figure 11–1), the client can perform a selected target response in a broad spectrum of life situations. As an adjunct, self-efficacy scaling may be employed to assess client expectations.

In outline form:

A. Teach or convince the client by means of:
  1. clinician live modeling and instruction,
  2. emotional appeal,
  3. verbal persuasion, and
  4. evidence from direct performance accomplishments,
B. that by invoking the three self-monitoring subfunctions of
  1. self-observation,
  2. self-judgment and evaluation, and
  3. self-reaction and reinforcement,
C. the client can perform the target response in a broad spectrum of life situations.
D. Client expectations may be assessed by means of self-efficacy scaling.

SCSE Models in Stuttering

In treatment of speech fluency disorders, success of the above described SCSE activities may depend first on operationally defining targeted fluency enhancing cognitive and motor speech skills, and then on the client's reliable identification of those features. These activities would ordinarily be conducted in the clinical environment accompanied by clinician-evaluated client performance. Extraclinical transfer may be facilitated by stimulus and response generalization procedures. Given that caveat, Bandura's theoretical framework, due to its breadth, seems to account for most other clinical activities that would be likely to take place in the treatment of stuttering.

However, many clinicians and scientists working in the specialty area of speech fluency disorders might question the applicability of some of the sources of efficacy expectation. For example, attempting to convince a client only through verbal persuasion and emotional appeal that stuttering does not matter, or that the client possesses a nonexistent fluency skill, might be looked upon with disfavor by some specialists. Other highly regarded clinicians and scientists might find persuasion and emotional appeal acceptable. However, given the previously stated cautions concerning the use of suggestion, exhortation, and attribution, it might be more suitable to instate a core fluency enhancing behavior first, by means of stuttering modification, fluency shaping, or a combination of the two (cf. Peters & Guitar, 1991). Having done that, the client could be convinced of fluency capability (however it is defined) through direct evidence from graduated extraclinical performance accomplishments.

A few published reports have considered SCSE in the treatment of stuttering. Prins (1993), for example, has argued that invoking the self-monitoring subfunctions may play a role in determining treatment outcome. Specifically, improved fluency has been found to result from creating in the client cognitive awareness of the planned contingency arrangement between a target behavior and a consequent signal (Siegel & Hanson, 1972). In this way, the client's response was modified by means of judgmental processes (Figure 11–1) rather than through operant manipulation alone. The power of another of the three self-monitoring subfunctions, self-reaction, is exemplified in at least two other investigations (R. Ingham, 1982; Martin & Haroldson, 1982). In these studies, generalization was described to occur when clients provided *self*-evaluation of stuttering occurrences rather than when the evaluation was provided by a clinician.

In a later discussion on the modification of reactive behavior in those who stutter, Prins (1997) traced the linkage of compatibility between philosophies and therapies for modifying reactive responses during stuttering (Johnson, 1946; Van Riper, 1973; Williams, 1957) and the SCSE theories of Bandura (1977, 1986). He pointed out that although the language of these two approaches may differ, they are clinically compatible. Additionally, Prins provided clinical illustrations of the compatibility between stuttering modification therapy and SCSE.

Self-efficacy scaling, another facet of SCSE, has been employed in different ways to assess client efficacy expectations for speech fluency and willingness to approach communicative situations. At the beginning of treatment sessions, Ladouceur, Caron, and Caron (1989) asked subjects to predict the percentage of stuttered syllables (%SS) that they would emit during the session. Self-efficacy expectations for five of nine subjects correlated moderately well ($r = .70$ to $.79$) with the observed %SS during each session across many sessions. The relationship between efficacy expectations and fluency was less impressive for the remaining four subjects. One subject attained a correlation coefficient of $r = .62$, and results for the remaining three were $r = .48$ or less.

In more comprehensive applications, self-efficacy scaling has been clinically employed to assess client-perceived ability to enter into successively challenging communicative situations (an Approach mode), and then to speak fluently in those situations (a Performance mode). Two assessment scales have been designed for this purpose: the Self-Efficacy Scale for Adult Stutterers—SESAS (Ornstein & Manning, 1985) and the Self-Efficacy for Adolescents Scale—SEA Scale (Manning, 1994). Each of these scales contains a list of communicative situations, for example: "Introducing two friends at a shopping mall," or "Asking a person of the opposite sex to go with you to a school dance." For the Approach Mode in the SESAS, the client responds to each item on the list by stating the number of times out of 100 (in decade intervals of 0 to 100) that he or she would be willing to talk in that or a similar situation even though stuttering might occur. For the Performance Mode, the client states the number of times out of 100 (also in decade intervals) that he or she could speak in that or a similar situation without a listener knowing that the client has a history of stuttering. Responses are averaged across all items to obtain a score between 0 and 100 for each response mode (Approach or Performance). Clients may respond to these scales on repeated occasions, and the resulting scores may be plotted in time series to measure client progress. Reported retest reliability for an earlier form of the SESAS is somewhat modest ($r = .84$, $N = 10$), but may be spuriously low due to instructions to clients in that early form to set their own definitions for what constitutes speaking "fluently." For the SEA Scale, Cronbach's *alpha* is high ($\alpha = .98$) indicating excellent internal consistency. These scales may serve as mediators in SCSE counseling as well as time-series measures of client efficacy expectations.

Critical Appraisal

As previously stated, the concepts of operationism and of generalization based on traditional learning theory are well established. Even the more recent SCSE concepts have provided a potentially useful model for selection of therapeutic goals and assessment of progress (Lee, 1989). However, the basic theoretical concepts underlying SCSE have yet to gain general acceptance as an explanation of human behavior. Although

SCSE allows description and prediction of behavior with reasonable accuracy, it does not offer a scientific explanation of behavior (Lee, 1989; Wolpe, 1989). Lee asserts that, as in the case of other cognitive models, variables are not well operationalized, making it difficult to determine how inputs such as sources of efficacy expectation and modes of induction relate to efficacy expectation.

Additionally, the issue of dependency has been cited by Lee as a cause for concern. That is, to what extent is performance outcome a cause or an effect of expectancy as measured by self-efficacy scales, or are they both parallel responses to other events in the environment? Both Hillis (1993) and Ornstein and Manning (1985) reported using the SESAS to measure what they considered a *dependent* variable, the client's efficacy expectations for life situations, presumably arising from fluent communicative experiences. Finn (P. Finn, personal communication, April 3, 1997) observed that this usage of self-efficacy scaling may be inconsistent with SCSE because it is not tied to the specific situation in which the performance occurs, and that normally in SCSE research, subjects scale their efficacy expectations just prior to entering the situation under investigation. Finn's observation concerning the conventional operation of self-efficacy scaling is correct (cf. Bandura et al., 1977; Ladouceur et al., 1989), and may well be shared by other readers of this chapter. However, the apparent purpose of administering the scales just prior to performance attempts is to determine if performance is dependent on efficacy expectation. In this regard, Bandura states that "expectations of personal efficacy determine whether coping behavior will be initiated, how much effort will be expended, and how long it will be sustained" (Bandura, 1977, p. 191), but "expectations of personal efficacy are [in turn] based on four major sources of information: *performance accomplishments* [emphasis added], vicarious experience, verbal persuasion, and physiological states" (p.195). These statements suggest that interdependency of efficacy expectation and performance may be viewed as reciprocal in some sense and that the research or clinical question being asked would determine the type of self-efficacy scale and the order of its administration.[3]

Models and theories of behavior in their formative stages are not necessarily meant to suggest or describe accepted principles of science or approaches to treatment. Instead they may serve to generate hypotheses for further examination and refinement of behavior theory. For example, in the previously cited tutorials by Bandura spanning a period

---

[3] The authors of this chapter employ the SESAS as a measure of client-perceived extraclinical fluency, which may be dependent on motor speech patterns that the client has learned to emit and self-monitor in clinical and life situations.

of nearly 15 years, over 200 references, many of them controlled research studies, either led to or were derived from SCSE. Although SCSE
is still, or should be regarded as, a work in progress, a useful purpose
may be served by demonstrating some parallels between this theory and
clinical practice in the management of stuttering.

The remainder of this chapter will provide clinical examples of
treatment based on the various theoretical models just discussed. The
treatment approach will be that of fluency shaping; that is, modifying
the client's total speech pattern with the goal that it should be perceived
externally by the client and others as fluent and natural in a variety of
situations.[4]

WHAT TO GENERALIZE

It is difficult to design a generalization plan for the goal just described
without specifying in operational terms what would be generalized. In
all likelihood "fluency" would not be the target of choice because fluency, including attendant cognitive beliefs and emotional states, is
multifaceted and defies valid assessment as a construct for generalization. One would presume that performance of some kind of fluency-
enhancing speech activity, as found in stuttering-modification and/or
fluency-shaping therapies (cf. Peters & Guitar, 1991), would constitute
a response to be generalized. Then the "fluency effect" of whatever is
generalized can be operationally assessed by other means. A rationale
for operationalizing the response pattern to be instated and generalized
will now be considered.

Fluency-Modifying Motor Speech Patterns

In recent decades, treatment approaches for stuttering have increasingly
reflected interest in modification of the motor speech pattern, focusing
on some aspect of speech physiology. Clinical and research reports (e.g.,
Azrin & Nunn, 1974; Curlee & Perkins, 1969, 1973; Goldiamond, 1965; R.
Ingham, 1975; Perkins, 1973; Webster, 1974) have led to the revival of a
previously held notion that certain perceptually determined motor be-

---

[4] *Client* satisfaction with the fluency and naturalness of resulting speech as well
as with the amount of effort and concentration required to sustain such an
outcome is a matter of major importance. Although presently available assessment routines are insufficient to measure the client's effort or concentration, a
body of work is beginning to emerge in that area (cf. Finn & Ingham, 1994;
Ingham & Cordes, 1997).

haviors of speech onset and flow appear to reduce concurrently the severity and frequency of stuttering. Among those presumed fluency enhancing motor behaviors, sometimes referred to as "prolonged speech" (PS), the following appear salient: gentle onset of phonation, prevoice exhalation, continued phonation (or continued speechflow), slow change of articulation, and adequate breath support.

Instating and reinforcing these elements of presumed fluency enhancing speech behavior may now be facilitated by the availability of electronic instrumentation. Real-time objective assessment is accessible for kinematic, aerodynamic, and acoustic equivalents of the perceptually identified speech patterns just named (Bakker, 1997). Much of this instrumentation has been specifically designed or configured to measure these physical aspects of speech output in clinical settings and to feed the information back to the client in real time during treatment (e.g., Dembowski & Watson, 1991; Goebel, 1986; Hillis, 1993; Webster, 1979). Dembowski and Watson (1991) have classified these objectively measured speech patterns as "subperceptual" to symbolize the notion that they are not easily characterized without physical instrumentation.

Continued Phonation

Although the modification of any of a number of presumed fluency enhancing speech behaviors (whether identified perceptually or by instrumentation) may improve speech fluency, only a behavior commonly referred to as "continued phonation"[5] has been shown to result in improved speech fluency when modified by itself as the independent variable in controlled experimentation. R. Ingham, Montgomery, and Ulliana (1983) and Gow and R. Ingham (1992) demonstrated dramatic improvements in speech fluency by reducing the frequency of brief phonated intervals (PIs) in the range of approximately 150 ms or less. The fluency-enhancing effect of continued phonation identified and investigated by R. Ingham and colleagues is all the more interesting in light of the fact that the reverse of the relationship they demonstrated also appears to exist. That is, speech fluency, even when resulting from a modification of the more traditional Van Riperian treatment approach (Van Riper, 1973), has produced greater continuity of phonation. This relationship was illustrated by Metz, Onufrak, and Ogburn (1979), Metz, Samar, and Sacco (1983), and Samar, Metz, and Sacco (1986). These

---

[5] As Bakker (1997) has pointed out, continued phonation is a relative term and not possible in an absolute sense during speech. However, technology is available to measure the *extent* of continuation for phonation or speechflow (to be defined).

researchers found that silence in the intervocalic interval (IVI) of voiced stops was significantly correlated with stuttering frequency prior to treatment, and also with the magnitude of stuttering reduction following treatment.

Continued Speechflow

"Continued phonation" and "continued speechflow" are similar constructs, but can be differentiated by the manner in which the speech energy is transduced. In measures of "continued phonation," speech energy is transduced by placement of a contact microphone, an accelerometer (R. Ingham et al., 1983), or sensors for electroglottograph (Gow & Ingham, 1992) on the external surface of the larynx. This method picks up glottal vibrations (or very similar activity depending on the transducer) but excludes all or virtually all energy of voiceless phonetic segments arising from supralaryngeal sources. In measures of "continued speechflow," on the other hand, a conventional microphone is placed near the speaker's mouth allowing transduction of acoustic energy emanating from the supralaryngeal structures as well as from the glottis. This procedure considers all acoustic energy radiating from the talker, including phonation and voiced/voiceless articulation. Both continued phonation and continued speechflow have been assessed in speech, and differences have been found between the perceptually fluent and the stuttered speech of people who stutter and/or the speech of people who do not (Gow & Ingham, 1992; R. Ingham et al., 1983; Love & Jeffress, 1971; Metz et al., 1979; Metz et al., 1983; Prosek & Runyan, 1983; Samar et al., 1986).

In a demonstration of clinical time-series assessment in the management of stuttering (Hillis, 1993), speech energy was transduced by a microphone placed near the mouth of the speaker, and the measure is therefore termed "continued speechflow." Just as improved speech fluency may accompany "continued speechflow" (see immediately preceding references), increased stuttering, in the speech of those who are prone to stutter, may accompany "discontinuous speechflow." These opposing classes of speech characteristics constitute sets of mutually exclusive competing behaviors. That is, as discontinuous speechflow decreases, continued speechflow proportionately increases. The fewer the number of discontinuities per minute, the greater the continuity of speechflow, and according to the previously cited research, the more fluent the speech should be. Hillis labeled two types of discontinuities in speechflow: "pauses" and "phrase junctures." Based on pause research in fluent and stuttered speech (Goldman-Eisler, 1968; Love & Jeffress, 1971; Umeda, 1977), Hillis defined a "pause" as any break in speech energy lasting between 200 and 400 ms inclusive. Because breathing was not measured in Hillis's analysis, the construct "phrase" was offered as an alternative to "breathgroup." Whereas a "breathgroup" is regarded as the speech contained in a single outflow of the breath-stream, a "phrase" was defined by Hillis as a unit of speech energy separated from other such units by silence exceeding 400 ms in duration. Hence a "phrase juncture" would be a silence exceeding 400 ms, followed at some point in time by renewed speech energy. These constants were employed to define pauses and phrase junctures in a clinical example presented later in this chapter.[6]

Acoustic data using the timing constants specified by Hillis may be analyzed to yield the following parameters of continued speechflow: (1) pauses per minute of acoustic energy (PPM), (2) mean phrase duration in seconds of acoustic energy (MPD), and (3) speech-time ratio (STR). The latter measure is the summed durations of acoustic energy taken as a ratio to the summed durations that the client is attempting to talk. The ratio is multiplied by 100 to yield a percentage. Preliminary normative ranges for these parameters obtained by Hillis (1993) for the 15th to 85th percentile of 20 normally speaking college students were PPM: 19–35; MPD: 2.4 s to 6.6 s; STR: 60% to 73%.

The first of these measurement parameters operationally defines the continuity of speechflow. In Hillis's (1993) procedure, an audible click is produced as feedback to the client each time the client emits a pause (in the range of 200–400 ms) during speech. Clients are instructed to reduce the frequency of these pauses. As they do this, the frequency of stuttering is concurrently reduced. A low PPM reflects increased continuity of speechflow within phrases. Although PPM is not a measure of stuttering, research cited earlier has demonstrated that pause rates covary with stuttering rates. In the case of Hillis (1993), stuttering was at or near 0 stuttered syllables per min (SSPM) when the pause rate reached 5 or less per min. The second and third of the above-listed parameters may not be fluency-enhancing, but it is apparent that they may relate to the overall naturalness of the speech sample.

Obstructions in Speechflow

The use of objective instrumentation during treatment sessions has the distinct advantage of allowing highly reliable identification and

---

[6] Although the speech modification procedure employed by Hillis (1993) and that employed by R. Ingham et al. (1983) and Gow and R. Ingham (1992) are both concerned with continuity of speech, the concept of continuity is differently defined in each case.

immediate feedback concerning speech productions believed to prop-
agate fluency. However, this very advantage can work to the detriment
of generalizing fluency enhancing speech patterns to life situations
where objective instrumentation is not available. That is, clients who
have acquired fluency passively through objective electronic feedback
rather than actively through the self-monitoring subfunctions described by Bandura (1991) may experience more adversity in generalizing that fluency to other environments. For example, Dembowski
and Watson (1991), Goebel (1986), and Hillis (1993) reported only partial generalization of clinical fluency attained subsequent to instrumental feedback without perceptual training for self-monitoring. Moreover, self-identification of stuttering by clients has been shown to
result in improved generalization and maintenance when compared to
external identification (R. Ingham, 1982; Martin & Haroldson, 1982). In
both instances these findings pertain to identification of occurrences
of stuttering and (in the case of Ingham) to broad estimates of speaking rate.

To enhance the likelihood of generalization of the target behavior
pattern under Bandura's self-monitoring subfunction, the authors of this
chapter devised an operational construct that would function somewhat
as a perceptual equivalent to the "pause" defined by Hillis (1993). This
construct was termed an "obstruction in speechflow," or simply
"obstruction."

> An obstruction in speechflow is the auditory perception of the
> closure of an articulatory valve (including the glottis) during
> speech (or during the speech attempt) for some other purpose than
> speech, or for longer than needed to produce speech. An obstruc-
> tion may be hardly noticeable, even by a trained listener, but
> should be counted as such if it meets the above criteria. Although
> some obstructions in speechflow may be perceived as part or all
> of a stuttering occurrence, most may be perceived as within ac-
> ceptable limits for fluency.

This weak operational definition poses a problem for interobserver reliability. The issue of interobserver reliability, which is important to begin
with, becomes even more consequential due to the fact that clients must
be able to identify obstructions reliably for effective generalization.
Therefore a technique for assessment and calibration of interobserver
agreement on perceived events will be examined in the next section on
operationalizing the self-monitoring process. But before moving on,
there is one more response pattern that should be given consideration
as a candidate for instatement and subsequent generalization.

"Can-Do" Attitude

A body of literature concerned with client cognitive structures and typified by SCSE has emerged over the past two decades (see Wolpe, 1989, for a succinct review). To summarize, aberrant behavior is believed, under cognitive theory, to be in a large measure cognitively based. For example the client may be thought to harbor irrational fears, incorrectly believing that there is danger in certain activities he or she may pursue. In these cases treatment would require the adjustment of aberrant cognitive structures. Addressing Bandura's sources of efficacy expectation (performance accomplishments, vicarious experience, verbal persuasion, and emotional arousal) through the previously described modes of induction is an example of how this treatment might be provided according to principles of SCSE. Manning (1996) has reviewed other cognitive restructuring therapies having more direct application to the treatment of stuttering.

Of course, "Expectation alone will not produce desired performance if the component capabilities are lacking" (Bandura, 1977, p. 194). Therefore, appropriate skills for identification, motor speech performance, and self-monitoring should be in place before modification of efficacy expectations would be likely to succeed in the treatment of stuttering. Moreover, even though all four sources of efficacy expectation may constitute acceptable treatment after appropriate skills are in place, the client's efficacy expectations may more readily derive from client performance accomplishments in clinical and directed extraclinical settings.

Cognitive change (i.e., a "can-do" attitude) could then be assessed by attitude scales augmented by behavior observation. The present choice of the authors for assessment in this regard is the Approach and Performance scales of the SESAS.

OPERATIONALIZING THE SELF-MONITORING PROCESS

In Hillis's (1993) previously described procedure for pause reduction, an audible click is produced as feedback to the client each time the client emits a pause during speech. In this procedure, discontinuities in speechflow are automatically identified by the instrumentation rather than by the clinician or by client self-monitoring. As a consequence, self-monitoring is not operationalized and there is no assurance that the client has attained self-monitoring skills.

On the other hand, a strategy for reducing obstructions in speechflow (previously defined) requires active client identification and self-monitoring of these obstructions. Three clinical procedures are applied by the authors in sequential order to operationalize self-monitoring and to train clients in this skill. Briefly, the procedures train the client in:

1. self-identification of obstructions in speechflow,
2. self-monitoring to reduce obstructions in speechflow, and
3. monitoring the self-monitoring process to facilitate extraclinical generalization.

These clinical procedures will now be described in further detail. The advancement criteria to be recommended were developed from clinical trial and error with 33 clients over a 5-year period.

Self-Identification

A computer-aided system, designated as "Reliability of Observation" (RelObs; Hillis, 1992a, 1992b) is employed by the authors to calibrate observers for perceptual identification of stuttering-related events, including obstructions in speechflow. Agreement is based on time-interval measurement somewhat similar to that employed by Cordes, Ingham, Frank, and Ingham (1992), but with smaller interval durations and different measures of agreement. In the case of RelObs, event identifications from different observers are registered as agreements if they differ in time by less than a second. Cohen's kappa (κ) (Cohen, 1960) is the primary measure of agreement. Several parameters of verbal output, here termed "speech features," are defined behaviorally for evaluation by RelObs. Some features of interest here are *moments of stuttering, stuttered syllables, obstructions in speechflow,* and *breathgroups*. RelObs allows data logging and online assessment of interobservation agreement for several measurement parameters including: (1) time available for speaking, (2) time speech is attempted, (3) total number of occurrences tallied for a specified speech feature, and (4) moment, to the nearest tenth of a second, that each occurrence of a specified speech feature was identified.

The user is invited to choose a speech sample, a speech feature, and an observe/compare routine from a menu. All speech features on the menu are behaviorally defined, and the user may call up the definition by pressing a help key. From this point, the user may log observational data or make comparisons of her/his own observations with observations of other users, or in some cases with observations logged by an "IDEAL" observer. In less than 10 s and without need for a written transcription, a complete interobserver agreement analysis can be performed for a behavior sample of up to 8 min.

Users may call for an animated audiovisual display of points of agreement between themselves and any other observer. The display (Figure 11–3) unfolds second by second, synchronized with the behav-

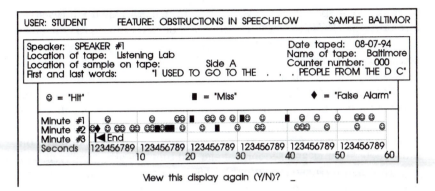

USER: STUDENT   FEATURE: OBSTRUCTIONS IN SPEECHFLOW   SAMPLE: BALTIMOR

Speaker: SPEAKER #1   Date taped: 08-07-94
Location of tape: Listening Lab   Name of tape: Baltimore
Location of sample on tape: Side A   Counter number: 000
First and last words: "I USED TO GO TO THE . . . PEOPLE FROM THE D C"

☺ = "Hit"   ■ = "Miss"   ◆ = "False Alarm"

Minute #1	☺ ☺ ☺☺ ■ ☺☺ ☺ ☺ ■☺ ☺ ■ ☺ ☺ ☺ ☺☺ ☺
Minute #2	☺◆ ☺ ☺☺ ☺☺ ☺☺■☺■ ☺ ☺ ■ ☺ ☺☺ ☺☺☺ ☺ ☺ ☺
Minute #3	◄ End
Seconds	123456789 123456789 123456789 123456789 123456789 123456789
	10 20 30 40 50 60

View this display again (Y/N)? _

Figure 11–3. Screen from computer program "Reliability of Observation" (RelObs). An animated audiovisual display of points of agreement between two observations of "obstructions in speechflow" from the same speech sample.

ior sample being played back from an audio or video system. A mark representing a tally by an observer pops up accompanied by a pulse tone during the second in the playback that the tally had previously been logged. A specialized mark (happy face) representing an agreement pops up each time tallies occur less than a second apart for both observers. This display is useful for calibration because it allows each observer to determine what kinds of behavioral events resulted in a tally by the IDEAL observer or any other observer who has logged observations for the same speech sample and feature.

The analysis includes a contingency matrix and a set of agreement indexes including total percentage agreement (the lesser/greater ratio), interval-by-interval percentage agreement, and Cohen's κ. Time intervals for defining units of agreement may be varied by the user from 0.2 to 2.0 s. The default time interval is 1.0 s. Additional information pertaining to reliability issues and agreement indexes, especially with regard to speech fluency disorders, is available in several recent publications (Cordes, 1994; Cordes & R. Ingham, 1994; Lewis 1994). Clients are trained to identify obstructions in their own speechflow in agreement with their clinician to a criterion of $\kappa \geq .70$ before progressing to monitoring exercises.

Self-Monitoring

At this point the clinician and client work together with a computer program for record keeping and audiovisual feedback during trials. This program assists clinician and client in evaluating successive 6-s intervals of continuous speech. Exercises range in a hierarchical GILCU-style format (Ryan, 1974) from the echoing of modeled phrases to conversation. During this procedure, the clinician presses a computer key contingent on each obstruction during the client's speech. The key press is registered as a beep and a blip on a moving bar at the top of the computer screen (Figure 11–4). The bar sweeps the screen every 6 s. If the client is perceived by the clinician to emit no obstructions in a given 6-s interval, that interval is defined as a continuous interval. With each 6-s screen sweep, a measure of percent continuous intervals is updated on the screen. Minutes and seconds of elapsed time are also displayed.

Throughout these activities the clinician continues to elevate the client's efficacy expectations by means of the various modes of induction associated with Bandura's sources of efficacy information as in Figure 11–2. The clinician and client may elect, at the end of each minute, to switch to a screen displaying a progress chart. Even while the client is emitting a low percentage of continuous intervals, evidence of improvement, as displayed on the progress chart, may elevate efficacy expectation through knowledge of performance accomplishments.

When the client achieves advancement criteria, say 70% continuous intervals, in conversational speech across any successive 10-min period (client's attempted speaking time), the client will probably be fluently speaking and it is assumed that an understanding of what it means to "self-monitor" has been achieved. Advancement criteria are:

1. at least 70% continuous intervals, [7,8]
2. less than one stuttered syllable per min of client's attempted speech time,
3. between 190 and 230 syllables per minute of client's attempted speech time, and
4. speech output judged as natural by client, clinician, and supervisor.[9]

---

[7]This criterion is essential. Clients may sometimes meet the other three criteria, even before beginning treatment. If, however, "stuttering" is the complaint and this criterion has not been met, treatment to reduce obstructions in speechflow will continue.

[8]If the client is not speaking fluently upon achievement of this criterion, assessment of interobserver agreement may show that criteria for identification of obstructions are too lax. In such case, client, clinician, and supervisor are recalibrated by agreement training (RelObs), or a higher level of percent continuous intervals is adopted.

[9]The judgment choices are "natural" or "unnatural." If the speech is judged as unnatural, speech characteristics seeming to result in the unnatural judgment are modified directly.

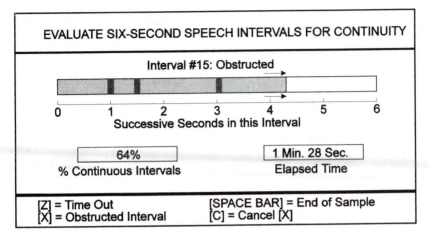

Figure 11–4. Screen from computer program for perceptual evaluation of successive 6-s intervals of speech. Online feedback of speech continuity to client.

Achievement of these criteria should be ultimately demonstrated in conversation having between 5 and 10 interchanges per minute. When the criteria are met, exercises in monitoring self-monitoring are initiated.

Monitoring the Self-Monitoring Process

The client is trained to invoke Bandura's self-monitoring subfunctions (Figure 11–1) through graduated self-monitoring activities. During self-monitoring activities, the client talks to the clinician in monologue and later in a hierarchy of conversation, role-playing activities and telephone while time sampling self-monitoring by pressing a key on a computer keyboard at random points in time. Randomly, about twice each min during the activity, a beep signal is issued from the computer and the client is asked the question on-screen (Figure 11–5), "Were you self-monitoring?" The client responds "Yes," "No," or "No response" by pressing an appropriate key.[10] The client may select the "No response" option if he or she was not talking at the time the question was asked. Failure to make one of the three selections within 1 s will also be registered as

---

[10]This is similar to a procedure described by Shames and Florance (1980) in which the client produces a hand signal continuously to indicate self-monitoring. The present time-sampling approach was designed to reduce the likelihood that the client will inadvertently continue with a hand signal even when no longer self-monitoring.

"No response." Each time the client selects a "Yes" or "No" response, a dot is placed or moved to a vertical position on the computer screen indicating the percentage of time monitored for the current block of 10 responses. At the conclusion of each block of 10 responses, the dot is permanently placed on the vertical line corresponding to that block of 10 responses, and a connecting line is drawn between the dot and the one preceding it on the chart. Throughout these activities, as before, the clinician continues to elevate the client's efficacy expectations through modes of induction associated with sources of efficacy information. Progress as charted on-screen may serve to raise the client's efficacy expectation, thereby increasing the likelihood of continued improvement, as predicted by SCSE.

As the client learns to monitor self-monitoring in conversation, telephone, and role-playing activities, other listeners—clinic staff, friends, family, etc.—may participate for stimulus generalization of continued speechflow and self-monitoring by means of associative shifting. Additionally, stimulus generalization is broadened to include extraclinical activities. These activities are derived from client responses to the SESAS Performance scale. For stimulus generalization by associative shifting, clients may take a laminated credit card-sized image of Figure 11–5 to serve as a discriminative stimulus during these outside assignments.

TRACKING PROGRESS AND ELEVATING EFFICACY EXPECTATIONS

Generalization can be reciprocally monitored and expedited for the client by simultaneous tracking of multiple fluency constructs throughout treatment. The client's efficacy expectations can be elevated by knowledge of performance accomplishments derived from continuous fluency tracking as well as from participant modeling (role-playing) and performance exposure (extraclinical assignments).

Tracking Client Progress

Throughout the course of treatment, principles of operationism are utilized to track client progress and generalization across as many measurement parameters, environmental settings, and weeks of treatment as economically feasible. The data obtained allow the clinician to monitor client progress and generalization and to modify treatment as necessary. It is also helpful for the client to observe the charted progress as a source for elevating efficacy expectations.

Probe-test data are acquired weekly or biweekly as conditions allow. Speech measures are obtained from audiotaped extraclinical

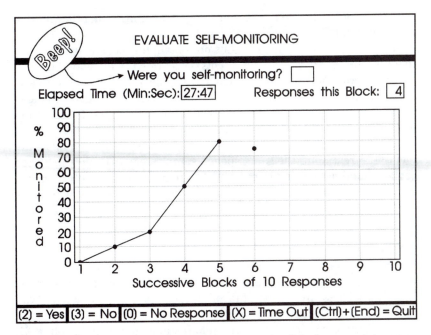

Figure 11–5. Screen from computer program "Monitor." Evaluates and charts percentage of time client claims to be self-monitoring speech continuity by randomly asking at 30-s variable intervals if the client is self-monitoring.

speech samples and/or from speech samples obtained in the clinic just before treatment sessions in order to minimize warm-up effect. For those clients whose speech samples are acoustically analyzed to obtain MPD, STR, and PPM, electronic analysis of the probe-test speech sample is performed live, on-line, in the clinic, and without immediate feedback to the client. Electronic analyses utilizing the timing constants specified by Hillis (1993), and summarized earlier in this chapter, allow the following acoustic measures of continued speechflow:

MPD: Mean "Phrase" Duration in seconds of acoustic energy per "phrase."
Normative range: 2.4 s to 6.6 s (Hillis, 1993).

STR: Speech-Time Ratio, summed durations of acoustic energy as a ratio to summed durations of attempted speech.
Normative range: 60%–73% STR (Hillis, 1993).

PPM: Pauses (200–400 ms) per minute of acoustic speech energy.
Fluency enhancing range: ≤ 5 PPM (Hillis, 1993).
Normative range (15th to 85th percentile): 19–35 PPM (Hillis, 1993).

The difference between the "fluency enhancing range" and the "normative range" for PPM (see above) is noteworthy. In the authors' clinical experience, consistent fluency does not obtain for those who are prone to stutter unless PPM is 5 or less. This pause rate is well below the 15th percentile of nonstuttering students from university public speaking courses—therefore below normal. Nevertheless, the speech of clients containing ≤ 5 PPM is perceived as natural by listeners if it is within normative ranges for MPD, STR, and SPM.

In those cases where electronic analysis is employed in measurement and treatment, the same speech samples electronically analyzed at the beginning of a treatment session are later perceptually analyzed by hand tallies from audiotape recordings and assessed for interobserver agreement after the treatment session. The perceptual measures are:

SPM: Speech rate in Syllables per Minute with syllables ignored that do not contribute to the transmission of information—that is, repeated words or phrases, stereotyped insertions (as "you know," "I mean"), and incomplete words.
Normative range: 190–230 SPM (estimated from Johnson, 1961; mean word rate of male and female nonstuttering speakers at 3rd and 7th deciles on Job Task; multiplied by 1.5 for syllable-rate conversion and reported to nearest decade).

SSPM: Stuttered Syllables per Minute defined as continuation, stopping, or repetition *within* words.
Normative range: < 1 SSPM (estimated from Johnson, 1961; mean of male and female nonstuttering speakers from 1st through 7th deciles on Job Task).

SPM and SSPM are also determined from presession audiotaped speech samples of clients whose speech is not electronically analyzed. Additionally, a perceptual analysis of obstructions in speechflow is performed for clients whose speech is not electronically analyzed. The unit of measure is:

%OTI: Percent On-target Intervals—the percentage of 6-s intervals of speech that are emitted without obstructions in speechflow as previously defined.
Fluency enhancing range: ≥ 70 %OTI (determined by trial and error in clinical practice).
Normative range: Unknown

These acoustic and perceptual measures are augmented for all clients by the Approach and Performance scales of the SESAS:

Appr: Approach scale of the SESAS as previously described.
Normative range: $\geq$ 75 (Ornstein & Manning, 1985).

Perf: Performance scale of the SESAS as previously described.
Normative range: $\geq$ 90 (estimated from Ornstein & Manning, 1985).

The fluency enhancing ranges of PPM or %OTI function as *essential* treatment goals. The authors of this chapter consider clinical fluency as questionable unless one of those target ranges is met, at least during in-clinic probe tests administered at the beginning of the session for two or three successive sessions. *Normative ranges* of the other measurement parameters, that is with exception of PPM or %OTI, serve as *ideal* goals. If the fluency enhancing ranges of PPM or %OTI have been attained, clinical fluency is then regarded as having been achieved to whatever extent the normative ranges of the other parameters can also be attained.

Ordinarily the client's speech is classified as "clinically fluent" when the following two criteria are met:

1. Client meets stated goal ranges for SPM and SSPM *and* for either %OTI *or* all of the following three: MPD, STR, and PPM.
2. Client's speech output is judged as natural (see Footnote 9) by the client, clinician, and supervisor or one other person.

Fluency treatment by reduction of PPM was conducted by the authors with a different set of clients than was treatment by increasing %OTI. Therefore no client received treatment by both of these procedures. In those cases where clinical fluency was acquired by reduction of PPM, generalization efforts were directly concentrated on extraclinical approach and performance as measured by Perf and Appr. If, on the other hand, clinical fluency had been acquired by increasing %OTI, extraclinical generalization was not attempted until the client had also demonstrated ability to monitor self-monitoring activities, as previously described.

Elevating Efficacy Expectations

Even considering its ambivalent status as a theory of human behavior, SCSE provides a potentially useful model for selection of therapeutic goals and assessment of progress. There are, however, two previously cited features concerning the clinical application of SCSE that bear repeating at this point: (1) Modes for elevating efficacy expectation based on persuasion without arranging conditions to facilitate performance may lead to failure, and (2) interdependency of efficacy expectation and performance should probably be viewed as reciprocal in some sense rather than as independent and dependent variables. Given these considerations, it would be a mistake to rely absolutely on elevation of efficacy expectations as a source of improved performance. Nevertheless, these two variables may reciprocate back and forth as dependent and independent, improving performance (speech fluency) through stimulus generalization in related situations. This relationship would justify attempts to improve speech fluency in extraclinical situations by elevating fluency expectancy through improved speech fluency in other similar situations.

Accordingly, the authors recommend selecting communicative situations from items on the SESAS for role-playing activities in the clinic. Where possible, clinical role-playing should be done at some point with someone other than the client's clinician. Typically, the authors have observed modest elevation of the self-efficacy score for a given SESAS situation after it has been successfully role-played in the clinic. For extraclinical trials, the authors select situations that occur with some regularity in the client's life and that show reasonably promising efficacy expectations after clinical role playing. Ordinarily the initial situation selected should be associated with an efficacy expectation (single-item SESAS score) exceeding 70 if possible. This caution is exercised because success or failure in an extraclinical trial may affect efficacy expectations with regard to related communicative situations. During the first week or so of these generalization activities, it may be best to select only one extraclinical situation. The time and place would be selected in advance where possible, and the situation should be practiced in the clinic by role playing as realistically as conditions will allow.

In a procedure recommended by the authors, the client is provided with a Single-Situation Transfer Plan on which the client will later record performance on a selected activity. An outline of the contents of the Transfer Plan appears in Table 11–1. In advance, the clinician and client log pretrial information: the intended date, listeners, time, place, and real-life purpose. The client's efficacy expectation is also stated as pretrial information. Efficacy expectation is listed as the client's perceived probability of fluency between 0 and 100. As with the SESAS, fluency is taken here to mean that the client will perceive that listeners would not be aware, based on the client's speech, of a history of stuttering. The fluency precursive target ($\leq$ 5 PPM or > 70 %OTI) is also stated as pretrial information. After completion of the assigned communicative situation, the client records success in remembering to self-monitor the fluency precursive target. Success in this regard is registered if the client

Table 11–1. Contents of Single-Situation Transfer Plan.

Pre-Event	Post-Event
Date	Remembering Self-monitoring
Listeners	Fluent vs. Stuttered
Time	Efficacy Expectation (Performance)
Place	Comments
Purpose	
Efficacy Expectation (Performance)	
Fluency Enhancing Target (PPM or %OTI)	

records having thought of self-monitoring for the target just before entering the situation and at least once during the situation. A posttrial efficacy expectation from 0 to 100 is also recorded by the client based on the situation just experienced. Additionally, comments may be added by the client.

More situations are planned based on the recorded outcome of the transfer assignment. As transfer activities meet with success and SESAS scores improve, up to four or five transfer activities may be assigned in a week. Selection of activities may be based on factors such as efficacy expectation scores, likelihood of generalization due to stimulus similarities, and importance of a given situation in the client's communicative lifestyle.

Inasmuch as a universal cure for stuttering has yet to be demonstrated, few clients may achieve SESAS Perf scores consistently in excess of 80. Even fewer may be expected to attain scores within the normal range ($\geq$ 90) during the course of formal treatment. For this reason, the clinician should consider the utilization of operational criteria for withdrawal from formal treatment. Some suggestions for treatment withdrawal are offered in the next brief section.

OPERATIONAL CRITERIA FOR TREATMENT WITHDRAWAL

Typically after 20 to 40 hr of treatment, clients should be able to maintain fluency precursive speech patterns, including self-monitoring, in role-playing and telephone activities within the clinical setting. At that point there is probably little to be gained from continued practice in the clinical environment. Criteria should therefore be established for introducing new in-clinic activities and reducing the frequency of clinical visits. The authors recommend changing clinical activities and placing the client on a reduced clinical schedule when the client meets goal ranges for clinical fluency as previously defined. If clinical fluency has been acquired by increasing %OTI, the client should also be able to monitor self-monitoring to a criterion of $\geq$ 80% (Figure 11–5). When these goals are achieved, clinic visits may be reduced from intensive therapy (several hours a week where possible) to one or two 1-hour visits a month.

Several activities are recommended for maintenance of clinical fluency and generalization during these monthly or bimonthly visits:

1. Probe testing to monitor current status of:
   (a) %OTI (or PPM, etc.), SPM, and SSPM in clinic, and at home or work via audiotape when available, and
   (b) SESAS Approach and Performance scores.
2. Practicing motor speech skills if above measures do not meet criteria for clinical fluency.
3. Review of success in previously assigned single-situation transfer plans.
4. Role-playing and assignment of new single-situation transfer plans based on SESAS scores and previous transfer success.

The authors recommend continuing with these semimonthly or monthly generalization sessions until SESAS Approach and Performance fail to show continued gains over any 6-month period after the client is clinically fluent. At the time of discharge, clients should be counseled very carefully concerning relapse, and they should be invited to return for annual checkups. They should be advised that in case of relapse, the same therapy that worked before is quite likely to work again, probably faster because all they should have to do is refresh a skill that they have already acquired.

CLINICAL EXAMPLES

The various data parameters previously described are presented as time-series charts synchronized with each other across successive calendar weeks (Figures 11–6 through 11–8). One to five pretreatment baseline measures are obtained for each parameter. Data in the body of each chart are acquired weekly or biweekly if possible, after completion of pretreatment baselines, but the pretreatment baseline data are telescoped into a shorter duration to reduce the waiting time between initial evaluation and treatment. That is, pretreatment data may be obtained daily, whereas data obtained during the course of treatment may be obtained weekly or biweekly. Any effect that this procedure may have on baselines and subsequent in-treatment records is unknown.

As the performance charts will show, problems in generalization are not uncommon. Operational precision and long-term, multiple-baseline tracking, allow identification of those sources of difficulty. Efforts can then be undertaken to manage problem sources through the use of clinical generalization procedures. Suggested generalization strategies are influenced by theoretical concepts previously described in this chapter: operationism, traditional learning theory, and SCSE. Especially of note are the following procedures embodied in those theoretical concepts:

1. Reliable measurement (operationism)
2. Operationalized self-monitoring (operationism and SCSE)
3. Stimulus generalization (traditional learning theory)
4. Inhibition of undesirable response generalization (operationism and traditional learning theory)
5. Tracking client progress (operationism)
6. Elevation of efficacy expectations (SCSE)

Individual clinical examples will now be described. In some instances, certain generalization procedures such as associative shift (described earlier in this chapter) and vicarious observation of treatment success were not available for clinical use due to client lifestyles and scheduling difficulties. These deficits and their possible effect will be pointed out. The names used in reference to clients are pseudonyms intended to link text narratives with corresponding charted data by a common designation.

As previously described, fluency treatment by reduction of PPM was conducted by the authors with a different set of clients than was treatment by increasing %OTI. The first client to be presented, "Dave," was treated only by reduction of PPM. The remaining two clients, "Ralph" and "John," were treated by increasing %OTI.

Dave

Dave is a 25-year-old structural engineer. He had received treatment for stuttering at various times throughout his life in the public schools and at four university speech and hearing centers. His charts appear as Figure 11–6.

Treatment Analysis

By the 3rd week of post baseline treatment, Dave's PPM had decreased from 60 to 5 with a corresponding dramatic decrease in SSPM as measured in the clinic. By the 6th week his syllable rate had doubled from a

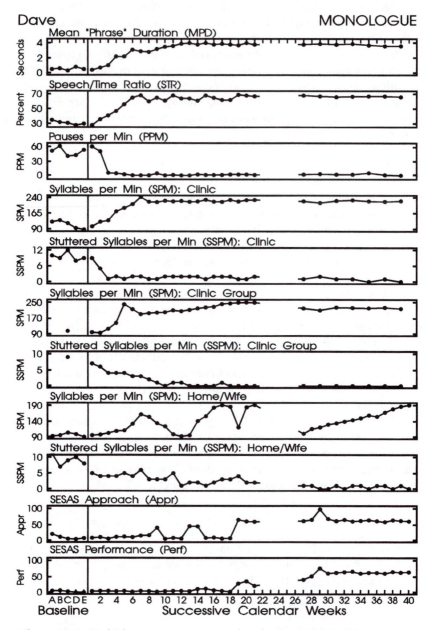

Figure 11–6. Multiple-parameter progress chart for Dave. PPM = Pauses per Min, MPD = Mean Phrase Duration, STR = Speech-time Ratio, SPM = Syllables per Min, SSPM = Stuttered Syllables per Min, Appr = SESAS Approach, Perf = SESAS Performance.

range approximating 100 SPM to over 200 SPM and his stuttered-syllable rate had decreased from 10 SSPM at baseline to about 2 SSPM. These changes in fluency levels are displayed in charts for Clinic (SPM and SSPM). Actually 5 of 16 measures of SSPM from the 3rd through the 18th week were less than 1 SSPM; the others were between 1 and 2 SSPM. This is quite fluent but slightly above the previously stated normative range of < 1 SSPM. During the first 18 weeks, shaping of clinical fluency continued with generalization efforts limited to improvement of efficacy expectations by allowing the client to review his charted performance progress.

Generalization to other environments, Home/Wife (SPM and SSPM) and SESAS (Appr and Perf), is apparent but not impressive during the first 18 weeks. On the other hand, the charts for Clinic Group (SPM and SSPM) illustrate a slow but apparently spontaneous and rather complete generalization during the first 18 weeks to a voluntary group role-playing session. The speaking mode in the group is a 3-min impromptu delivery while standing at a lectern in front of a group of clinicians and clients. Because the group meets only once a week, there is a pretreatment basepoint but no baseline. No deliberate effort was made toward improvement in the group performance during the first 18 weeks, but the observed generalization to the group was probably not spontaneous in the true sense of the word. Review of charts to improve efficacy expectation during this period has already been cited. Additionally, the client's clinician was present during the group meeting, which was held in a conference room across the hall from the individual treatment rooms. The similarity of this stimulus field to that in which clinical fluency was acquired seems to have been enough to facilitate generalization through associative shifting, a process described earlier in this chapter. Clinical fluency may have spontaneously generalized but weakly to other environments as demonstrated in charts for Home/Wife (SPM and SSPM) and SESAS (Appr), but some kind of active promotion is nearly always required for a more complete generalization than that shown during the first 18 weeks.

In Week 18 more deliberate generalization efforts were initiated. The client's wife attended two of the treatment sessions, during which she and the client conversed in the presence of the clinician while pause-contingent feedback was provided by the monitoring instrumentation. As expected, stuttering rate concomitantly varied with pause rate during these treatment sessions. At first the client could not reduce the pause rate in the clinic in the presence of his wife without stretching syllabic nuclei and consequently reducing SPM. Stimulus generalization of this speech pattern, presumably by associative shifting, did occur as evidenced by the Home/Wife (SPM and SSPM) charts. This is especially apparent beginning in Week 27 after a 5-week summer break. Unfortunately the undesirable slow syllable rate (SPM) generalized to the home as well as the desirable reduction of stuttering (SSPM). The client was in-

structed to push the envelope of SPM upward week by week while attempting to maintain the low SSPM in the home recordings. Each week, onward
from Week 27, efforts to elevate the client's efficacy expectations were
continued by reviewing his charted progress on the home recordings as
well as on other measurement parameters including SESAS.

Other generalization activities were initiated on Week 18. The major
activities involved efforts to improve efficacy expectation through clinical role playing and extraclinical assignments as described previously
under the heading of Elevating Efficacy Expectations. As evidenced by
SESAS Appr and Perf charts, generalization did occur. The improvement
is robust, increasing from 0 (or slightly higher in Appr) at Week 18 to
about 65 seven treatment weeks later and continuing to the conclusion
of treatment. This level falls short of the normative ranges previously
described for these parameters, but the client was pleased with the results and elected to terminate treatment after Week 40, which coincided
with the break between the fall and winter/spring semesters.

Note that between Weeks 8 and 14 inclusive, sporadic increments
in Appr may be seen even though Perf remains at or near 0. Some might
interpret the observed precedence of Appr as evidence that speech performance is dependent on attitudes. Actually the observed precedence
appears to be an artifact associated with the difference in definition
between Appr and Perf. A positive Appr experience requires only willingness to enter into a situation even though the client believes stuttering might occur. On the other hand, a positive Perf experience requires
that the client enter into the situation *and* leave with the belief that
anyone listening was not aware that the client had ever stuttered. Perf,
as it is measured by SESAS, is more difficult to attain and would therefore be expected to lag Appr by that fact alone.

The lower end of the normative range for Perf, as previously stated, is
90, well above the client's Perf level of 65 at termination. Nevertheless, the
client's terminal Perf level indicates that he believes he would be so fluent
on the average in 65% of the SESAS situations that listeners would not know
that he had ever stuttered. As one might expect, the client was not cured of
stuttering. Even so, at the end of 35 weeks of treatment by supervised
graduate students, he had changed from a person who reported stuttering
and avoidance in nearly all communicative situations to one who reported
participation and full fluency in well over half of the same situations.

Cross-Correlational Analysis

It is clearly evident from inspection of Figure 11–6 that there is considerable covariation among the measures employed even though they are
of different physical, perceptual, and attitudinal parameters. To test the
extent to which these measures covaried, cross-correlational analyses

were computed for each possible combination of two measurement parameters for the complete data array in Figure 11–6. Cross-correlational analysis produces Pearson product-moment correlation coefficients (r) that predict how well one variable (e.g., PPM) predicts performance of another variable (e.g., SESAS Perf) several weeks into the future. Available space does not permit a detailed description of this procedure, but interested readers are referred to an account by Box and Jenkins (1970) for further explanation.

The number of weeks into the future that one variable predicts another is termed "lag." Although it may be expected that one variable may predict another best under conditions of 0 lag, that is not always the case. In the example to be presented, based on Dave's progress charts, some predictions were maximized at 0 lag, but most were maximized when the predictor variable lagged the predicted variable—in cases of extraclinical generalization by as much as 15 to 22 weeks.

For noncyclical data as in Dave's case, if one variable predicts the future status of another variable, the correlation coefficients more or less monotonically increase with each increase in lag until a maximum obtained value is reached. At that point the correlation coefficients tend to decrease monotonically until they approximate $r = 0.00$. Conventionally, this time-series relationship between any two variables under investigation is displayed by plotting the values of all of the correlation coefficients in sequence as a function of lag time on the horizontal scale. The comparisons of 55 parameter pairs made in this example would necessitate 55 graphic displays. The information is abridged in this presentation by displaying in Table 11–2 only the maximum obtained value of r and its corresponding lag time for each of the 55 sets of paired parameters. The predictor variable is abbreviated on the left side of the table and the predicted variable is designated by letter at the top of the table.

Autocorrelations (correlating a variable with itself) with a lag of 1 measurement week were computed for each variable to obtain estimates of retest reliability for the client and parameter under consideration. The boldface values on the diagonal of the table represent these estimates of reliability. Retest reliability of these measures will be underestimated by this procedure for values that undergo quantum shifts associated with treatment, relapse, or extraneous client variables such as emotional trauma or illness. Typical of such a shift is the reduction in speaking rate (Home/Wife, SPM) between the 21st and 27th weeks. It was largely this shift, following treatment, that resulted in the relatively low retest reliability estimate of $r = .73$ for the SPM parameter at home. Note that the estimated retest reliability for the same parameter measured in the clinic is $r = .96$. Even though treatment and client variables may result in shifts of client performance, they would be unlikely to produce measurement error. Despite these spurious influences, the ob-

Table 11–2. Cross-Correlational Analysis for Dave.

Variables	A	B	C	D	E	F	G	H	I	J	K
A. PPM	**.90**	−.93	−.93	−.93	.92	−.87	.90	−.54	.76	−.86	−.89
B. MPD	1	**.97**	.96	.96	−.85	.91	−.96	.60	−.83	.82	.94
C. STR	1	0	**.96**	.98	−.89	.90	−.96	.62	−.84	.81	.96
D. SPM (Cl)	1	0	0	**.96**	−.86	.90	−.96	.63	−.86	.82	.96
E. SSPM (Cl)	0	0	0	0	**.90**	−.86	.88	−.57	.85	−.81	−.94
F. SPM (Gr)	2	0	0	0	2	**.89**	−.92	.61	−.88	.86	.94
G. SSPM (Gr)	6	3	3	3	6	4	**.97**	−.45	.73	−.52	−.51
H. SPM (H)	0	1	1	0	1	1	18	**.73**	−.68	.64	.65
I. SSPM (H)	17	0	18	18	21	19	15	7	**.85**	−.70	−.87
J. Appr	16	14	15	15	17	18	10	6	11	**.82**	.89
K. Perf	20	15	17	17	20	19	10	17	22	0	**.96**

Note: The cross-correlational procedure is based on Box and Jenkins (1970). The data on the diagonal (underlined in boldface) were obtained by cross-correlational analysis using a lag time of 1 week. They represent estimates of product-moment retest reliability on all variables for this client from one week to the next on the measures employed. The data below the diagonal represent lag times (in weeks) at which maximum correlation coefficients were obtained between corresponding variables at the top and left margin. The resulting correlation coefficients at these optimum lag times are aligned with their corresponding variables above the diagonal. PPM = Pauses per Min, MPD = Mean Phrase Duration, STR = Speechtime Ratio, SPM = Syllables per Min, SSPM = Stuttered Syllables per Min, Appr = SESAS Approach, Perf = SESAS Performance, (CL) = Clinic, (Gr) = Group, (H) = Home.

tained estimates of retest reliability for time-series assessment in Dave's case are most encouraging.

The maximum product-moment correlation coefficients, obtained by comparing each possible pair of parameters in cross-correlation, are presented above the diagonal of Table 11–2. The lag times corresponding to each maximum correlation coefficient for a given pair of parameters appear below the diagonal. The maximum cross-correlations between many of the data sets are high, supporting the concurrent and construct validity of the measurement procedures for the client under consideration. Of particular interest is the fact that the attitudinal scales, SESAS Appr and Perf (Variables J and K in Table 11–2), are predicted best (and exceptionally well) by acoustic measures of motor performance obtained in the clinic 14 to 20 weeks earlier. It would be a mistake, however, to conclude that there is necessarily a direct and totally causal relationship between the measures of motor performance and the presumably reactive measures of the SESAS several weeks later. A lag of 14- to 20-measurement weeks is a long time, allowing known and unknown intervening variables to affect the outcome. The most obvious of the known intervening variables is the previously described generalization activity initiated in Week 18 of treatment. Furthermore, clients often express agony and doubt during generalization, even as they may during the period of clinical-fluency establishment. Attention to these reactive responses requires careful and insightful counseling. Therefore, one should not assume that changes in Appr and Perf are simply the result of maturation during a gestation period of several weeks after having learned a set of fluency-precursive speech targets.

Clinic probe tests with consequent increase in efficacy expectations, accompanied by associative shift, may well be the most parsimonious explanation for the client's improved Group performance. Note that three of the five correlation coefficients between Clinic probe tests and Group performance are $r = -.96$ (sign in predicted direction) with a lag of 3 weeks. The other two correlation coefficients between these two sets of measures are high also, with both lag times at 6 weeks.

All totaled, 1,244 product-moment correlation coefficients were computed for this cross-correlational analysis of Dave's performance data. Clearly, the results obtained in this analysis cannot be extrapolated beyond Dave. Replications of these observations with different clients would be required for that purpose. However, as shown in examples to follow, there is often too much missing information in clinically acquired data arrays to allow a satisfactory cross-correlational analysis. Nevertheless, this example may serve as a useful prototype for consideration in developing models for the study of generalization under more ideal conditions. The procedure enhances information contained in time-series charts where adequate data are available. It is easily performed by computer analysis (Hillis, 1991) in less than 2 min complete with a print-out of Table 11–2.

The remaining two clients were treated by means of the procedure described earlier in this chapter for modifying the total speech pattern through reduction of obstructions in speechflow (increasing %OTI). To review the procedure, first clients are taught to identify the previously defined obstructions in agreement with their clinician to a criterion of $\kappa \geq .70$. Then they progress through a hierarchical series of increasing and maintaining "percent on-target speech intervals" (%OTI) to a criterion of $\geq 70\%$ while expanding length and complexity of speech utterances. In these cases, an on-target speech interval is defined as a 6-s segment of speech evaluated by the clinician to be perceptually natural and free of obstructions. On achievement of the 70% criterion in 15 min of monologue each session, the client and clinician continue with monologue and conversation while the client records self-monitoring success in response to randomly presented computer prompts (Figure 11–5). Some variations in this procedure have been implemented in treatment for these clients due to continuing software modifications and diversity of client responses.

The next clinical example illustrates again the potential of concepts pertaining to operationism, stimulus and response generalization, and SCSE in effecting extraclinical generalization. The possible role of operationism in controlling undesirable response generalization in relapse is of particular interest in this example.

Ralph

"Ralph," age 39, is employed as an in-house computer consultant for a management firm. His goal in therapy was to improve oral-verbal communication skills, thereby increasing the likelihood of his promotion to a supervisory position. On initial evaluation, Ralph's speech was characterized by frequent hesitations resulting in a low speech rate ranging from approximately 70 to 150 SPM during a pretreatment baseline under monologue conditions. His pretreatment stuttering was infrequent, mostly in the range of 4 to 5 SSPM, and consisted of brief effortless prolongations and single repetitions of word-initial segments. As Ralph's charts in Figure 11–7 indicate, his on-target (obstruction-free) speech intervals increased from a pretreatment baseline of 20 %OTI to 50 %OTI in the 6th week of treatment. Corresponding improvement can be seen in SSPM for both reading and monologue during the same period. The prolonged times without data (Weeks 7 to 17 and 27 to 31) are a result of absence due to the client's employment responsibilities coupled with semester breaks in the university clinic.

A relapse in %OTI to pretreatment levels in both reading and monologue can be seen in Week 18 upon return from a semester break of 10 weeks. This relapse is accompanied to a lesser extent by concomitant relapses in SSPM which, nevertheless, remain better than pretreatment levels. Earlier in this chapter a form of response generalization was described in which a previously acquired motor speech pattern may deteriorate over time. In the client's case, reinforcement had not been provided for on-target speech during the 10-week absence from treatment. A consequent drift off-target resulting from response generalization may account for the observed relapse that occurred. Because the client's speech behavior had been operationalized and tracked while the clinic was in session, it was possible to observe the extent of drift in the presumably fluency enhancing %OTI and to modify it upward again when the client returned. As this modification took place, SSPM returned also to its prerelapse levels.

Although percent on-target intervals did not improve beyond 50 %OTI except in reading during the first semester, stuttered syllable rates did improve to 0 SSPM in both reading and monologue during Week 25 in the second semester. Given these improved fluency levels, single-situation extraclinical transfer assignments, as previously described,

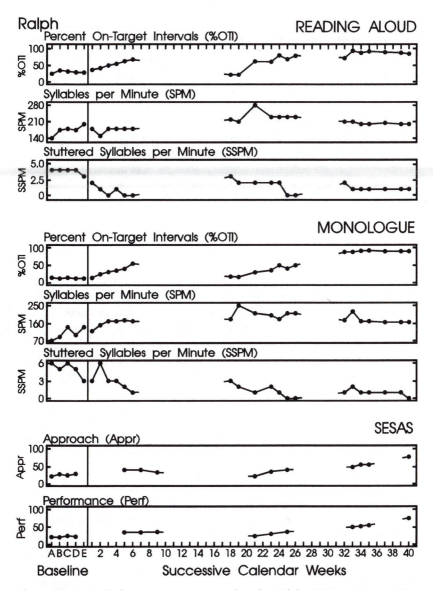

Figure 11–7. Multiple-parameter progress chart for Ralph. %OTI = Percent "On-Target" (continuous) Intervals. Other abbreviations are the same as in Figure 11–6.

were initiated in Week 26. Due to an impending semester break, the client was given several such assignments to complete before returning for the next semester. For the most part, the client succeeded in these assignments, and corresponding improvements in SESAS Appr and Perf were noted from Weeks 33 to 40. SESAS scores had increased from about 30 pretreatment to 75 at Week 40. Speech continuity also improved in both reading and monologue in the last semester to 90 %OTI. Finally, the client reported, 3 months after the last charted data in Figure 11–7 that he had changed employment settings successfully to one requiring more frequent oral-verbal communication.

The last clinical example, below, illustrates rapid acquisition and consistent maintenance of *clinical* fluency across a time span of 59 weeks. Additionally, a high degree of covariation between %OTI and SSPM may be observed. Even with these positive aspects of treatment, generalization of clinical fluency to extraclinical situations is far from complete. This circumstance and possible reasons for its occurrence will be discussed.

John

"John" is a 23-year-old third-year law student. At the 59th week of treatment, which has encompassed 30 sessions, he is in his final week of law school and interning with a law firm. His progress charts in Figure 11–8 illustrate exceptionally rapid acquisition of clinical fluency, after 2 weeks (4 hr) of treatment, while reading aloud. Clinical fluency in monologue occurred 2 weeks later, and, except for a brief upward spike in SPM at Week 14, no clinical relapses occurred. As evidenced by SESAS Appr, John denies virtually any avoidance of communicative situations. Interviews with him concerning his communicative lifestyle and activities confirmed the validity of these Appr scores. However, examination of the client's SESAS Perf scores for the pretreatment baseline and first 8 weeks of treatment suggest the possibility of artifact in the client's responses. All responses show a score of 50 without variability. In response to inquiries concerning these responses, the client replied that he was unable to speculate on his likelihood of fluency during the situations represented on the SESAS. He further explained that his best estimate of fluency probability during those situations was between 0 and 100 and that the best he could do was to respond with 50, the midpoint of those values. At Week 18 single-situation contracts were assigned for extraclinical performance. Also at that time, the client reported a clearer understanding of what it means to be fluent in life situations. Five weeks later, his Perf score peaked at 70, indicating his belief that he would be perceived as fluent on the average in 70% of the situations depicted on the SESAS. This represents a fair level of generalization in the authors' experience, especially considering the client's apparent willingness to encounter difficult and threatening situations. However, as the progress charts indicate, the Perf score of 70 in Week 23 is a high-water mark.

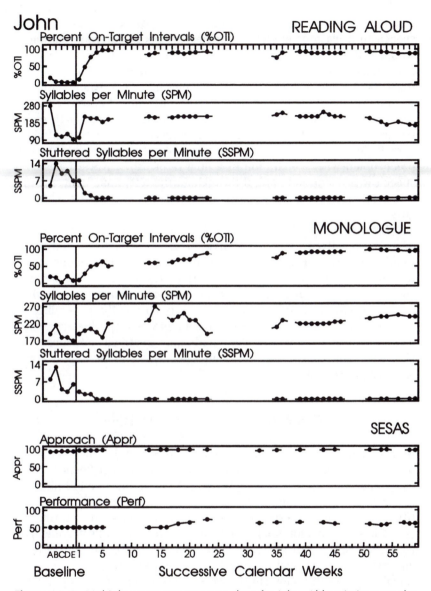

Figure 11–8. Multiple-parameter progress chart for John. Abbreviations are the same as in Figures 11–6 and 11–7.

As this chapter is being written, the client is still in treatment and reports much good feeling and success with regard to his fluency in life situations. He is able to converse fluently and naturally with other clients whom he does not know well. Within the last 3 weeks, he gave a 10-min speech to a class of graduate students in speech-language pathology whom he did not know. The presentation was entirely fluent and natural. A week later, accompanied by his graduate-student clinician, he visited the student center of the university and engaged, fluently and naturally, in a prearranged debate with a student that he did not know. Still later, to the client's surprise, one of the authors of this chapter (JWH) called him at home in Week 59 to ask for his most recent SESAS scores, which were 95 for Appr and 60 for Perf. It was late in the evening and he was preoccupied with preparation of a final term paper. Nevertheless, his speech was fluent and natural throughout the telephone conversation. When asked about this, he replied, "Yes, I'm always fluent with you guys."

Efforts to generalize the fluency just described to a wider spectrum of communicative situations may have been hampered by limited opportunities for transfer by associative shift. This client lives alone and is therefore not able to record his speech routinely with a listener at home. Due to scheduling problems he is unable to make probe-test recordings in the workplace or other settings. This ruled out the generalization effects often attained by having clients obtain weekly probe-test recordings at home or in the workplace. Additionally, treatment activities could not be scheduled for associative shift, either in the clinic or at external sites with the client's associates.

SUMMARY AND CONCLUSION

In this chapter theoretical concepts were reviewed that may pertain to problems encountered in the generalization of clinical fluency to life situations. Among these concepts are: (1) operationism and reliability, (2) traditional learning theory as it pertains to generalization, and (3) social cognitive and self-efficacy theory, including self-monitoring and self-efficacy. Also addressed was the unresolved issue of selecting operational constructs for generalization, including motor speech patterns and attitudes. Additionally, clinical strategies were suggested for operationalizing the self-monitoring process and tracking client progress and efficacy expectations. Finally, clinical illustrations were provided of obstacles encountered during the establishment and generalization of clinically acquired fluency. These deterrents and possible solutions were discussed in terms of the theoretical concepts reviewed at the beginning of the chapter.

This review and report of clinical experiences suggest a need for continued research in at least two related areas concerning the establishment and generalization of speech fluency. First is the issue of what behavioral parameters should be established and generalized. "Fluency" in all of its complex manifestations is probably not the target of choice. This broader concept of fluency would be more appropriately assessed in efficacy studies of treatment outcome by whatever measures are deemed appropriate. As previously suggested, some fluency enhancing speech gesture or pattern, perhaps as found in preparatory sets (Van Riper, 1973) or in PS treatment and its variants (R. Ingham, 1984), might very likely constitute a response to be generalized. Presently most fluency-shaping treatment procedures train clients simultaneously in several supposed fluency enhancing speech patterns which may include prolonged speech, gentle onset of phonation, pre-voice exhalation, continued phonation (or continued speechflow), slow change of articulation, and adequate breath support. These concepts, depending on the clinical delivery system in use, may or may not have been operationalized or evaluated for their reliability. Fluency may result, but in such a multifaceted approach, one cannot determine if a single motor speech pattern or some combination of patterns produced the consequent speech fluency. Moreover, the sheer number of targets presented for self-monitoring and generalization presents a daunting task for the client and may increase treatment time unnecessarily. Initial efforts directed toward isolating fluency enhancing speech patterns (Gow & R. Ingham, 1992; R. Ingham et al., 1983) suggest that some measure of continued phonation or continued speechflow may offer the best opportunity for easy establishment and generalization of speech fluency. Additional effort should be directed toward discovering one or a limited number of reliably observable motor speech constructs determined to be necessary and sufficient for the enhancement of fluent and natural speech in those who are prone to stutter.

Attitudinal parameters including their assessment and modification are also in need of further investigation. Time-series assessment of attitudes, especially concerning client-perceived ability to function as an effective speaker, fluent or otherwise, in life situations should be a matter of prime concern. The SESAS provides for time-series assessment of the client's efficacy expectations across a broad spectrum of communicative situations. It does not, however, isolate client attitudes toward particular types of situations (telephone, strangers, authority figures, etc.) nor does it provide for linkage between the client's efficacy expectation and actual performance.

Certainly, further investigation into these physical/perceptual and attitudinal parameters would do much to help clients with the acquisition and generalization of speech fluency.

REFERENCES

Azrin, N. H., & Nunn, R. G. (1974). A rapid method of eliminating stuttering by a regulated breathing approach. *Behavior Research and Therapy, 12*, 279–286.

Bakker, K. (1997). Instrumentation for the assessment and treatment of stuttering. In R. F. Curlee & G. M. Siegel (Eds.), *Nature and treatment of stuttering: New directions* (2nd ed., pp. 377–397). Needham Heights, MA: Allyn & Bacon.

Bandura, A. (1977). Self-efficacy: Toward a unifying theory of behavioral change. *Psychological Review, 84*, 191–215.

Bandura, A. (1986). *Social foundations of thought and action: A social cognitive theory.* Englewood Cliffs, NJ: PrenticeHall.

Bandura, A. (1991). Social cognitive theory of self-regulation. *Organizational Behavior and Human Decision Processes, 50*, 248–287.

Bandura, A., Adams, N. E., & Beyer, J. (1977). Cognitive processes mediating behavior change. *Journal of Personality and Social Psychology, 35*, 125–139.

Bekhterev, V. M. (1932). *General principles of human reflexology.* New York: International Press.

Boberg, E. (Ed.). (1981). *Maintenance of fluency.* New York: Elsevier.

Boberg, E., & Kully, D. (1994). Long-term results of an intensive treatment program for adults and adolescents who stutter. *Journal of Speech and Hearing Research, 37*, 1050–1059.

Box, G. E. P., & Jenkins, G. M. (1970). *Time series analysis.* San Francisco: Holden-Day.

Bridgman, P. W. (1927). *The logic of modern physics.* New York: Macmillan.

Cohen, J. (1960). A coefficient of agreement for nominal scales. *Educational and Psychological Measurement, 20*, 37–46.

Cooper, E. B. (1986). Treatment of disfluency: Future trends. *Journal of Fluency Disorders, 11*, 317–327.

Cordes, A. K. (1994). The reliability of observational data. I: Theories and methods for speech-language pathology. *Journal of Speech and Hearing Research, 37*, 264–278.

Cordes, A. K., & Ingham, R. J. (1994). The reliability of observational data. II: Issues in the identification and measurement of stuttering events. *Journal of Speech and Hearing Research, 37*, 779–788.

Cordes, A. K., Ingham, R. J., Frank, P., & Ingham, J. C. (1992). Time-interval analysis of interjudge and intrajudge agreement for stuttering event judgments. *Journal of Speech and Hearing Research, 35*, 483–494.

Costello, J. M. (1983). Generalization across language settings: Language intervention with children. In D. Yoder, J. Miller, & R. L. Schiefelbush (Eds.), *Language intervention* (pp. 275–297). ASHA Reports No. 12. Rockville, MD: The American Speech-Language-Hearing Association.

Craig, A., Hancock, K., Chang, E., McCready, C., Shepley, A., McCaul, A., Costello, D., Harding, S., Kehren, R., Masel, C., & Reilly, K. (1996). A controlled clinical trial for stuttering in persons aged 9 to 14 years. *Journal of Speech and Hearing Research, 39*, 808–826.

Culatta, R., & Goldberg, S. A. (1995). *Stuttering therapy: An integrated approach to theory and practice.* Needham Heights, MA: Allyn & Bacon.

Curlee, R. F., & Perkins, W. H. (1969). Conversational rate control therapy for stuttering. *Journal of Speech and Hearing Disorders, 34,* 245–250.

Curlee, R. F., & Perkins, W. H. (1973). Effectiveness of a DAF conditioning program for adolescent and adult stutterers. *Behaviour Research and Therapy, 11,* 395–401.

Dembowski, J., & Watson, B. C. (1991). An instrumented method for assessment and remediation of stuttering: A single-subject case study. *Journal of Fluency Disorders, 16,* 241–273.

Finn, P., & Ingham, R. J. (1994). Stutterers' self-ratings of how natural speech sounds and feels. *Journal of Speech and Hearing Research, 37,* 326–340.

Garrett, H. E. (1958). *Great experiments in psychology.* New York: Appleton-Century-Crofts.

Goebel, M. D. (1986). *Computer-aided fluency establishment trainer: User's manual for installation and therapy.* Annandale, VA: Annandale Fluency Clinic.

Goldiamond, I. (1965). Stuttering and fluency as manipulatable operant response classes. In L. Krasner & L. P. Ullmann (Eds.), *Research in behavior modification* (pp. 106–156). New York: Holt, Rinehart & Winston.

Goldman-Eisler, F. (1968). *Psycholinguistics: Experiments in spontaneous speech.* London: Academic Press.

Gow, M. L., & Ingham, R. J. (1992). Modifying electroglottograph-identified intervals of phonation: The effect on stuttering. *Journal of Speech and Hearing Research, 35,* 495–511.

Hillis, J. W. (1991). CrossCor: A procedure for cross-correlation of clinical time-series data [Computer program]. Unpublished.

Hillis, J. W. (1992a). Computer-aided assessment and training of ability to identify behavioral events: Second prize winner. [Abstract]. *Zenith Data Systems Masters of Innovation IV, 1992 Competition* (p. 60). Buffalo Grove, IL: Zenith Data Systems.

Hillis, J. W. (1992b). *Interobserver reliability for behavioral events: A system for assessment and calibration (RelObs users' guide).* Bethesda, MD: The author.

Hillis, J. W. (1993). Ongoing assessment in the management of stuttering: A clinical perspective. *American Journal of Speech-Language Pathology: A Journal of Clinical Practice, 2,* 24–37.

Hovland, C. I. (1937). The generalization of conditioned responses. I: The sensory generalization of conditioned responses with varying frequencies of tone. *Journal of General Psychology, 17,* 125–148.

Ingham, J. C. (1989). Generalization in the treatment of stuttering. In L. V. McReynolds & J. E. Spradlin (Eds.), *Generalization strategies in the treatment of communication disorders* (pp. 63–81). Toronto: B. C. Decker.

Ingham, R. J. (1975). Operant methodology in stuttering therapy. In J. Eisenson (Ed.), *Stuttering: A second symposium* (pp. 333–399). New York: Harper & Row.

Ingham, R. J. (1982). The effects of self-evaluation training on maintenance and generalization during stuttering treatment. *Journal of Speech and Hearing Disorders, 47,* 271–280.

Ingham, R. J. (1984). *Stuttering and behavior therapy: Current status and experimental foundations.* San Diego: College-Hill Press.

Ingham, R. J. (1993a). Current status of stuttering and behavior modification— II. Principal issues and practices in stuttering therapy. *Journal of Fluency Disorders, 18,* 57–79.

Ingham, R. J. (1993b). Transfer and maintenance of treatment gains of chronic stutterers. In R. F. Curlee (Ed.), *Stuttering and related disorders of fluency* (pp. 166–178). New York: Thieme Medical Publishers, Inc.

Ingham, R. J., & Cordes, A. K. (1997). Self-measurement and evaluating stuttering treatment efficacy. In R. F. Curlee & G. M. Siegel (Eds.), *Nature and treatment of stuttering: New directions* (2nd ed., pp. 413–437). Needham Heights, MA: Allyn & Bacon.

Ingham, R. J., Montgomery, J., & Ulliana, L. (1983). An investigation of the effect of manipulating phonation duration on stuttering. *Journal of Speech and Hearing Research, 26,* 579–587.

Johnson, W. (1946). The Indians have no word for it. In W. Johnson, *People in quandaries: The semantics of personal adjustment* (pp. 439–466). New York: Harper & Brothers.

Johnson, W. (1961). Measurements of oral reading and speaking rate and disfluency of adult male and female stutterers and nonstutterers. In W. Johnson (Ed.), *Studies of speech disfluency and rate of stutterers and nonstutterers* (pp. 1–20). ASHA Monograph Supplement 7. Rockville, MD: The American Speech-Language-Hearing Association.

Kerlinger, F. N. (1964). *Foundations of behavioral research.* New York: Holt, Rinehart and Winston.

Koegel, R. L., & Koegel, L. K. (1988). Generalized responsivity and pivotal behaviors. In R. H. Horner, G. Dunlap, & R. L. Koegel (Eds.), *Generalization and maintenance: Lifestyle changes in applied settings* (pp. 41–66). Baltimore: Paul H. Brookes.

Ladouceur, R., Caron, C., & Caron, G. (1989). Stuttering severity and treatment outcome. *Journal of Behavior Therapy and Experimental Psychiatry, 20,* 49–56.

Lee, C. (1989). Theoretical weaknesses lead to practical problems: The example of self-efficacy theory. *Journal of Behavior Therapy and Experimental Psychiatry, 20,* 115–123.

Lewis, K. E. (1994). Reporting observer agreement on stuttering event judgments: A survey and evaluation of current practice. *Journal of Fluency Disorders, 19,* 269–284.

Lick, J., & Bootzin, R. (1975). Expectancy factors in the treatment of fear: Methodological and theoretical issues. *Psychological Bulletin, 82,* 917–931.

Love, L. R., & Jeffress, L. A. (1971). Identification of brief pauses in the fluent speech of stutterers and nonstutterers. *Journal of Speech and Hearing Research, 14,* 229–240.

Manning, W. H. (1994, November). *The SAE-scale: Self-efficacy scaling for adolescents who stutter.* Paper presented at the meeting of the American Speech-Language-Hearing Association, New Orleans, LA.

Manning, W. H. (1996). *Clinical decision making in the diagnosis and treatment of fluency disorders.* Albany, NY: Delmar Publishers.

Martin, R. R. (1993). The future of behavior modification of stuttering: What goes around comes around. *Journal of Fluency Disorders, 18,* 81–108.

Martin, R. R., & Haroldson, S. K. (1982). Contingent self-stimulation for stuttering. *Journal of Speech and Hearing Disorders, 47,* 407–413.

Martin, R. R., & Siegel, G. M. (1966). The effects of simultaneously punishing stuttering and rewarding fluency. *Journal of Speech and Hearing Research, 9,* 466–475.

Metz, D. E., Onufrak, J. A., & Ogburn, R. S. (1979). An acoustical analysis of stutterers' speech prior to and at the termination of therapy. *Journal of Fluency Disorders, 4,* 249–254.

Metz, D. E., Samar, V. J., & Sacco, P. R. (1983). Acoustic analysis of stutterers' fluent speech before and after therapy. *Journal of Speech and Hearing Research, 26,* 531–536.

Onslow, M., Andrews, C., & Lincoln, M. (1994). A control/experimental trial of an operant treatment for early stuttering. *Journal of Speech and Hearing Research, 37,* 1244–1259.

Onslow, M., Costa, L., Andrews, C., Harrison, E., & Packman, A. (1996). Speech outcomes of a prolonged-speech treatment for stuttering. *Journal of Speech and Hearing Research, 39,* 734–749.

Onslow, M., & Packman, A. (1997). Designing and implementing a strategy to control stuttered speech in adults. In R. F. Curlee & G. M. Siegel (Eds.), *Nature and treatment of stuttering: New directions* (2nd ed., pp. 364–365). Needham Heights, MA: Allyn & Bacon.

Ornstein, A., & Manning, W. H. (1985). Self-efficacy scaling by adult stutterers. *Journal of Communication Disorders, 18,* 313–320.

Paul, G. L. (1966). *Insight vs. desensitization in psychotherapy.* Stanford, CA: Stanford University Press.

Perkins, W. H. (1973). Replacement of stuttering with normal speech. II: Clinical procedures. *Journal of Speech and Hearing Disorders, 38,* 295–303.

Perkins, W. H. (1983). An alternative to automatic fluency. In J. F. Gruss (Ed.), *Stuttering therapy: Transfer and maintenance* (pp. 63–74). Memphis: Speech Foundation of America.

Perkins, W. H. (1990). What is stuttering? *Journal of Speech and Hearing Disorders, 55,* 370–382.

Peters, T. J., & Guitar, B. (1991). *Stuttering: An integral approach to its nature and treatment.* Baltimore: Williams & Wilkins.

Prins, D. (1993). Models for treatment efficacy studies of adult stutterers. *Journal of Fluency Disorders, 18,* 333–349.

Prins, D. (1997). Modifying stuttering—the stutterer's reactive behavior: Perspectives on past, present, and future. In R. F. Curlee & G. M. Siegel (Eds.), *Nature and treatment of stuttering: New directions* (2nd ed., pp. 335–355). Needham Heights, MA: Allyn & Bacon.

Prosek, R. A., & Runyan, C. M. (1983). Effects of segment and pause manipulations on the identification of treated stutterers. *Journal of Speech and Hearing Research, 26,* 510–516.

Quesal, R. W. (1989). Stuttering research: Have we forgotten the stutterer? *Journal of Fluency Disorders, 14,* 153–164.

Ryan, B. P. (1974). *Programmed therapy for stuttering in children and adults.* Springfield, IL: Charles C. Thomas.

Ryan, B. P., & Ryan, B. V. K. (1995). Programmed stuttering treatment for children: Comparison of two establishment programs through transfer, maintenance, and follow-up. *Journal of Speech and Hearing Research, 38,* 61–75.

Samar, V. J., Metz, D. E., & Sacco, P. R. (1986). Changes in aerodynamic characteristics of stutterers' fluent speech associated with therapy. *Journal of Speech and Hearing Research, 29,* 106–113.

Shames, G. H., & Florance, C. L. (1980). *Stutter-free speech: A goal for therapy.* Columbus, OH: Charles E. Merrill.

Sheehan, J. G. (1983). Relapse and recovery from stuttering. In J. F. Gruss (Ed.), *Stuttering therapy: Transfer and maintenance* (pp. 87–97). Memphis: Speech Foundation of America.

Siegel, G. M. (1987). The limits of science in communication disorders. *Journal of Speech and Hearing Disorders, 52,* 306–312.

Siegel, G. M., & Hanson, B. (1972). The effect of response-contingent neutral stimuli on normal speech disfluency. *Journal of Speech and Hearing Research, 15,* 123–133.

Starkweather, C. W. (1980). A multiprocess behavioral approach to stuttering therapy. *Seminars in Speech, Language, and Hearing, 1,* 327–337.

Stevens, S. S. (1935). The operational basis of psychology. *American Journal of Psychology, 47,* 323–330.

Stokes, T. F., & Baer, D. M. (1977). An implicit theory of generalization. *Journal of Applied Behavior Analysis, 10,* 349–367.

Thorndike, E. L. (1937). *The fundamentals of learning.* New York: Bureau of Publications, Teachers College, Columbia University.

Umeda, N. (1977). Consonant duration in American English. *The Journal of the Acoustical Society of America, 61,* 846–858.

Underwood, B. J. (1957). *Psychological research.* New York: Appleton-Century-Crofts.

Van Riper, C. (1973). *The treatment of stuttering.* Englewood Cliffs, NJ: Prentice-Hall.

Webster, R. L. (1974). *The precision fluency shaping program: Speech reconstruction for stutterers.* Roanoke, VA: Hollins Communication Research Institute.

Webster, R. L. (1979). Empirical considerations regarding stuttering therapy. In H. H. Gregory (Ed.), *Controversies about stuttering therapy* (pp. 209–239). Baltimore: University Park Press.

Williams, D. E. (1957). A point of view about stuttering. *Journal of Speech and Hearing Disorders, 22,* 390–397.

Wolpe, J. (1989). The derailment of behavior therapy: A tale of conceptual misdirection. *Journal of Behavior Therapy and Experimental Psychiatry, 20,* 3–15.

Yates, A. J. (1970). *Behavior therapy.* New York: John Wiley & Sons.

CHAPTER

Influence of Nontreatment Variables on Treatment Effectiveness for School-Age Children Who Stutter

PATRICIA M. ZEBROWSKI, Ph.D.,
and
EDWARD G. CONTURE, Ph.D.

The purpose of this chapter is to assess various nontreatment factors which may influence, or be related to, the overall efficacy of stuttering therapy for school-age children who stutter. It is certainly important to consider the individual and combined contributions of the child, the child's environment, the clinician's training and skill, and the service delivery models typically employed in school; however, these variables have been considered elsewhere (e.g., Blood & Conture, 1998; Conture, 1996; Conture & Guitar, 1993; Costello, 1983; Ingham, 1993). Instead, in this chapter we would like to focus on several key variables specific to the child, his or her constitution, and his or her skills and abilities.

There are a number of nontreatment variables that are likely to have some influence on therapy effectiveness for the school-age child who stutters. In this chapter, we will briefly discuss several which have been recently discussed in both the clinical and research literature in childhood stuttering. These include the existence of concomitant phonological problems, a Family History Positive (FHP) of stuttering, and three different but interrelated phenomena: the child's attitudes toward speaking and stuttering, the child's sensitivity to stuttering, and specific aspects of the child's temperament. We want to emphasize that both preliminary research and clinical observation permit reasonable speculation that these factors in some way effect the extent and rate of progress a child experiences in therapy; however, the functional relationship of these factors to overall treatment efficacy is in need of additional empirical support.

THE PROBLEM OF DEFINING THERAPEUTIC EFFECTIVENESS IN COMMUNICATION DISORDERS

The definition and measurement of therapy effectiveness are fundamental issues in any clinical profession, and speech-language pathology is no exception. In some health-related professions, such as physical and occupational therapy, whether not a particular treatment "works" can be more readily determined and measured. One reason for this is that improvements in performance in physical activity more often have a readily perceived utility to the client and his family (Conture & Guitar, 1993). Furthermore, specific behaviors or functions having a relationship to this improved physical performance are easier to delineate and sample. For example, when exercising specific leg and back muscles leads to greater ease of mobility, an individual might regard the treatment as extremely effective due to the strong impact improved mobility can have on daily activities.

In contrast, practitioners in fields such as clinical psychology and speech-language pathology often find it more challenging to define "effectiveness" and to obtain samples of factors related to the efficacy of a particular therapy approach. In speech-language pathology, this problem is related, in part, to the fact that communication is a multidimensional phenomenon comprised of "an infinite number of behaviors" (Olswang, 1993, p. 128). Further, the specific speech and language behaviors targeted for therapy may be interrelated (for example, fluency and language), and in and of themselves they are often unlikely to have a one-to-one correspondence with the larger goal of overall improvement in communicative competence.

For these and other reasons, the definition and measurement of treatment effectiveness for disorders of speech and language is a complex task. When combined with the challenges inherent in implementing efficacy research designs (see Moscicki, 1993; Schiavetti & Metz, 1996, pp. 120–148, for excellent reviews in this area), this complexity creates a significant challenge to clinical researchers interested in studying therapy effectiveness. As a consequence, while a relatively large number of treatment programs are described in the literature (see Bloodstein, 1995, pp. 437–447, for a detailed description), relatively few of them enjoy empirical support based on controlled clinical studies. Presently, limited availability of published, data-based studies documenting the effectiveness of therapy quite accurately reflects the state of affairs in the treatment of a wide variety of speech and language problems, including stuttering in children.

THE EFFECTIVENESS OF TREATMENT FOR CHILDREN WHO STUTTER: BASIC ISSUES

Although there exists a relatively limited research base in stuttering therapy effectiveness for school-age children (see Conture & Guitar, 1993, for review), it is probably not the case that there is similarly a limited number of treatment programs or approaches which are effective. It is true, however, that only a relatively small number of approaches have been proven effective through rigorous scientific methods. Over the years, clinical researchers have provided numerous written descriptions of the treatment approaches they use or recommend for school-age children who stutter (e.g., Conture, 1990; Costello, 1983; Dell, 1993; Gregory, 1991; Healey & Scott, 1995; Ingham, 1993; Peters & Guitar, 1991; Ramig & Bennett, 1997; Runyan & Runyan, 1993). The therapy approaches described by these and other authors are presumably based on a combination of clinical expertise and experience, which involves treating children who stutter and then observing and documenting the results in a wide variety of ways. Further, we can safely assume that many such therapy approaches are effective to some extent. The problem, however, is that in most cases efficacy has *not* been shown through rigorous experimental evidence, but instead has been concluded from anecdotal reports of outcome. The basic problem of defining and measuring the phenomenon of "treatment effectiveness" (see Conture, 1996), along with the complexities of service delivery, are among the primary roadblocks to conducting efficacy research in the treatment of childhood stuttering.

When considering a particular stuttering treatment approach to be "effective," the subjective views or perspectives of a number of individuals, including the child who stutters, his family and close associates, as well as the clinician, should be considered. As discussed by Conture and Wolk (1990), the effectiveness of stuttering therapy is reflected by both *subject-independent* and *subject-dependent* variables. Subject-independent factors are those overt behaviors which external observers can more readily observe and objectively measure (e.g., frequency and duration of stuttered disruptions). Subject-dependent measures, on the other hand, are typically those which may not be visually or auditorally apparent, and therefore are relatively difficult for an external observer to objectively measure and analyze. These subject-dependent factors are likely to include the thoughts, feelings, and attitudes which children who stutter possess about talking, stuttering and related behaviors, their use of "avoidance" strategies while talking, and so forth. In addition, for children who stutter, subject-dependent variables also include the observations and judgments made by the child's significant caregivers (parents, teachers, speech-language pathologist) regarding how effective treatment is or has been.

For a particular child, then, a combination of subject-dependent and subject-independent factors is likely to be related to the overall perception that he "is better" or has been helped by receiving stuttering therapy. Indices of improvement may include: (1) reduced frequency of disfluency and associated behaviors across time and contexts; (2) the child's perception that he can talk the way he wants, at any time, to anyone (Conture & Wolk, 1990; Williams, 1979); (3) the parents' perception that the child "stutters less" and "seems happier"; (4) the parents' own feelings of reduced stress or anxiety about the child and his stuttering; (5) the classroom teacher's subjective impression that the child "doesn't seem so nervous," along with the objective observation that the quality of his classroom work has improved; and (6) the clinician's objective assessment that the child produces fewer disfluencies overall, and more physically "easy," shorter duration stutterings when he does stutter. Presently, there is general agreement that some of these variables are more difficult to measure objectively than others. More important, however, there is no general agreement regarding which measures are the most closely associated with the effectiveness of a particular treatment approach. The assessment of treatment effectiveness for children who stutter is further complicated by the likely presence of individual variation in the factor or combination of factors most closely related to therapy outcome.

TREATMENT EFFECTIVENESS WITHIN THE CONTEXT OF COMMUNICATIVE EFFECTIVENESS

Therapy for the school-age child who stutters can be considered "effective" if it is shown to be related to improvement in overall communicative competence or ability. While apparent with adults who stutter, the extent to which naturalness (e.g., Ingham, Gow, & Costello, 1985; Ingham, Costello Ingham, Onslow, & Finn, 1989), and suitability (e.g.,

Franken, van Bezooijen, & Boves, 1997) of speech and communication relate to treatment effectiveness for children who stutter is unknown. As such, in order to evaluate therapy efficacy, the clinician needs to determine which behaviors (both subject-independent and subject-dependent) best reflect the phenomenon of effective communication for a particular child, as well as those which interfere with that process and how they might be adequately sampled. Obviously, for a large proportion of children who stutter, the most salient behavior impeding effective communication is the frequency with which they produce stuttered speech; therefore, therapy which leads to a reduction in the overall frequency of stuttering will have a major impact on communicative effectiveness. For other children, the most pertinent obstacle to effective communication may be the extent to which they initiate or respond in verbal interaction with others, or feel comfortable or confident saying what they want, when they want, to whomever they want (Williams, 1979). And for still others, the perceptions of parents and other listeners, and their comfort level concerning the child's fluency and related speech and language skills, may be the most important hindrances to effective communication. Within this orientation, then, stuttering therapy which targets those behaviors which most represent obstacles to communicative competence is likely to be efficacious for individual children who stutter.

NONTREATMENT FACTORS RELATED TO THE EFFECTIVENESS OF STUTTERING THERAPY

In the following section we will discuss specific nontreatment factors which have recently been identified in the literature as possible contributors to treatment outcome for children in stutter. These include the presence of concomitant phonological delay or disorder, a family history of stuttering, the child's attitudes towards both speaking and stuttering, and the child's temperament.

Concomitant Phonological Problems

In recent years, the relationship between a child's phonological ability and the onset, development, and treatment of stuttering has received attention in the literature. For example, Paden and Yairi (1996) observed that young children whose stuttering persisted (i.e., 36 months or more postonset) exhibited a higher percentage of phonological errors than did either their normally disfluent peers, or a matched group of children who recovered from stuttering anywhere from 18 to 36 months postonset. They concluded that for some children who stutter, coexisting deficits in phonological ability in the beginning stages of their stuttering problem are associated with nonrecovery. In a related vein, a number of recent studies and reviews of the pertinent literature (e.g., Louko, Edwards, & Conture, 1990; Nippold, 1990; Wolk, Edwards, & Conture, 1993) have shown that there is a relatively high prevalence of phonological delay or disorder within the population of children who stutter, as compared to their nonstuttering peers. Further, Conture, Louko, and Edwards (1993), and Bernstein Ratner (1995), have described the clinical observation that children who stutter and exhibit coexisting phonological problems sometimes make little or no progress in therapy, or take longer to show improvements in speech fluency over the course of treatment. These children may also demonstrate qualitatively different stuttering behavior than their stuttering counterparts who exhibit normal phonological systems.

Presently, it has been suggested that the simultaneous treatment of stuttering and disordered phonology is the preferred therapy route, because such an approach best reflects the interacting processes by which children acquire speech, fluency, and language. In addition, it has been speculated that sequential treatment, in which the focus on fluency is delayed, may result in a protracted stuttering problem which can lead to "significant social, emotional, and educational consequences" (Bernstein Ratner, 1995, p. 182).

In a published account of an experimental, simultaneous treatment approach for this population, Conture et al. (1993) extended Kolk and Postma's (1997) "covert repair hypothesis" theory of stuttering to speculate that the relationship between stuttering and disordered phonology is rooted in the child's "slow-to-activate" (p. 73) system for phonological encoding. They proposed that therapy which simultaneously emphasizes (1) the elimination of phonological processes through clinician modeling, auditory discrimination, the use of minimal and modified pairs, and facilitating contexts, and (2) rate reduction and increased turn-switching pause duration, would result in decreased stuttering and age-appropriate phonology. Results from a group of four children indicated that phonological goals were met for three out of the four. Fluency goals were met for only two of four children, while the other two children showed no observable change in stuttering behavior over the course of treatment.

Findings from this study support the notion that for some children who stutter, simultaneous treatment of stuttering and concomitant phonological deficits is beneficial, while for some children this approach may result in little or no improvement in either domain. On the other hand, it should be noted that this approach, at least for the children in this study, did not exacerbate or increase stuttering, which is something of concern when treating disordered phonology in children who stutter. Regardless, it is clear that sequential treatment did not result in both reduced stuttering and improved phonology for these children; perhaps sequential treatment would have produced such an outcome. At the very least, there is a need for replication of this study with school-age children who stutter. Further, additional work examining the effectiveness of similar and different treatment approaches (e.g., using either a sequential or cycles schedule) provided to stuttering children exhibiting delayed or disordered phonology is warranted.

Family History of Stuttering

In a recent review, Felsenfeld (1997) called for the investigation of possible relationships between family history of stuttering and a variety of epidemiological factors such as (1) stuttering severity and other characteristics of stuttering behavior, (2) the probability of spontaneous recovery, and (3) the likelihood of relapse following successful or "effective" stuttering therapy. Some headway has been made toward achieving at least one of these goals in that recent work in the behavioral genetics of stuttering has uncovered a relationship between spontaneous remission in young children who stutter and the recovery patterns observed in affected family members (Yairi, Ambrose, Paden, & Throneburg, 1996). That is, children who recover from stuttering without receiving intervention tend to have more relatives who also recovered than do children who continue to stutter (Curlee & Yairi, 1997). Unfortunately, while it has been assumed that FHP status may also predict whether children who do not recover either show relapse following treatment or exhibit stuttering which is resistant to therapy (Boberg, Howie, & Woods, 1979; Yairi, 1997), there is no conclusive evidence of a relationship between these variables.

We support Felsenfeld's (1997) appeal to study the influence of family history on therapy effectiveness. Specifically, such factors as relapse and resistance to stuttering, or the appearance of a chronic stuttering problem nonresponsive to conventional stuttering treatment approaches, should be studied in stuttering children with and without an FHP of stuttering. Of course if such studies do reveal a relationship between a genetic predisposition to stuttering and treatment outcome or therapy effectiveness, we would still need to uncover the specific behaviors, characteristics or factors through which different stuttering profiles (e.g., family patterns of recovery vs. nonrecovery) are expressed, and that are more directly related to treatment responsiveness. These may include such variables as oral motor ability, temperament, language, and language processing status.

The Child's Attitudes Towards Speaking and Stuttering

The clinical significance of speech attitudes has been extensively studied in the adult population. Overall, adults who stutter have been shown to exhibit more negative attitudes about talking than their nonstuttering counterparts (e.g., Andrews & Cutler, 1974; Silverman, 1980), and an individual's negative perceptions of the process of talking are predictably related to his or her speech performance (Ulliana & Ingham, 1984). More important, however, is the relationship between speech attitudes and treatment effectiveness. For example, Guitar (1976) showed that for adults who stutter, therapeutic success was related to pretreatment speech attitudes, such that more negative attitudes prior to the initiation of therapy were correlated with less improvement in fluency at dismissal. In addition, for adults who stutter, posttreatment attitudes have been shown to be valid predictors of fluency maintenance up to 1 year posttherapy (Guitar & Bass, 1978).

Presently, there are few data which directly assess the speech attitudes exhibited by children who stutter. In 1991 DeNil and Brutten published the results of a study in which they administered a Dutch version of *The Communication Attitude Test* (Brutten & Dunham, 1989) to a group of school-age (7–14 years old) Belgian children who stutter and a control group. Results indicated that the stuttering children exhibited significantly more negative attitudes toward speech than did their non-stuttering counterparts, and that speech-related attitudes became more negative with increasing age for the stuttering children (the nonstuttering group showed the opposite trend). As well, similar to Ulliana and Ingham (1984), DeNil and Brutten (1991) observed that those children judged to exhibit "severe" stuttering possessed the most negative speech attitudes, while children whose stuttering was judged to be "mild" and "moderate" displayed more positive attitudes about talking.

Because the limited speech attitude data available from children who stutter appears similar to that obtained from adults, it seems reasonable to speculate that as with adults, the pre- and posttreatment attitudes of children who stutter may serve to predict therapy success or effectiveness. In order to facilitate our understanding of this relationship, we need to continue to develop valid ways of measuring children's perceptions of their communication abilities, as well as how both stuttering and successful stuttering treatment affect their quality of life.

The Child's Sensitivity to Stuttering

In a recent chapter, Guitar (1997) contended that some children who stutter may be particularly resistant to treatment because they experience "a strong emotional response to stuttering" (p. 280). In addition, he suggested that children who exhibit such a heightened emotional sensitivity to their own stuttering are at risk for dropping out of therapy, and may in fact account for some of the roughly 33% of children who discontinue participation in treatment efficacy studies prior to the completion of the therapy protocol.

Guitar speculated that some children who stutter may display a greater emotional reactivity in general. Accordingly, an exacerbating cycle takes place, where heightened reactivity may lead to increased muscular tension, which in turn precipitates speech disruptions in the form of stuttering. These episodes of stuttering may lead to additional increases in emotional response, which may be manifest more specifically as frustration or fear related to talking. Finally, Guitar suggested that children with heightened sensitivity to certain fear or anxiety-inducing stimuli may experience increased difficulty in working on their speech and speech fluency, because they may be more likely to respond to talking, stuttering, or overt attempts by the clinician to highlight or discuss with either a "conditioned flight or avoidance response" (p. 282).

To illustrate the aforementioned relationship, Guitar provided two case studies of boys who stuttered, who displayed reluctance to participate in stuttering therapy, regardless of the form it took (e.g., fluency-shaping or stuttering modification). According to Guitar, these children both showed signs of avoidance, withdrawal, and frustration directly related to speech and speaking activities, but they also displayed more generalized avoidance and withdrawal patterns as well. Through his description of their treatment, Guitar concluded that children who show evidence of strong emotional reactivity to stuttering experience limited success in "traditional" stuttering therapy, and have difficulty generalizing and maintaining fluency beyond the clinic.

The Child's Temperament

As Bloodstein (1995) noted, "there is considerable inconsistency in the findings resulting from research on the stutterer's personality" (p. 236). Clearly, both adults and children who stutter, as a group, are not markedly different from their nonstuttering counterparts in terms of psychosocial adjustment; that is, there is little evidence to suggest that people who stutter, as a group, are neurotic, psychotic, or severely maladjusted. However, as Bloodstein also noted, there "is some justification for the inference that stutterers on the average are not quite as well adjusted as are typical normal speakers" (1995, pp. 236–237). Bloodstein points out, however, that such "lack of adjustment" is more related to social adjustment than emotional health; put in colloquial terms, perhaps these are normal ways to react to abnormal speech. That is, it is more likely that adults and children who stutter may exhibit relatively low self-esteem as a result of their reactions to their stuttering, rather than their stuttering resulting from a lack of social adjustment. Obviously, there are other plausible explanations; for example, it may be the case that the same home environment which contributes to the perpetuation of stuttering in children, also results in reduced social adjustment. For the purposes of this discussion, however, we will consider the more obvious notion that adjustment concerns result from, rather than cause, stuttering. For children who stutter, there may be specific personality characteristics which contribute to the ways in which they react to their stuttering, as well as to other self-produced behaviors and environmental stimuli. For example, when considering the previous discussion, some children's heightened emotional reactivity to stuttering may be related to specific temperamental characteristics. Temperament has been defined as inherited personality traits which appear early in life (see Goldsmith et al., 1987; Kagan & Snidman, 1991, for excellent reviews of temperament).

Temperament, like many such variables in the area of personality, is a multifaceted construct which is used to describe a child's general disposition, and involves the range of moods that typify his emotional life. Unlike some constructs, however, temperament is considered to be largely inherited (Goldsmith et al., 1987). Further, temperament is also believed to be mutable as a result of environmental influences. More specifically, one salient aspect of temperament relates to *reactivity* and *self-regulation*. As suggested in the prior discussion, reactivity refers to the excitability of the autonomic or central nervous system to behavioral responses or external stimuli. Self-regulation refers to the processes that either facilitate or inhibit reactivity, including attention, approach or avoidance strategies or tendencies, and so forth (Derryberry & Rothbart, 1984). Further, individual differences in a child's temperament relate to differences in *emotionality* (e.g., minimal to maximal emotional responses to novel stimuli), *activity* (e.g., lethargic to almost hyperactive levels of activity), and *sociability* (e.g., a preference for being alone as opposed to being with others). Whichever aspect of temperament we focus upon at any given time, most workers believe that temperament is the attribute which mediates the influence of the environment on the child (Goldsmith et al., 1987).

Presently, relatively little is known about the specific temperamental characteristics of children who stutter and how they compare to those expressed by nonstuttering children. Even less is known about the influence of temperament on the child's performance in stuttering therapy, although Guitar has proposed a hypothetical model of this relationship (Guitar, 1997; see above). Glasner (1949) provided some insight into this phenomenon when he reviewed the case files of 70 young stuttering children under the age of 5. He reported that the parents of these children routinely described their child's most common temperamental characteristic as a distinct "hypersensitivity." Based on these limited data, as well as our own clinical experience, it seems that the possible role of temperamental variables in the perpetuation of stuttering in children warrants exploration, as does its relationship to treatment effectiveness or lack of same.

The work of Kagan (1984, 1994) seems particularly germane to this exploration. In particular, Kagan has described the "behaviorally inhibited" (BI) child as one type of temperamental profile. The BI child is one who appears timid around the unfamiliar, shy around strangers, overly sensitive and prone to self-reproach, and who exhibits higher levels of reactivity and lower thresholds of excitability when compared to other children. Kagan (1984) estimated that approximately 15–20% of children can be characterized as BI, a temperamental profile that would appear to markedly influence the ways in which the child interacts with the environment. It should be emphasized here that BI in and of itself is not abnormal; instead, it is considered to lie somewhere on the normal continuum or distribution of temperamental characteristics which children exhibit. It is very possible that those children, who stutter and who tend to exhibit BI, may interact with their environment in ways that are appreciably different from those children who are behaviorally uninhibited. Further, such differences may hold important implications for either the perpetuation or recovery from stuttering in very young children, or for the effectiveness of treatment in nonrecovering stuttering children.

Recently, Oyler (1996a, 1996b) and Oyler and Ramig (1995) have begun to explore such possibilities. Specifically, they have examined the relationship between stuttering, sensitivity, and BI in children. To do so, Oyler developed two paper-and-pencil scales which were completed by parents: the Temperament Characteristic Scale (TCS) and the Parent Perception Scale (PPS). Based on parental responses as assessed by these scales, Oyler observed that children who stutter ($n = 25$) are significantly more behaviorally inhibited and temperamentally sensitive than nonstuttering children between 1 and 4 years of age. Further, stuttering children are significantly less likely to take risks than nonstuttering children, an observation which supports Bloodstein's (1995) conclusion based on his review of the literature that "many stutterers are low . . . in willingness to risk failure" (p. 237).

What does all this mean? First, of course, Oyler's research will need replication with more children who stutter, at different ages, and with additional objective measures based on behavioral observations rather than relying solely on parents' judgments. Second, Oyler's work lends support to Glasner's and other's observations that some children who stutter may be somewhat "hypersensitive," and may be distinctly sensitive to interpersonal stress (e.g., Greiner, Fitzgerald, Cooke, & Djurdic, 1985). Third, if temperament is inherited, and behavioral inhibition is a variation of temperament, it is quite possible that children who stutter who inherit such characteristics might respond to both their environment and treatment regimens in ways that differ markedly from children who are not behaviorally inhibited. Whether such response patterns in any way, shape, or form influence stuttering, recovery, or treatment effectiveness is quite unknown; however, the possibility remains that some children who stutter possess genetically determined temperamental characteristics which contribute to the susceptibility to begin, as well as recover from, stuttering. That is, they have a lower threshold for arousal and a more intense reaction to behavioral responses or environmental stimuli. It behooves us to consider such temperamental characteristics, at least on an individual basis, for those children for whom therapy is either less than successful or protracted in nature.

FUTURE RESEARCH

While we have limitless opportunities for future research in this area, we have limited resources with which to meet these opportunities. Thus, choices must be made, priorities set. What follows, therefore, are those issues that would seem to need top priority when examining the influence of nontreatment variables on treatment effectiveness with school-age children who stutter.

First, in addition to measuring various facets of stuttering, researchers should be strongly encouraged to thoroughly document the pretreatment characteristics and behaviors of school-age children who stutter (this does not suggest that previous workers have never done so, only that present and future researchers should continue such efforts). And then, subsequently, researchers should be encouraged to correlate these conditions and behaviors (e.g., expressive language behavior, scores on paper and pencil assessments of temperament, etc.) with posttreatment changes in stuttering frequency, duration, type, etc. Perhaps, a select number of these nontreatment behaviors are highly correlated with short-, medium-, and long-term improvement in stuttering, but only through a series of single as well as group study designs will such correlations, if any, emerge. Of course, a correlation does not a cause and effect make, but obtaining such correlations would be a beginning, a door through which future researchers could enter to explore potentially fruitful areas of investigation.

Second, there is a strong need for systematic study of how treatment for stuttering is influenced by concomitant problems such as disordered phonology, delays in expressive and receptive language abilities, neuromotor control for speech, and so forth. Conversely, there is an equally strong need to study how treatment for stuttering is influenced by concomitant expressive and receptive language abilities which are superior. That is, while we tend to be "deficit oriented" when examining disorders like stuttering, we have evidence that speech disfluency can be associated, for *some* children, with advanced speech and language development, or communication skills which are above normal limits (e.g., Enger, Hood, & Shulman, 1988). In essence, as long as speech (dys)fluency in (pre)school-age children is considered in essential isolation from other aspects of syntactic, semantic, phonologic and motoric ability and development, it will be extremely difficult, if not impossible, to integrate stuttering practically or theoretically into the wider realm of human communication processes and disorders.

Third, future researchers should be encouraged to explore the influence of less than easy to objectify variables, for example, temperament, and their possible influence on treatment effectiveness. That tremendous advances in understanding are obtainable without ratio level of measurement documentation can be seen by examining Kagan and colleagues' careful, systematic, but often times perceptual-based observations of temperament in preschool children. We hasten to point out that there is nothing, at this point, to suggest that these variables *cause* stuttering; however, one can reasonably speculate that these variables might *exacerbate* stuttering, at least for some children. It is quite possible, therefore, that until we better understand and account for these variables during treatment, their presence may make it difficult for school-age children who stutter to receive maximum short-, medium-, or long-term therapeutic benefit.

Finally, treatment studies, whether single-subject or group designs, are needed where identical type, length, and course of treatment are administered to children who stutter with and without delays in expressive language. With such study, the emphasis should not only be on short- and medium-term, but long-term change in stuttering as well. Such information would be invaluable to practicing clinicians who frequently must treat stuttering that is bundled together, for some children, with several other concerns that may limit the child's ability to receive maximum, long-term benefits from treatment.

CONCLUSIONS

We have explored some nontreatment variables that may have significant potential for influencing treatment effectiveness for stuttering in children. Such variables include, but are not limited to, disorders in phonology, a family history of recovery from stuttering, emotional sensitivity towards stuttering, and temperament. While there are a limitless number of nontreatment variables that may influence treatment, there are limits to the resources we would need to explore such variables. Therefore, we will need to set our priorities and only assess, at least to begin, those topics seemingly having the most potential recovery from stuttering, heterogeneity among clients, language issues, and temperament may have considerable potential.

Recovery From Stuttering that Runs in Families

The past, it is said, is the best predictor of the future. Thus, when we find a school-age client whose relatives stuttered but did not recover, we may suspect the same regarding the child in front of us. Why? Well, obviously, we don't know in any precise way, but whatever the child may have inherited in terms of the problem of stuttering itself, as well as other variables, may make his or her problem less than tractable.

Heterogeneity Among Children

While perhaps platitudinous, it is nevertheless true that every child is an individual. The presence of such individuality may make it difficult to prescribe a one-size-therapy-fits-all approach, or at least to expect one-size therapy to result in equal benefit across all children. At present, results of a series of single-subject studies might help us better understand what individual differences are more or less salient when assessing treatment efficacy. In essence, researchers who study treatment effectiveness should be encouraged to carefully document pretreatment individual characteristics, for example, history of recovery from stuttering in the client's family, expressive language skills, and so forth, and study how these variables correlate with short-, medium-, and long-term improvement in stuttering.

Syntactic, Semantic, Phonologic, and Motor Development

The influence of language formulation (syntactic, semantic, and phonologic) on treatment effectiveness for stuttering is an area seriously in need of systematic study by means of single-subject and/or group designs. Treating stuttering as an isolate, separate from syntactic, semantic, phonologic, and motoric processes is neither wise nor appropriate. There is much to be gained and little to be lost from trying to integrate, whenever possible, stuttering theory and therapy into the broader realm of linguistic and psycholinguistic knowledge.

Temperament

Anecdotes and clinical observations make apparent that more than a few of our young clients are overly reactive, sensitive, responsive, etc., to environmental change, differences, and transitions. Whether these temperamental variables influence treatment effectiveness is, of course, completely unclear. Perhaps temperamental characteristics have no appreciable bearing on treatment effectiveness for childhood stuttering. However, given the pervasiveness of informal observations of "hypersensitivity" among children who stutter (e.g., Glasner, 1949), the fact that such temperamental states have a strong inherited component (e.g., Goldsmith et al., 1987), and that such states have real potential for significantly mediating almost every aspect of the child's interaction with his or her environment, it seems more than reasonable to suggest that temperament should be studied relative to treatment of stuttering in school-age children.

In recent years, the fields of speech-language pathology in general and stuttering in particular have made some, albeit imperfect, attempts to objectively compare pre-, short-, medium-, and long-term posttreatment behaviors (with appropriate nontreatment control groups, in some instances) and to standardize diagnostic and treatment procedures. Without a doubt, much work remains in terms of refining, documenting, and assessing treatment procedures and efficacy. We suggest that variables not directly involved with treatment be considered in parallel with treatment variables. The fruits of such labors, we believe, should improve our ability to serve the entire range of children who stutter.

REFERENCES

Andrews, G., & Cutler, J. (1974). Stuttering therapy: The relation between changes in symptom level and attitudes. *Journal of Speech and Hearing Disorders, 39*, 312–319.

Bernstein Ratner, N. (1995). Treating the child who stutters with concomitant languages or phonological impairment. *Language, Speech, and Hearing Services in Schools, 26*(3), 180–186.

Blood, G., & Conture, E. (1998). Measurement issues in fluency disorders. In C. Frattali (Ed.), *Measuring outcomes in speech-language pathology.* New York: Thieme Medical Publishers.

Bloodstein, O. (1995). *A handbook on stuttering* (5th ed.). San Diego, CA: Singular Publishing Group.

Boberg, E., Howie, P., & Woods, L. (1979). Maintenance of fluency: A review. *Journal of Fluency Disorders, 4*, 93–116.

Brutten, G. J., & Dunham, S. (1989). The Communication Attitude Test: A normative study of grade school children. *Journal of Fluency Disorders, 14*, 371–377.

Conture, E. G. (1990). *Stuttering* (2nd ed.). Englewood Cliffs, NJ: Prentice-Hall.

Conture, E. (1996). Treatment efficacy: Stuttering. *Journal of Speech and Hearing Research, 39*, S18–S26.

Conture, E. G., & Guitar, B. E. (1993). Evaluating efficacy of treatment of stuttering: School-age children. *Journal of Fluency Disorders, 18*, 253–287.

Conture, E., Louko, L., & Edwards, M. L. (1993). Simultaneously treating stuttering and disordered phonology in children: Experimental therapy, preliminary findings. *American Journal of Speech-Language Pathology, 2*(3), 72–81.

Conture, E., & Wolk, L. (1990). Efficacy of intervention by speech-language pathologists: Stuttering. *Seminars in Speech and Language, 11*, 200–211.

Costello, J. M. (1983). Current behavioral treatments for children. In D. Prins and R. J. Ingham (Eds.), *Treatment of stuttering in early childhood* (pp. 69–112). San Diego: College-Hill Press.

Curlee, R. F., & Yairi, E. (1997). Early intervention with early childhood stuttering: A critical examination of the data. *American Journal of Speech-Language Pathology, 6* (No.2), 8–18.

Dell, C. W., Jr. (1993). Treating school-age stutters. In R. F. Curlee (Ed.), *Stuttering and related disorders of fluency* (pp. 45–67). New York: Thieme Medical Publishers.

De Nil, L. F., & Brutten, G. J. (1991). Speech-associated attitudes of stuttering and nonstuttering children. *Journal of Speech and Hearing Research, 34*, 60–66.

Derryberry, D., & Rothbart, M. (1984). Emotion, attention, and temperament. In C. E. Izard, J. Kagan, & R. Zajonc (Eds.), *Emotion, cognition, and behavior* (pp. 132–166). New York: Cambridge University Press.

Enger, N., Hood, S., & Shulman, B. (1988). Language and fluency variables in the conversational speech of linguistically advanced preschool and school-age children. *Journal of Fluency Disorders, 13*, 163–172.

Felsenfeld, S. (1997). Epidemiology and genetics of stuttering. In R. F. Curlee & G. M. Siegel (Eds.), *Nature and treatment of stuttering* (2nd ed., pp. 3–23). Needham Heights, MA: Allyn & Bacon.

Franken, M. C., van Bezooijen, R., & Boves, L. (1997). Stuttering and communicative suitability of speech. *Journal of Speech and Hearing Research, 40*, 83–94.

Glasner, P. (1949). Personality characteristics and emotional problems in stutterers under the age of five. *Journal of Speech and Hearing Disorders, 14*, 135–138.

Goldsmith, H., Buss, A., Plomin, R., Rothbart, M., Thomas, A., Chess, S., Hinde, R., & McCall, R. (1987). Roundtable: What is temperament? Four approaches. *Child Development, 58*, 505–529.

Gregory, H. (1991). Therapy for elementary school-age children. *Seminars in Speech and Language, 12*, 323–335.

Grenier, J., Fitzgerald, H., Cooke, P., & Djurdic, S. (1985). Assessment of sensitivity to interpersonal stress in stutterers and nonstutterers. *Journal of Communication Disorders, 18*, 215–225.

Guitar, B. (1976). Pretreatment factors associated with the outcome of stuttering therapy. *Journal of Speech and Hearing Research, 19*, 590–600.

Guitar, B. (1997). Therapy for children's stuttering and emotions. In R. F. Curlee & G. M. Siegel (Eds.), *Nature and treatment of stuttering* (2nd ed., pp. 280–291). Needham Heights, MA: Allyn & Bacon.

Guitar, B., & Bass, C. (1978). Stuttering therapy: The relation between attitude change and long-term outcome. *Journal of Speech and Hearing Disorders, 43*, 392–400.

Healey, E. C., & Scott, L. A. (1995). Strategies for treating elementary school-age children who stutter: An integrative approach. *Language, Speech, and Hearing Services in Schools, 26*, 151–161.

Ingham, R. J. (1993). Current status of stuttering and behavior modification. II: Principal issues and practices in stuttering therapy. *Journal of Fluency Disorders, 18*, 57–79.

Ingham, R. J., Costello Ingham, J. M., Onslow, M., & Finn, P. (1989). Stutterers' self-ratings of speech naturalness: Assessing effects and reliability. *Journal of Speech and Hearing Research, 32*, 419–431.

Ingham, R. J., Gow, M., & Costello, J. M. (1985). Stuttering and speech naturalness: Some additional data. *Journal of Speech and Hearing Disorders, 50*, 217–219.

Kagan, J. (1984). *The nature of the child.* New York: Basic Books, Inc.

Kagan, J. (1994). *Galen's prophecy.* New York: Basic Books, Inc.

Kagan, J., & Snidman, N. (1991). Temperamental factors in human development. *American Psychologist, 48*, 856–862.

Kolk, H., & Postma, A. (1997). Stuttering as a covert repair phenomenon. In R. F. Curlee & G. M. Siegel (Eds.), *Nature and treatment of stuttering* (2nd ed., pp. 182–203). Needham Heights, MA: Allyn & Bacon.

Louko, L., Edwards, M. F., & Conture, E. (1990). Phonological characteristics of young stutters and their normally fluent peers: Preliminary observations. *Journal of Fluency Disorders, 15*, 191–210.

Moscicki, E. (1993). Fundamental methodological considerations in controlled clinical trials. *Journal of Fluency Disorders, 18*, 183–196.

Nippold, M. (1990). Concomitant speech and language disorders in stuttering children: A critique of the literature. *Journal of Speech and Hearing Disorders, 55*, 51–60.

Olswang, L. B. (1993). Treatment efficacy research: A paradigm for investigating clinical practice and theory. *Journal of Fluency Disorders, 18*, 125–131.

Oyler, M. E. (1996a). *Vulnerability in stuttering children.* (No. 9602431). Ann Arbor, MI: UMI Dissertation Services.

Oyler, M. E. (1996b, December). *Temperament: Stuttering and the behaviorally inhibited child.* Seminar presented at the American Speech-Language-Hearing Association Annual Convention, Seattle, WA.

Oyler, M. E., & Ramig, P. R. (1995, December). *Vulnerability in stuttering children.* Seminar presented at the American Speech- Language-Hearing Association Annual Convention, Orlando, FL.

Paden, E., & Yairi, E. (1996). Phonological characteristics of children whose stuttering persisted or recovered. *Journal of Speech and Hearing Research, 39*(5), 981–990.

Peters, T. J., & Guitar, B. (1991). *Stuttering: An integrated approach to its nature and treatment.* Baltimore, MD: Williams & Wilkins.

Ramig, P. R., & Bennett, E. M. (1997). Clinical management of children: Direct management strategies. In R. F. Curlee & G. M. Siegel (Eds.), *Nature and treatment of stuttering* (2nd ed., pp. 292–312). Needham Heights, MA: Allyn & Bacon.

Runyan, C. M., & Runyan, S. E. (1993). Therapy for school-age stutterers: An update on the fluency rules program. In R. F. Curlee (Ed.). *Stuttering and related disorders of fluency* (pp. 101–114). New York: Thieme Medical Publishers.

Schiavetti, N., & Metz, D. (1996). *Evaluating research in speech pathology and audiology* (3rd ed.). Boston: Allyn & Bacon.

Silverman, F. H. (1980). Dimensions of improvement in stuttering. *Journal of Speech and Hearing Research, 23*, 137–151.

Ulliana, L., & Ingham, R. J. (1984). Behavioral and nonbehavioral variables in the measurement of stutterers' communication attitudes. *Journal of Speech and Hearing Research, 49*, 83–93.

Williams, D. E. (1979). A perspective on approaches to stuttering therapy. In H. Gregory (Ed.), *Controversies about stuttering therapy* (pp. 241–268). Baltimore, MD: University Park Press.

Wolk, L., Edwards, M. L., & Conture, E. G. (1993). Coexistence of stuttering and disordered phonology in young children. *Journal of Speech and Hearing Research, 36*, 906–917.

Yairi, E. (1997). Disfluency characteristics of childhood stuttering. In R. F. Curlee & G. M. Siegel (Eds.), *Nature and treatment of stuttering* (2nd ed., pp. 49–78). Needham Heights, MA: Allyn & Bacon.

Yairi, E., Ambrose, N., Paden, E., & Throneburg, R. (1996). Predictive factors of persistence and recovery: Pathways of childhood stuttering. *Journal of Communication Disorders, 29*, 51–77.

INDEX

SSPM. *see* Stuttered syllables per
     minute
Stimulus generalization, 247–248
STR, *see* Speech-time ratio
Structure of treatment, 226
Stutter-free utterances of children,
     acoustic analyses of
  comparisons of speech, studies,
     145–148
  discussion, 155–159
  method, 148–151
  results, 151–155
Stuttered syllables per minute
     (SSPM), 270–271
Stuttering
  cerebral dominance theory, 104
  diagnosogenic theory, 105–106
  operant behavior approach,
     106–107
  research agenda, 107–1110
     clinic, 109
     puzzle-solving research, 110
     technology and, 110
  summary, 110–111
  technology, and future of research,
     110
Stuttering, applications to, 12–20 *see
     also* Recovery without
     treatment
  model of recovery, 18–20
     alternative model, 19
     genetic-based factor, 18–19
     summary, 19–20
     traditional model 18, 19
  terminology and definition, 13–15
  verification of recovery, 15–18
     drawbacks, 17–18
     strengths, 16–17
Stuttering, behavioral data language
     of, *see* Behavioral data
     language of stuttering
Stuttering Foundation of America
     (SFA), 215
Stuttering treatment literature, *see*
     Literature on stuttering
     treatment
Stuttering Treatment Rating Recorder,
     180

Stuttering-like disfluency (SLD), 33,
     35, 36
Success in treatment outcome,
     defining, 215–217, 228–229
  complaint as stuttering disorder, 216
  complaint as stuttering events, 216
Superfluous behaviors, 40, 42
Supplementary motor area (SMA)
     model on stuttering, 77–80
  frequency-altered feedback, 79–80
  prolonged speech, 76–79
  respiration, 79
Syllable repetition, 29, 30, 31, 32, 33,
     40, 41, 43, 46
Syllables
  per minute, 206
  percent stuttered, 203–206
Syllables per minute (SPM), speech
     rate in, 269, 270–271
Syntactic development of school-age
     child, 306
Systemic Disfluency Analysis (SDA)
  diagnostic evaluation procedures
     of, 224–225
  transcription system, 225–226

T

Temperament of school-age child,
     301–304, 306–307
Tense pause, 29, 30, 32
Test of Language Development
     (TOLD), 164, 165
  cross-sectional study scores, 166
  longitudinal study scores, 167
  picture vocabulary test of, 173–174
Therapy for stuttering
  defining effectiveness in
     communication disorders,
     problem of, 294–295
  factors related to effectiveness of,
     297–304
Theory of stuttering, *see* Behavioral
     data language of stuttering;
     Generalization; Genetic
     research; Recovery without
     treatment; Speech motor
     control research; Stuttering